Acclaim for *The Mother of All Pregnancy Books* and Ann Douglas

"*Mother* knows! Start reading this treasure trove even before you get pregnant so you can make it through every jam-packed page before your baby arrives."
—Paula Spencer, author of *Everything ELSE You Need to Know When You're Expecting: The New Etiquette for the New Mom*

"*The Mother of All Pregnancy Books* is a comprehensive and incredibly informative resource about pregnancy (and what comes before and after!). Ann Douglas tells all in her witty style, entertaining readers along the way. Unlike other pregnancy books, Douglas combines thorough research and reporting with the human touch, offering her own experiences and insight while educating her readers at one of the most important times in their lives. This book is not to be missed!"
—Elisa Ast All, Editor-in-Chief, iParenting.com, *Pregnancy* magazine, and *Baby Years* magazine

"An extremely comprehensive and even-handed volume that provides just about everything but the baby! *The Mother of All Pregnancy Books* is an amazing resource and Ann Douglas is a reassuring and savvy guide."
—Cecelia A. Cancellaro, author of *Pregnancy Stories: Real Women Share the Joys, Fears, Thrills and Anxieties of Pregnancy from Conception to Birth*

"At long last, a new pregnancy bible for women of my generation and younger has emerged in the form of *The Mother of All Pregnancy Books*. With humor, sensitivity, an easy, no-jargon style and a million "extras" that the leading pregnancy books on the shelves don't cover, Ann Douglas holds nothing back. Not only do I love this book, but I will use it as a valuable tool in my own work as a women's health author."
— M. Sara Rosenthal, author, *The Pregnancy Sourcebook* and *The Breastfeeding Sourcebook*, and founder, www.sarahealth.com

"This is truly 'the mother of all pregnancy books' — an intelligent resource that covers every pregnancy-related topic imaginable in a fun, reassuring way. Ann Douglas has done an exceptional job of arming parents-to-be with the facts they need to make the healthiest possible choices from preconception through postpartum. A must-have!"
—Susan Newman, Ph.D., author of *Parenting An Only Child: The Joys and Challenges of Raising Your One and Only*

"The must-read pregnancy book! Ann Douglas has created the most comprehensive guide to pregnancy we've ever seen."
—Denise & Alan Fields, authors, *Baby Bargains*

"Finally, a pregnancy book that includes essential pre-pregnancy concerns, such as planning and physical and emotional preparation! Ann Douglas has written her masterwork, *The Mother of All Pregnancy Books* in the same unpretentious, concise style as her *Unofficial Guide*. She also stays true to her goal of informing parents and prospective parents as completely as possible, so they will be well-equipped to sort through the pros and cons of their own life choices as they see them. Not one to forgo difficult issues, her chapter entitled 'When Pregnancy Isn't Perfect' is one of the best I've read, both for its sensitivity and for its emphasis on coping and prevention. This is a book that will serve women and their families well."

—Christine Harris, Ph.D., author of *The Pregnancy Journal*,
Baby's First Year Journal, and *The Toddler Journal*

"Here's a book that's packed with up-to-date information and practical advice on almost every aspect of pregnancy — from prenatal testing to proper nutrition, from infertility procedures to financial planning, from bedrest to breastfeeding. Yet despite its breadth and depth, the text is not dry or dull. Instead, Ann Douglas's reassuring style and insightful anecdotes make readers feel like they're chatting with a savvy, smart, sympathetic friend."

—Tamara Eberlein, coauthor of *When You're Expecting Twins, Triplets,or Quads*
and *Program Your Baby's Health*

"If you're looking for an all-in-one 'tell me everything and tell it like it is' book on pregnancy, *The Mother of All Pregnancy Books* is it. Not only is this hefty volume filled with facts about fertility, pregnancy and birth, but it also contains hundreds of anecdotes from moms who lived — and maybe even loved — pregnancy. Author Ann Douglas knows her stuff, and is wise but not preachy, friendly but not overbearing. Keep this book close at hand for instant guidance through the highs and lows of this extraordinary time!"

— Nancy Price, ePregnancy.com

the
mother
of all
pregnancy
books

the
mother
of all
pregnancy
books

ANN DOUGLAS

WILEY

Wiley Publishing, Inc.

To Joan and Robert,
for believing in my "baby"
and for serving as midwives
during its delivery

About the Author

Ann Douglas is one of North America's foremost pregnancy and parenting writers. She is the author of 18 books, including the highly popular *The Unofficial Guide to Having a Baby* (co-authored with John R. Sussman, M.D.); *Trying Again: A Guide to Pregnancy After Miscarriage, Stillbirth, and Infant Loss* (co-authored with John R. Sussman, M.D.); and *Family Finance: The Essential Guide for Parents* (co-authored with Elizabeth Lewin). Her books have been spotlighted in such magazines as *Parenting, Parents, Working Mother,* and *Good Housekeeping*.

Ann's syndicated pregnancy column, "The Mother Load," appears in newspapers and magazines across North America. She also writes on pregnancy-related issues for WebMD.com and a number of other Web sites.

Ann is the mother of four children, ages four through thirteen. She also has experienced infertility, miscarriage, and stillbirth. She can be contacted via her Web site at www.having-a-baby.com.

Acknowledgments

While my name may be the one that's splashed on the front cover of this book, *The Mother of All Pregnancy Books* was anything but a solo effort. Writing a book of this size and scope requires assistance from a huge number of people — people I'd like to take a moment to thank right now.

First of all, I'd like to thank the parents who agreed to share intimate details about their lives with me while I was researching this book: Stephanie Anderson, Mike Arless, Kim Arnott, Rita Arsenault, Claudia E. Astorquiza, Gustavo F. Astorquiza, Josie Audet, David Austin, Sadia Baig, Aubyn Baker, Ken Barker, Nicole Barker, Christina Barnes, Kristi-Anna Beaudry, Michael Beaudry, Kim Becker, Lorinda Beler, Lori Bianco, Janelle Bird, Janet Bolton, Susan Borkowsky, Carolin Botterill, David Botterill, Lanny Boutin, Alison Briggs, Julie Burton, Rosa Caporicci, Stacey Couturier, Alex Crump, Jennifer Crump, Julie Cunningham-Marrows, Elvi Dalgaard, Marguerite Daubney, Marinda deBeer, Claudio Dinucci, Julie Dufresne, Rod Dufresne, Don Estabrook, Stephanie Estabrook, Maria Ferguson, Susan Fisher, Jane Fletcher, Cyndie Forget, Deirdre Friedrich, Jiri Fuglicek, Anne Gallant, Daniel Gallant, Sean Gallaway, Shannon Gallaway, Carrie Gallo, Monique Gibbons, Susan Gibson, Cheryl Gilleshammer, Andrea Gould, Jeff Gould, Joyce Gravelle, Susan Gray, Line Hamelin, Bonnie Hancock-Moore, Terri Harten, Lynn Hawrys, Jennifer Henderson, Kevin Henderson, Charlie Hendren, Mark Higgins, Richard Higgins, Brian Holmes, Lisa Holmes, Tracey Hrvoyevich, Kathy Ireland, Mark Ireland, Jodi Jaffray, Robert Jaffray, Debbie Jeffery, Jennifer Johnston, Teagan Jones, Chris Kapalowski, Maria Latham-Foley, Brian Lavender, LeeAnne Lavender, David Lindensmith, Kimberly Long, Janis Louie, Liz Luyben, Lana Luzny, Warren Luzny, Jeff MacDonald, Jennifer MacDonald, Myrna MacDonald,

Stephanie MacDonald, Lara MacGregor, Pandora D. MacMillan, Alexandra Marocchino, Heather McElroy, Melanie McLeod, Colleen Melsted, Jennifer Millenor, Kirk Millenor, Christopher Moore, Carissa Nicholson, Chris Nicholson, Erika Nielsen, Beverley North, Tammy Oakley, Chrystelle Pasquet, Yves Pasquet, Ken Pawlitzki, Maria Phillips, Tina Pilon, Heather Polan, Julie Pyke, Angelina Quinlan, Scott Ridley, Jennifer Kathleen Roos, Regan Ross, Lynn Rozon, Donna Sanders, Russ Sanders, Chris Schneider, Denice Schneider, Brenda Scott, Collin Smith, Jennifer Smith, Charlie Sousa, Elizabeth Sousa, Jenna Stedman, Ben Stephenson, Bevin Stephenson, Elizabeth Taylor, Jasmine Taylor, Lori Voth, Jane Walden, Amanda Walker, Darci Walker, Garth Walker, Jennifer Walker, Dorothy Williamson, Henry Williamson, Chrystal Workman, Laura Young, and Susan Yusishen.

I'd also like to thank the technical reviewers who agreed to review relevant portions of the manuscript of this book to ensure that my facts were bang-on: nutritionist Susan Hubay, high risk pregnancy expert Kathryn MacLean, fitness consultant Jenna Stedman, and Candace Hurley, founder of Sidelines National High-Risk Pregnancy Support Network

I owe a huge debt of gratitude to obstetricians John R. Sussman, M.D., and Margaret Lightheart, M.D., for reviewing the manuscript for accuracy and offering countless helpful suggestions. Their detailed comments on the book arrived by fax and e-mail at all hours of day and night — basically anytime they found themselves with a lull between deliveries! I am also forever indebted to my husband, Neil, for the countless hours he spent holding down the fort and entertaining a tribe of wild children so that I could (almost) meet my book deadline.

Finally, I'd like to thank all the people who played an important role behind the scenes while I was researching and writing this book: my research assistant Janice Kent; my U.S. editors Tracy Boggier and

Tim Gallan; and the numerous unsung heroes on the editorial, production, and marketing teams at Wiley. Last but not least, I wish to thank two very special people who are responsible for not just this book, but for my entire career as an author: Robert Harris, who gave me the opportunity to write my very first book and who's still one of my greatest supporters as I put book number 18 to bed; and Joan Whitman, who believed in this book from the moment the idea was first "conceived" and who served as its midwife right through delivery day — even when the "baby" ended up being 50% bigger than expected and a little overdue!

Writing this book has been a dream come true for me. Thank you all for helping to make it possible.

About the Medical Reviewer

John R. Sussman, M.D., is one of North America's most respected pregnancy authors. His first book, *Before You Conceive: The Complete Prepregnancy Guide,* has been a consistent best-seller since it was first published more than a decade ago; and his subsequent books, *The Unofficial Guide to Having A Baby* and *Trying Again: A Guide to Pregnancy After Miscarriage, Stillbirth, and Infant Loss,* have also received much critical acclaim.

Dr. Sussman is a frequent contributor to such parenting and health Web sites as WebMD.com and BabyCenter.com, most recently co-hosting two pregnancy courses through WebMD University. He founded the highly popular Preparation for Pregnancy program at New Milford Hospital in New Milford, Connecticut, more than 15 years ago.

A graduate of the Cornell University Medical College, Dr. Sussman completed his residency in gynecology and obstetrics at Johns Hopkins Hospital. He is a fellow of the American College of Obstetricians and Gynecologists and has been certified by the American Board of Obstetrics and Gynecology. He is currently serving as the chief of obstetrics and gynecology at New Milford Hospital and as an assistant clinical professor in obstetrics and gynecology at the University of Connecticut School of Medicine. During his 19 years in private practice, he has delivered more than 2,000 babies, including one of his own two children.

Table of Contents

CHAPTER 9
To Test or Not to Test? 317

CHAPTER 10
Lights, Camera, Action! 331

Introduction

The bookstore shelves are overflowing with books on conception, pregnancy, and birth. In fact, the last time I was in one of the big chain superstores, there were no fewer than four bookcases devoted to the business of making babies. (Clearly, the pregnancy book world is experiencing a population explosion of its own!)

While some folks might argue that the last thing the world needs is another pregnancy book, I beg to differ. You see, what's been missing from bookstore shelves (at least until now) is an informative guide to pregnancy that's both fun to read and packed with nitty gritty information on that amazing roller-coaster ride called pregnancy.

That's why I decided to write this book.

A One-of-a-Kind Pregnancy Book

As you've no doubt noticed by now, pregnancy books tend to fall into one of two distinct categories: bossy books that treat pregnancy as a nine-month exercise in deprivation and that leave you feeling like a bad person if you ingest so much as a single Tylenol during your entire pregnancy; and humorous books that treat pregnancy and birth as one big joke. (Hey, I enjoy a laugh as much as the next gal, but there are times when I'd prefer a hefty serving of hard medical facts!)

The Mother of All Pregnancy Books doesn't fall into either of these classic pregnancy book traps. It doesn't pretend to know what's best for you (like preaching to you about the evils of eating junk food during pregnancy, as one best-selling pregnancy book likes to do). Nor does it waste pages and pages discussing such inane topics as your fantasies about your obstetrician (the type of subject that another best-selling pregnancy book takes particular delight in talking about). Instead, *The Mother of All Pregnancy Books* arms you with the facts so that you can make up your own mind about such important issues as nutrition during pregnancy, prenatal testing, pain relief during labor, circumcision, and breastfeeding.

Why *The Mother of All Pregnancy Books?*

It isn't difficult to figure out why we chose to call this book *The Mother of All Pregnancy Books.* This is one comprehensive book, after all! If you take a quick flip through its pages, you'll discover a lot of valuable information packed between the covers, including

- a frank discussion of what it's really like to have a baby — the emotional and physical challenges of pregnancy, the career and financial costs of starting a family, and other important issues that most pregnancy books don't touch upon; a concise summary of what you need to know about preparing your body for pregnancy (including a discussion of the latest research about the father's role in ensuring a healthy conception); helpful tips on deciding whether or not you and your partner are good candidates for genetic counseling

- practical advice on what you can do to increase your chances of conceiving quickly

- the latest news about treatments for infertility and what it takes to successfully make your way through the fertility treatment maze (including tips on arm-wrestling with your insurance company, if necessary)

- up-to-date information on the costs and success rates for various high-tech methods of treating infertility

- useful tips on choosing a caregiver and a place to give birth (assuming, of course, that you have the luxury of choice)

- detailed information about making the healthiest possible choices for your baby

- the top ten worries for each trimester served up with a hefty side dish of reassurance

- the inside scoop on coping with a smorgasbord of pregnancy-related aches and pains

- fascinating facts about fetal development and how your body changes during pregnancy

- helpful advice on coping with a high-risk pregnancy

- detailed information on what it's like to give birth vaginally and through cesarean section

- the facts you need to make up your mind about such important issues as circumcision and breastfeeding

- practical advice on weathering the highs and lows of the postpartum period

- helpful insights on how your relationship with your partner may change during pregnancy and after the birth

- a sneak peek at "life after baby"

- a frank discussion of the joys and challenges of welcoming a baby who has special needs

- a detailed look at the latest research concerning miscarriage, stillbirth, and infant loss

- a glossary of pregnancy- and birth-related terms

- a sample birth plan

- emergency childbirth instructions

- a directory of organizations of interest to new or expectant parents

- a directory of Internet resources of interest to parents-to-be

- a summary of important pregnancy-related statistics

- a prenatal record

- a list of recommended readings for parents-to-be who are eager to do more cramming before it's time for "the final exam."

What makes this book really special, however, is the fact that it's based on interviews with more than 100 parents and parents-to-be. These folks passed on their best advice on a variety of different pregnancy-related topics — everything from keeping the romance in your relationship while you're trying to conceive to keeping your breakfast down after you manage to get pregnant. It's this real-world perspective that makes *The Mother of All Pregnancy Books* such a fun book to read. After all, who better to talk about the ins and outs of conception, pregnancy, and birth than real people who've been there, done that, and lived to tell.

You'll also find a few other bells and whistles as you make your way through the book:

Mom's the Word: insights and advice from new and expectant parents

 Mother Wisdom: little-known facts about pregnancy — including some really fun pop culture tidbits about giving birth

 Facts and Figures: medical breakthroughs and noteworthy statistics related to pregnancy

 From Here to Maternity: leads on a variety of pregnancy-related resources that you and your partner will definitely want to know about — 1-800 numbers, Web sites, freebies, and more!

Please note that throughout the book, measurements are provided in standard units. And please consult the glossary section at the end of the book for a comprehensive listing of medical and technical terms used in the text.

As you've no doubt gathered by now, *The Mother of All Pregnancy Books* is unlike any other pregnancy book you've ever read. It's comprehensive, it's fun to read, and, best of all, it's packed with useful information you won't find anywhere else.

I hope you enjoy the book.

—Ann Douglas

P.S. My editors and I are determined to make *The Mother of All Pregnancy Books* the best pregnancy book on the market today. If you have any comments to pass along — good, bad, or ugly — we'd love to hear what you have to say. You can e-mail me directly at pageone@kawartha.com, or you can contact me in care of my publisher at www.hungryminds.com.

CHAPTER 1

Are You Really Ready to Have a Baby?

"There's never a 'perfect' time to have a baby. Realistically, some times are better than others, but if you keep waiting for the perfect time, you'll be waiting forever."
— *Lori, 29, mother of four*

"There's never a truly 'right time' to have a baby. Something always comes up. Simply hold each other's hands, smile, and jump on the train!"
— *Alexandra, 33, mother of two*

So you're thinking of having a baby — of trading your relatively sane and orderly life for the chance to hop on board what can best be described as an 18-year-long roller coaster ride. (Actually, friends of mine who have kids in their 20s tell me that the ride lasts a heck of a lot longer than 18 years, but I have to confess, I'm still in denial.)

Well, before you do anything rash, like tossing the birth control pills out the window or reaching for the thermometer and the temperature graph, put on the brakes for a moment. After all, don't you owe it to yourself to find out what it's really like to become a parent before you agree to sign on the dotted line?

If it's the scoop on parenthood that you're after, you've come to the right place. I mean, if there's one thing I've learned over the past 12 years, it's what it's really like to be a parent: the good, the bad, and the ugly. And, lucky for you, I'm prepared to spill the beans. (Just pour me a hot, steaming cup of decaf and I'm all yours.)

We're going to start out by bravely going where no other pregnancy book has dared to go until now: by considering the plain, unvarnished truth about parenthood. We'll begin by looking at the financial fallout associated with becoming a parent as well as the career costs of having a baby. Then we'll tackle the age issue — whether or not there's an "ideal age" to become a parent. We'll wrap up the chapter by talking about how you may feel about starting a family and what to do if you and your partner aren't exactly on the same page when it comes to the whole babymaking issue.

Just one small footnote before we move on to the real nitty-gritty: There are a number of important health-related issues to consider when you're planning a pregnancy. Rather than starting out with a heavy-duty biology lecture that might evoke frightening flashbacks to your ninth-grade health class, I thought I'd ease you into the book gently. That's why I've chosen to postpone the discussion of preconception health issues until Chapter 2. (Don't touch that dial!)

MOM'S THE WORD

"Truthfully, we didn't spend a lot of time talking about having a baby — we actually talked a lot about reasons why we shouldn't have a baby!"

— *Myrna, 32, mother of one*

A Question of Timing

If you're waiting for some sort of magical signal that will tell you in no uncertain terms that this is really-and-truly-without-a-doubt "the right time" to have a baby, you could find yourself in for a pretty lengthy wait. You see, there are always more reasons not to get pregnant than there are reasons to start a family. In fact, if you and your partner were to sit down with a pot of coffee and a pad of paper, you'd be bound to come up with a whole laundry list of reasons why you'd be insane to even think about getting pregnant right now. Here are a few of the reasons that might very well find their way onto your list:

- You've just bought a house and you're up to your eyeballs in debt. (You figure that if you scrimp and save and do without unnecessary frills like groceries and clothes, you just might manage to pay for the damned thing before it's time to retire.)

- You've just sprung for a hot new sports car — and the interior isn't exactly baby friendly. Even worse, there's no place to attach a car seat tether strap.

- You've just booked one of those truly decadent couples cruise-ship vacations and you know your partner would be less than thrilled if you were to spend most of the vacation holed up in the washroom, battling morning sickness.

- You've just changed jobs and you don't want to have to announce to your new employer that you're "in the family way" before you even get your first paycheck.

- You're approaching the busy season at work and you don't want to risk having to take any time off just because your stomach starts churning every time you come within 20 feet of the coffee pot.

- You and your partner are getting along so famously that you're reluctant to risk ruining a perfectly good relationship by adding a baby to the mix. (There's an alternative scenario to consider, just in case the phrase "marital bliss" isn't the first thing that comes to mind when you think of your partner. If you and your mate aren't getting along at all, you may wonder if having a baby would ultimately end up driving you to divorce court.)

- You've agreed to serve in your best friend's wedding party eight months from now and you know she wasn't counting on having you looking mega-pregnant in all the wedding photos.

- If you were to conceive tonight, you could end up giving birth in the midst of a midwinter blizzard or a midsummer heat wave — or, perhaps even worse from your partner's perspective, during the Super Bowl or the NHL playoffs.

- You need to lose weight and you'd like to drop those extra pounds before you start your family. (Or, conversely, you've just finished losing a ton of weight and you'd like to enjoy the sensation of having a flat stomach before you agree to sublet your belly.)

- You find the sound of children screaming in restaurants to be annoying rather than endearing — which makes you question whether you've really got what it takes to become a parent. (Of course, this experience can sometimes elicit the opposite reaction: It can convince you that you'd be bound to do a better job at parenting than that imbecile sitting next to you!)

Yes, there are always a million-and-one reasons not to have a baby. And some of them actually make a lot of sense. I mean, if you and your partner are thinking about calling it quits, a positive pregnancy test may not be exactly welcome at this stage of the game. Likewise, it's probably not a great idea to announce you're pregnant when you're just a week or two into a new job — unless, of course, you happen to be self-employed. But as for waiting until your financial affairs are in order, your calendar is clear for the next nine months, you've reached your ideal weight, and you feel psychologically fit to become a parent (whatever that means!), you could find yourself waiting a very long time. (Heck, I've got four kids and I'm still not 100% sure that I'm up to the challenge.)

What it really costs to raise children

There's no denying it: Government statistics about the cost of raising children are enough to convince you to put your baby-making plans on hold for at least the foreseeable future. According to the U.S. Department of Agriculture, you can expect to spend somewhere between $117,390 and $233,700 to raise a child from birth to age 18. (See Table 1.1 for a breakdown of expenses on a year-by-year basis.)

MOM'S THE WORD

"Don't plan your family around finances. Personally, I think a woman's internal clock is a more reliable guide to family planning! If you have access to free used baby stuff — perhaps from friends or older siblings — babies are not that expensive. I spent less than $2,400 on my pregnancy and my baby's first year of life."

— *Maria, 31, mother of two*

Statistics like these are further proof that a little knowledge can be a dangerous thing. Not only do they fail to remind you that you're not required to have the entire $160,000 on hand before you lose the birth control, they also neglect to point out that there are ways of paring down your childrearing costs without practically guaranteeing that your child will end up on the talk show circuit singing the "I Had a Deprived Childhood" blues.

As you've no doubt noticed by now, prospective fathers tend to be particularly shell-shocked by these types of statistics. In fact, the vast majority of men I know would rather reach for the condoms than risk finding themselves shacked up in some unheated shanty with a wife and a brood of children they can't afford to feed. (Clearly this provider thing is hot-wired into men's brains.)

TABLE 1.1

ANNUAL EXPENDITURE PER CHILD BY HUSBAND-WIFE FAMILIES BY FAMILY INCOME AND EXPENDITURE TYPE: 1999

Age of Child	Total	Housing	Food	Transportation	Clothing	Health Care	Child care/Education	Misc.(1)
Income: Less than $36,800								
Less than 2 years old	6080	2320	860	730	380	430	760	600
3 to 5 years old	6210	2290	960	700	370	410	860	620
6 to 8 years old	6310	2210	1240	820	410	470	510	650
9 to 11 years old	6330	2000	1480	890	460	510	310	680
12 to 14 years old	7150	2230	1560	1000	770	510	220	860
15 to 17 years old	7050	1800	1680	1350	680	550	360	630
Income: $36,800–61,900								
Less than 2 years old	8450	3140	1030	1090	450	560	1250	930
3 to 5 years old	8660	3110	1190	1060	440	530	1380	950

Income: $36,800–61,900

6 to 8 years old	8700	3030	1520	1180	480	610	890	990
9 to 11 years old	8650	2820	1790	1250	530	660	580	1020
12 to 14 years old	9390	3050	1800	1360	900	670	420	1190
15 to 17 years old	9530	2620	2000	1720	800	700	730	960

Income: More than $61,900

Less than 2 years old	12500	4990	1370	1520	590	640	1880	1560
3 to 5 years old	12840	4960	1550	1500	580	620	2050	1580
6 to 8 years old	12710	4880	1870	1610	630	700	1410	1610
9 to 11 years old	12600	4670	2170	1680	690	760	980	1650
12 to 14 years old	13450	4900	2280	1800	1140	760	750	1820
15 to 17 years old	13800	4470	2400	2180	1030	800	1330	1590

(1) Expenses include personal care items, entertainment, and reading material.

Source: Department of Agriculture, Center for Nutrition Policy and Promotion, Expenditures for Children by Families 1998 Annual Report

Myrna, a 32-year-old mother of one, remembers her partner experiencing these very types of money-related worries before they decided to take the plunge. "My husband is very practical," she explains. "He's very much into saving money and paying off our mortgage — so every time we thought about having kids, he'd get anxious about how much money it was going to cost to send them to college!"

While you don't want to embark on a pregnancy without giving any thought to how you're going to pay for a car seat, baby clothes, and other first-year essentials, you don't necessarily have to start sweating about how on earth you're going to finance Junior's Ph.D. studies at Harvard. (Heck, there will be plenty of time to worry about that after the baby is born.) A more sensible approach is to ensure that you'll be able to afford to take some time off work and that you'll have enough cash on hand to pay for your immediate baby-related expenses.

That's the route that Marinda, 30, and her husband chose when they started planning for their first pregnancy. "Although we didn't have much money, we both believed that if we waited to be completely financially stable before having children, we might never have them," she recalls. "Being self-employed, I knew I wouldn't receive any financial compensation from anyone for taking a maternity leave, so during my pregnancy I saved enough money to cover half the rent for exactly one year. This allowed me to stay home for an entire year with my baby."

Note: We'll be revisiting the money issue in Chapter 7, when we talk about ways to save on baby-related gear.

Career considerations

As if money-related worries weren't enough, many women find themselves worrying about the impact that having a baby will have on their careers.

While it would be nice to think that only a few Neanderthal employers still take the view that switching to the "Mommy Track" is proof that you're no longer as committed to your career as your childless counterparts, most women find there are still some career costs associated with having a baby. Bottom line? If you're no longer willing to put in 60 or more hours a week to prove to the powers-that-be that you're still on the career track, you could find yourself being overlooked come promotion time, particularly if you work in a profession such as law, where billable hours are king.

And then there are all the intangible opportunities that may be lost if you choose to work less-than-full-time hours or if you decide to drop out of the workforce altogether for a couple of years after your baby's arrival — career costs that can be very difficult to measure in dollars and cents.

Does this mean the situation is hopeless? That switching to the Mommy Track will automatically derail your career?

Not necessarily, says Lori M. Bamber, author of *Financial Serenity: Successful Financial Planning and Investment for Women*. She argues that the career hit can be lessened if both parents help to cushion the blow: "Having a child does mean sacrificing a degree of career advancement and financial well-being, but the damage can be lessened dramatically by applying the power of two — two loving partners who work together to share the costs."

FACTS AND FIGURES

According to the U.S. Labor Department, almost half of people who qualified for family leave under the Family and Medical Leave Act failed to take their leave because they were afraid of losing ground in their jobs; and one-quarter of those who did take such leave were worried that this brief timeout from the workforce might short-circuit their careers.

Does this mean that working parents should wave the white flag and leave the workforce entirely? Not necessarily — although that's certainly a solution for some. Most families find, however, that they have to bring two paychecks home in order to keep the bill collectors at bay: In 68% of households headed by married couples, both partners work in the paid labor force.

Bamber offers these words of wisdom to women who are trying to decide whether to return to work after their babies arrive: "I wish I had known that the period in which I was consumed by motherhood would be such a relatively short one relative to my career. At the time, it seemed like I was giving up so much and as if those sacrifices were forever. My children are already at an age (12 and 22) where they are as much a help to me as a responsibility, and I am only now entering my prime career years. If I could have known then what I know now, I think I would have relaxed a bit and enjoyed things all the more."

The age issue

Another issue that many prospective parents find themselves grappling with is whether or not there's a "perfect age" at which to have a baby.

Some parents choose to start their families when they're still in their 20s, believing that the physical demands of parenting will be less difficult to handle if they have their babies sooner rather than later. Others prefer to wait until they're a little older and more established so that they'll have fewer financial worries and a lot more life experience to bring to the parenting table.

Jennifer, a 31-year-old mother of two boys, ages 3 and 1, decided to start her family early: "I had visions of my child being 20 and me seeming really old," she recalls.

While most women, like Jennifer, choose to start their families before age 30, a growing number of women are opting to postpone motherhood until after they pass that particular milestone. According to the National Center for Health Statistics, birth rates for women in their 30s are now at their highest level in at least three decades. And, what's more, in 1997, 9% more women between the ages of 35 and 39 and 21% more women between the ages of 40 and 44 became pregnant than did a year earlier.

MOM'S THE WORD

"I wouldn't presume to try to tell any other couple when it's best to have a baby. I've heard all the arguments about young parents being better able to keep up with their energetic little ones, and that children should be born close together so they'll be friends and grow up together, but you can't always neatly plan your family life as carefully as you might have intended. Nature has a way of intervening in such plans. Furthermore, in my experience, older parents are more patient and less likely to get frazzled at the antics of children, so their so-called lesser energy — which isn't necessarily so — is balanced by these abilities."

— *Pandora, 45, mother of two children (ages 13 and 1) as well as a baby girl who died of SIDS-related causes at 1 month*

So, is postponing motherhood until your late 30s or early 40s in the best interests of both mother and baby? Not according to the American College of Obstetricians and Gynecologists, which is trying to spread the word that waiting too long to become pregnant may mean missing out on motherhood entirely.

You see, unlike men, who have the ability to manufacture sperm throughout their reproductive lives, women are born with all the eggs they will ever have. The quality of those eggs deteriorates over time — something that can lead to fertility problems and an increased chance of pregnancy loss as a woman ages. By the time a woman reaches 40, for example, nearly half of her eggs will be chromosomally abnormal — a dramatic increase over age 35 when just one-third of a woman's eggs are abnormal. What's more, according to a study reported in the *British Medical Journal*, by age 45, her odds of having her pregnancy end in miscarriage are close to 75%.

While you might not consciously choose to postpone your pregnancy until you're into your 40s, you could find yourself on the wrong side of 40 by accident. You might find, for example, that after going into babymaking mode at age 35 it takes you a couple of years to conceive, or that an undiagnosed medical condition (e.g., a sexually transmitted disease, fibroids, or endometriosis) has unexpectedly wreaked havoc on your fertility. While many of these problems can be resolved, fertility treatments take time — time that may no longer be on your side if you've postponed motherhood too long.

Here are some other things you should know about if you're planning to put your babymaking plans on hold for now:

- Your odds of conceiving decrease as you age. According to the American Society for Reproductive Medicine, while a woman in her early 20s has a 20% chance of conceiving during a particular menstrual cycle, a woman over 40 has just a 5% chance of becoming pregnant during any given cycle. Or, to look at it another way, while approximately one-third of couples in which the female partner is age 35 or older can expect to experience problems with fertility, fully two-thirds of women can expect to experience fertility problems by age 40. (See Chapter 4 for a more detailed discussion of the effect of aging on a woman's fertility.)

- Women who become pregnant later in life are more likely to conceive multiples. Given the higher rate of complications in multiple pregnancies and the fact that multiples are more likely to be born prematurely and to weigh less than five pounds at birth, this can be a mixed blessing indeed.

FACTS AND FIGURES

The biological clock doesn't just tick for the female partner. According to the American Society for Reproductive Medicine, a man's fertility and sexual functioning decline as he ages, something that can impact upon his and his partner's efforts to conceive. And according to a group of researchers at Bristol and Brunel Universities in England, the odds of a man's partner conceiving after a year of trying drop from 92% when the male partner is age 25 to 85% when the male partner is age 35.

- Older mothers are more likely to give birth to babies with chromosomal problems than younger mothers. While a 25-year-old woman faces 1/476 odds of giving birth to a baby with a chromosomal problem such as Down syndrome, a 45-year-old woman faces 1/21 odds.

- Some preliminary research from the Harvard Medical School indicates that babies born to older mothers tend to have higher blood pressure than babies born to younger mothers. Researchers found that for every five-year increase in a mother's age beyond age 20, there is a 1.5 point increase in her baby's systolic blood pressure — something that could have noteworthy implications for the lifelong health of that child.

- Women who become pregnant after age 40 are more likely to develop such potentially serious pregnancy-related complications as pre-eclampsia (extremely high blood pressure), placenta previa (when the placenta blocks the exit to the uterus), placental abruptions (the premature separation of the placenta from the uterine wall), gestational diabetes (a form of diabetes that's triggered during pregnancy), premature birth (birth before the 37th completed week of pregnancy), and intrauterine growth restriction (when the fetus is significantly smaller than what would be expected at a particular gestational age). Women over 40 are also more likely to have pre-existing health problems (e.g., coronary artery disease) that can complicate their pregnancies.

FACTS AND FIGURES

Women over the age of 40 may face a greater risk of experiencing problems with the placenta simply because they're more likely to be giving birth for the second or subsequent time. The risk of developing these types of problems increases with the number of babies you've had.

- Older mothers are more likely to require an operative vaginal delivery (e.g., a delivery in which forceps or a vacuum extractor are used) or an induction (when labor is induced artificially). What's more, according to a recent article in *Obstetrics and Gynecology*, women over the age of 44 are 7.5 times as likely to require a cesarean delivery as younger women.

FROM HERE TO MATERNITY

Looking for a more detailed discussion of the effects of delaying motherhood on your fertility? The American Society for Reproductive Medicine has published a patient information booklet entitled *Age and Fertility: A Guide for Patients*. You can download your copy from the ASRM Web site: www.asrm.com.

The message from the obstetrical community is painfully clear: If having children is important to you, you should give serious thought to starting your family sooner rather than later. While there are some things you can do to increase your odds of conception when the moment of truth arises, unlike a fine wine, your fertility does not improve with age. If motherhood isn't in the cards for you in the immediate future, but you're hoping to have a baby at some point down the road, you should plan to take the following steps to help safeguard your fertility:

🔊 **MOM'S THE WORD**

"I've had six miscarriages and have always struggled with infertility problems. That's why it's taken me 20 years to have four children. If you're willing to wait until you're older to start a family, then you must also be willing to deal with the possibility of fertility problems. I'm so glad that I started my family at 20."

— *Liz, 40, mother of four*

- Choose a birth control method that is fertility-enhancing rather than one that could cause you problems when you start trying to conceive. Most experts agree that the birth control pill is a good choice because it changes the consistency of your cervical mucus, thereby reducing the likelihood that bacteria will get into the uterus and tubes. Pill use has been proven to prevent ovarian cysts, to arrest the progression of endometriosis (a condition that can result in progressive scarring of the fallopian tubes), to decrease the incidence of ovarian and uterine cancer, and to restore a normal hormonal balance in women who don't ovulate. The intrauterine device (IUD), on the other hand, isn't attracting such rave reviews. It's been linked to an increased incidence of pelvic inflammatory disease (a major cause of infertility in women).

- Pay attention to your gynecological health. Don't neglect any problems just because you're not planning to have a baby in the immediate future. The time to resolve these problems is when they arise — not years after the fact. If, for example, you have a milky discharge from your breasts, you don't menstruate at all unless you're on the pill, or you experience increasing facial hair and acne into your 20s, you may not be ovulating regularly or you may have some sort of hormonal imbalance (e.g., polycystic ovarian disease). Likewise, if you experience unusual pain and bleeding, you may be developing ovarian cysts (generally non-cancerous growths that can disrupt your menstrual cycles), endometriosis, or fibroids (non-cancerous growths in the uterus that can prevent pregnancy or increase your likelihood of miscarriage). The sooner you seek out treatment for these conditions, the greater your odds of being able to start your family when you finally decide it's time.

- Find out about any reproductive red flags in your family tree. If you have a close female relative who had trouble conceiving or if there's a history of endometriosis, uterine fibroids, early menopause, or uterine anomalies in your family, it's possible that you could experience these problems too. Many of these conditions are treatable, so find out now which, if any, of them may be in the cards for you.

- Choose your sexual partner with care. If there's a baby in your future, you should plan to practice safe sex now. Be monogamous or limit your number of partners. Use condoms and spermicide (in addition to killing sperm, spermicides can help ward off viruses like HIV). And make a point of being tested regularly for sexually transmitted diseases (STDs) such as chlamydia, gonorrhea, syphilis, human papilloma virus (HPV), which can cause genital warts and which has been linked to both pre-cancerous and cancerous conditions of the cervix, herpes, HIV, and hepatitis B and C. These diseases can cause infertility by either contaminating the pelvic cavity or altering your body's immunological defenses, something that can trigger pelvic inflammatory disease. And, of course, the last four diseases could lead to some very serious health problems for both you and your baby-to-be.

- Quit smoking. Women who smoke are 30% less fertile than women who don't smoke. What's more, they're at increased risk of developing pelvic inflammatory disease — one of the greatest threats to a woman's fertility. There are also a number of other excellent reasons for kicking your cigarette habit — a subject we'll be discussing at great length in Chapters 2 and 6.

- Encourage your partner to safeguard his fertility, too. A man's reproductive system can be damaged as a result of sports injuries, from cycling long distances (e.g., more than 100 miles a week), through exposure to toxic chemicals or radiation, and through the use of anabolic steroids and certain types of medications that may hamper sperm production and/or reduce sperm counts. If he's serious about becoming a father someday, he should also plan to get rid of his spare tire: Men who are significantly overweight tend to have an oversupply of the female sex hormone estrogen — something that can scramble the messages passing between the testes and the pituitary gland. Finally, he should also give up alcohol, drugs, and cigarettes: These vices may hamper his ability to ejaculate and/or affect his fertility. Bottom line? Let him have all the sex and rock and roll he wants, but not the drugs!

Other health considerations

Sometimes there are other health considerations that need to be taken into account when you're deciding on the timing of a pregnancy.

Heather wasn't in any particular hurry to start her family until her doctor gave her a bit of a push. "I have celiac disease and had struggled with poor immune function, extremely low weight, and poor nutritional status for many years," the 37-year-old mother of one explains. "So in early 1996, when my gynecologist told me, 'This is as healthy as I've ever seen you, and if you want to have a child, this is probably the time to do it,' we decided it was now or never. I was in the midst of completing doctoral studies and we hadn't bought a house yet — one of our goals before having a baby — but we knew it was the right time. Given my health, it might be the only time that would be right, so we both agreed that starting our family was the thing to do."

Jenny, a 31-year-old mother of one, had a similar experience: "I have a pre-existing medical condition called Alport's syndrome, a form of hereditary kidney disease," she explains. "My nephrologist advised that if we wanted to have children, we should do so sooner rather than later. My husband and I agreed that we wanted children and acknowledged the seriousness of my doctor's recommendations."

Emotional readiness

Your age and your physical health aren't the only factors you need to consider in assessing whether this is the right time for you to have a baby. You need to think about your emotional readiness for parenthood as well.

MOM'S THE WORD

"I always knew that I wanted children, but it wasn't a burning need. Once we'd been married for a few years, I started thinking about babies. Having them, holding them, and wanting one really badly. My husband was the same. That's when we knew that we were ready: We just thought about it all the time."

—*Jennifer, 31, mother of two*

Some parents report that, after years of not feeling any burning desire to have children, they're suddenly hit with a powerful urge to go forth and multiply. That was certainly the case for

32-year-old Jennifer, who recently gave birth to her first baby: "Two years before, I couldn't see myself as anything but a career person and graduate student. A year before, I was comfortable with becoming a wife, but not a mother. Then, almost overnight, motherhood felt right."

Others are concerned because they don't experience any discernible gut feeling telling them that it's time to switch into babymaking mode. "We really had to make a conscious decision to have a baby," explains Mark, 32, whose wife, Debbie, 31, is expecting their first child. "Our lives are quite comfortable now and there was no real drive within us. We were kind of waiting to be hit by this uncontrollable urge, but it never came. Age was probably the biggest consideration for us, both for the baby's health and not wanting to be too old as the child was growing up."

Myrna, a 32-year-old mother of one, found herself experiencing similar feelings of ambivalence throughout her 20s. It took a family crisis to encourage her to give serious thought to having a baby: "What started me thinking about having a child was watching my father go through a very serious, acute illness," she recalls. "My parents have six children, and it really was a time that brought out the strengths in all our family members. I think it also reinforced in me the importance of family and the bond that I share with my parents and brothers and sisters. I finally became more aware of how much I would miss if I didn't have a child and experience that deep feeling of being a parent. I can't speak for Scott, but I think he was much more ready than I was: He had been secretly 'kid-watching' for quite a few months. So when we finally decided, it was actually a pretty quick decision."

When you and your partner don't agree

While Myrna and Scott arrived at their decision at roughly the same time, some couples find they're operating on entirely different timelines when it comes to embarking on that weird-yet-wonderful voyage to parenthood.

MOM'S THE WORD

"Our only reason for waiting a bit was to give us time to adjust to being a couple. It was our belief that parenting is a challenge requiring a definite team effort, and we wanted to strengthen our team with some practice since we'd both been single for so long."

—*Jennifer, 32, mother of one*

It's a phenomenon that author Marni Jackson describes in her book, *The Mother Zone: Love, Sex, and Laundry in the Modern Family*, when she recalls how she felt about her partner's reluctance to commit to starting a family: "I wanted him to want [a baby] in exactly the same way, and to the same degree, as I did," she writes. "It didn't occur to me that men might come at the idea of fatherhood from a different angle. Perhaps for men babies are just an idea, an abstraction until they hold them in their arms. But the initial urge, the detailed, irresistible, and irrational longing, was mine. It was physical, like hunger."

Jennifer, 26, remembers feeling impatient when it became obvious that her husband, Kirk, was less ready to start a family than she was. "Kirk took a little longer than me to feel that it was the 'right time,'" she explains. "He said that he wanted to learn to be a good husband before he also had to become a good father. Also, at the time, he was in a contract position that wasn't necessarily secure. His reasons were more logical than emotional, and they were very good reasons that needed to be considered.

"I have to be truthful and admit that it made me sad that he wasn't ready. I probably pressured him more than I meant to. I worried about waiting too long, as I'd had a bout of cervical cancer in my early 20s and didn't want scarring to prove too formidable an obstacle to conception. If we did have trouble conceiving, I really wanted to leave myself enough time to follow other options like assisted conception and adoption."

Fortunately for Jennifer, it didn't take Kirk very long to come around. The couple is currently expecting their first child. Jennifer offers these words of wisdom to other couples who may find themselves at different points on the journey to parenthood: "Deciding you're ready to have a baby is a monumental decision in the relationship of a couple. Although it's hard to wait for your partner to be 'ready,' it's imperative that you give him the opportunity to get used to the idea, too. It's important to remember that your partner's reasons for waiting are just as valid as your own. You'll never be happier than when you first make love after agreeing that the time is right: That feeling alone is worth waiting for."

If you find that you and your partner are ready to do battle on the babymaking issue, it may be time to call a temporary truce. Here are a few quick tips:

- Keep the lines of communication open. While it may be difficult — even painful — for you to hear your partner talk about his reluctance to start a family, it's important to encourage him to say what's holding him back. Is he worried about the effect that having a child may have on your financial situation? Is he not sure he's ready to be saddled with the responsibilities of caring for a tiny human being? The more you can find out about his concerns, the easier it will be for you to help him to address them.

- Focus on other aspects of your relationship. Try to remember what it was about your partner that attracted you to him in the first place — something that's easier said than done, of course, if you're feeling angry and frustrated with him right now! — and make a point of having fun together on a regular basis so that you can stay connected as a couple while you weather this difficult period in your relationship.

- Accept the fact that you can't force someone to want a baby any more than you can force them to fall in love with you. All you can do is give your partner the space and time he needs and hope for the best.

MOM'S THE WORD

"It was my husband who got the ball rolling. I always knew I wanted children, but was still a bit nervous about the whole thing. I wasn't sure I was ready. We were married when I was 25, and when I was 27 he gave me a card on Mother's Day that said, 'I'm ready when you are.' I think we talked about it for about six months after that."

—Jane, 33, mother of two

When Mother Nature has other plans

For some couples, the whole concept of planning a pregnancy is a moot point. Long before they get the chance to sit down to have "the big talk," the pregnancy test comes back positive.

That's what happened to Ken and Nicole, who welcomed their first baby 2 ½ years ago. Ken was thrilled at the prospect of becoming a father, but Nicole didn't initially share his enthusiasm. "I had a lot of adjusting to do," she recalls. "I wasn't sure if I was ready to be a mom yet, and I had to adjust to all the changes my life was about to undergo. Fortunately, time, love, and patience resolved the issues of readiness for me."

Bevin and Ben, parents of a 5-month-old baby girl, found themselves faced with a similar surprise. "Ben and I had actually decided that about four years from now would be the right time to have a baby," Bevin recalls. "Unfortunately, someone else had other plans! We were just starting the process of purchasing our first home, I was toiling away at university correspondence courses, Ben was very involved with his weekend passion of sky-diving, and we were both working to get debts paid off before having kids. Still, if you pledge to love and care for the child and to do the best you can, then if the timing is off, it's not the end of the world."

LeeAnne, a 29-year-old mother of three, feels that it can actually be a blessing to not have to consciously plan a pregnancy. "I never did decide it was the 'right time' to have a baby: They just sort of arrived on their own schedule. That was probably for the best. I don't think we would have decided on our own to have children as early in our 20s as we did, but we're both very glad that it turned out that way. The kids are great ages in relation to one another (7, 5 ½, and 3 ½), and we both feel we have more energy and focus now than we might in our late 30s or early 40s. (I could be wrong on that! Guess I'll find out when I get there, for sure!)"

Assuming you have the luxury of time and are actually able to plan your pregnancy, you'll want to do everything you can to ensure that you're in the best possible health before you conceive. That's what we'll be talking about in the following chapter.

CHAPTER 2

Your Pre-Game Plan

I f you had called your doctor's office to schedule a preconception checkup 20 years ago, your doctor would have thought you were completely out of your mind. After all, back then it was unusual for a woman to be seen by her doctor at any time prior to the end of her first trimester, let alone before she'd even started trying to conceive!

A generation later, the thinking is entirely different. Most doctors now encourage their patients to schedule a preconception checkup before starting to work on Project Baby. The reason is obvious: It's a lot easier to deal with any health-related problems if those problems are detected prior to pregnancy rather than after the fact.

In this chapter, we're going to talk about preconception health planning. We'll start out with what you can do right now to increase your odds of conceiving and giving birth to a healthy baby — everything from modifying your diet to avoiding hazardous substances to kicking any bad habits you may have. Then we'll wrap up by discussing what you can expect your preconception checkup to be like.

MOTHER WISDOM

Don't wait for the pregnancy test to come back positive before you start leading a healthy lifestyle. The key period in your baby's development occurs during the first days and weeks after conception — a time when many women aren't even aware they're pregnant! So rather than waiting for the official word that there's a baby on board, pretend you're already pregnant the moment you start trying to conceive. That way, you'll be able to give your future baby-to-be the healthiest possible start in life.

Training for the Big Event

Ready to sign up for the mother of all of marathons — that nine-month-long endurance event that culminates with the birth of a baby? Before you slip into your running shoes and head for the starting line, you'll want to be sure you're up for the race. Here are some things you can start doing right now to ensure the happiest and healthiest possible outcome to your pregnancy:

Watch your weight — but not too carefully

While it's always a good idea to get to a healthy weight prior to attempting a pregnancy, the key word is "healthy," not "body of a supermodel." Believe it or not, the extra padding on your hips and thighs that drives you crazy on a day-to-day basis will serve you well as you embark on Project Baby. Women who have too little body fat tend to stop ovulating, which can wreak havoc on their plans to conceive, and those who do manage to conceive face an increased risk of having a low-birthweight baby (one who weighs in at less than five pounds and who may be at increased risk of experiencing some potentially serious health problems).

That said, when it comes to body fat, you *can* have too much of a good thing. Women who start their pregnancy significantly overweight or who gain too much weight during pregnancy face a higher-than-average risk of experiencing pre-eclampsia (a serious medical condition characterized by extremely high blood pressure) or gestational diabetes (a form of diabetes that occurs during pregnancy and that puts a woman at increased risk of developing diabetes later in life), and of requiring a labor induction and/or a cesarean section (two medical interventions that aren't without risk). What's more, overweight women are more likely to give birth to excessively large babies, babies with neural tube defects, and babies who are at increased risk of developing diabetes later in life.

Now before you do anything drastic, like bidding a fond goodbye to cheesecake or swearing off French fries and all your other favorite foods for the next nine months, make sure you've actually got some weight to lose. Studies have shown that 97% of women who consider themselves to be slightly overweight are actually within the normal weight range for their height.

Since most of us tend to be less than objective when sizing up our own bodies, rather than merely looking in the mirror it's better to see how your weight measures up on the Body Mass Index (BMI). (See Table 2.1: Are You at a Healthy Weight?) Here's how to interpret the BMI figure that you'll find in the table for someone of your particular height and weight:

- If your BMI falls between 20 and 25, you're already at a healthy weight.

- If your BMI is greater than 25 but less than 27, you're in the "overweight warning zone" (in other words, those few extra pounds may or may not be a problem for you).

- If your BMI is greater than 27 but less than 30, you're at risk of developing some weight-related health problems.

- If your BMI is 30 or greater, you're classified as obese and consequently face an even greater risk of experiencing weight-related health problems.

TABLE 2.1
ARE YOU AT A HEALTHY WEIGHT?

Weight categories (by BMI): Ideal Weight · Overweight · Obese

Body Weight (pounds)

Height (inches) / BMI	19	20	21	22	23	24	25	26	27	28	29	30	31	32	33	34	35	36	37	38	39	40	41	42	43	44	45	46	47	48	49	50	51	52
58	91	96	100	105	110	115	119	124	129	134	138	143	148	153	158	162	167	172	177	181	186	191	196	201	205	210	215	220	224	229	234	239	244	248
59	94	99	104	109	114	119	124	128	133	138	143	148	153	158	163	168	173	178	183	188	193	198	203	208	212	217	222	227	232	237	242	247	252	257
60	97	102	107	112	118	123	128	133	138	143	148	153	158	163	168	174	179	184	189	194	199	204	209	215	220	225	230	235	240	245	250	255	261	266
61	100	106	111	116	122	127	132	137	143	148	153	158	164	169	174	180	185	190	195	201	206	211	217	222	227	232	238	243	248	254	259	264	269	275
62	104	109	115	120	126	131	136	142	147	153	158	164	169	175	180	186	191	196	202	207	213	218	224	229	235	240	246	251	256	262	267	273	278	284
63	107	113	118	124	130	135	141	146	152	158	163	169	175	180	186	191	197	203	208	214	220	225	231	237	242	248	254	259	265	270	278	282	287	293
64	110	116	122	128	134	140	145	151	157	163	169	174	180	186	192	197	204	209	215	221	227	232	238	244	250	256	262	267	273	279	285	291	296	302
65	114	120	126	132	138	144	150	156	162	168	174	180	186	192	198	204	210	216	222	228	234	240	246	252	258	264	270	276	282	288	294	300	306	312
66	118	124	130	136	142	148	155	161	167	173	179	186	192	198	204	210	216	223	229	235	241	247	253	260	266	272	278	284	291	297	303	309	315	322
67	121	127	134	140	146	153	159	166	172	178	185	191	198	204	211	217	223	230	236	242	249	255	261	268	274	280	287	293	299	306	312	319	325	331

BMI	19	20	21	22	23	24	25	26	27	28	29	30	31	32	33	34	35	36	37	38	39	40	41	42	43	44	45	46	47	48	49	50	51	52
	Ideal Weight						Overweight					Obese																						
												Body Weight (pounds)																						
68	125	131	138	144	151	158	164	171	177	184	190	197	203	210	216	223	230	236	243	249	256	262	269	276	282	289	295	302	308	315	322	328	335	341
69	128	135	142	149	155	162	169	176	182	189	196	203	211	216	223	230	236	243	250	257	263	270	277	284	291	297	304	311	318	324	331	338	345	351
70	132	139	146	153	160	167	174	181	188	195	202	209	216	222	229	236	243	250	257	264	271	278	285	292	299	306	313	320	327	334	341	348	355	362
71	136	143	150	157	165	172	179	186	193	200	208	215	222	229	236	243	250	257	265	272	279	286	293	301	308	315	322	329	338	343	351	358	365	372
72	140	147	154	162	169	177	184	191	199	206	213	221	228	235	242	250	258	265	272	279	287	294	302	309	316	324	331	338	346	353	361	368	375	383
73	144	151	159	166	174	182	189	197	204	212	219	227	235	242	250	257	265	272	280	288	295	302	310	318	325	333	340	348	355	363	371	378	386	393
74	148	155	163	171	179	186	194	202	210	218	225	233	241	249	256	264	272	280	287	295	303	311	319	326	334	342	350	358	365	373	381	389	396	404
75	152	160	168	176	184	192	200	208	216	224	232	240	248	256	264	272	279	287	295	303	311	319	327	335	343	351	359	367	375	383	391	399	407	415
76	156	164	172	180	189	197	205	213	221	230	238	246	254	263	271	279	287	295	304	312	320	328	336	344	353	361	369	377	385	394	402	410	418	426

Height (inches)

Adapted from a similar chart at the National Heart, Lung, and Blood Institute: www.nhlbi.nih.gov/guidelines/obesity/bmi_tbl.htm

*To convert your height from inches to meters, divide the number of inches by .39370, and then divide by 100; to convert your weight from pounds to kilograms, divide the number of pounds by 2.2046.

If your BMI is higher than it should be and you'd like to lose a few pounds before you become pregnant, the last thing your body needs or wants is to be forced to follow the Fad Diet du Jour. Not only do you run the risk of depleting your body of the very types of nutrients it will need to build a healthy baby, your body may actually stop ovulating. (When your body is faced with famine-like conditions, it goes into self-preservation mode. After all, if there's barely enough food around to sustain you, your body isn't about to do anything crazy like embark on a pregnancy.)

A far more sensible approach to losing those unwanted pounds is to eat sensibly and exercise regularly. It may not be the quick fix or magic little pill that you're after, but it's a much more body-friendly alternative to crash dieting.

Here are a few tips on losing weight before you start trying to conceive:

- Limit the number of servings that you consume each day from each of the four food groups found in The Food Guide Pyramid. (See Table 2.2.) If you're used to eating 11 servings from the grain-products food group, try cutting back to 6 servings instead. If you go with the minimum number of servings for each group, you'll be consuming about 1,600 calories per day, depending, of course, on the types of food choices that you make within each food group. (Hint: Eating bacon at each meal isn't going to do much to help you kiss those extra pounds goodbye.)

- Zero in on foods that pack the greatest possible nutritional punch. After all, you're trying to get your body ready for the greatest nutritional challenge it will ever experience: sustaining another human being throughout the entire nine months of pregnancy (and beyond, should you decide to breastfeed).

- Watch your portion size. A bagel is a bagel is a bagel, right? Wrong! Studies have shown that bagels can weigh as little as two to three ounces or as much as six ounces or more. That bagel you're counting as two servings of grain products may actually be a six-serving bagel in disguise. (A word to the wise: If an innocent-looking little serving of grain products can get you into this much trouble, just imagine the damage that miscalculating a serving size of ice cream can do!)

- When you're designing your meals, give fruits and vegetables star billing. Grain products, milk products, and meat and alternatives should play supporting roles. A good rule of thumb is to divide your dinner plate into quarters: Two of the quarters should be filled with vegetables, one quarter with grain products (e.g., rice), and one quarter with meat or alternatives.

- Don't overlook the importance of being physically active. It's a lot easier to lose weight if you're exercising at the same time as cutting back on your caloric intake. Here's why: Exercise helps your body to burn calories, boosts your metabolic rate during and after a workout, encourages your body to build muscle tissue (which helps it to burn more fat), curbs your appetite, and can even help you to maintain your weight loss once you reach your goal weight. (One study showed that 90% of women who successfully maintained their weight loss for five years or more exercised three times each week for at least 30 minutes.)

TABLE 2.2
THE FOOD GUIDE PYRAMID

Food Group	Why You Need This Type of Food	Number of Servings You Need in a Day	What Constitutes a Serving
Bread, cereal, rice, and pasta group	Foods in this group play a critical role in converting food to energy and for maintaining a healthy nervous system. They also provide vitamins, minerals, and fiber.	Five to eleven servings	1 slice of bread 1 ounce of ready-to-eat cereal 1/2 cup. of cooked cereal, rice, or pasta
Vegetable group	Vegetables are a good source of fiber, vitamins A and C, folate, and minerals.	Three to five servings	1 cup of raw leafy vegetables 1/2 cup of other vegetables, cooked or raw 3/4 cup of vegetable juice
Fruit group	Fruits are a good source of fibre and an provide important amounts of vitamins A and C and potassium.	Two to four servings	1 medium apple, banana, orange 1/2 cup of chopped. cooked, or canned fruit 3/4 cup of fruit juice

Food Group	Why You Need This Type of Food	Number of Servings You Need in a Day	What Constitutes a Serving
Milk, yogurt, and cheese group	Milk products provide protein, vitamins, and minerals. Milk, yogurt, and cheese and the best sources of calcium.	Two to three servings (Note: Consume three when you're pregnant or breastfeeding)	1 cup of milk or yogurt 1 1/2 ounces of natural cheese 2 ounces of process cheese
Meat, poultry, fish, dry beans, eggs, and nuts group	Meat, poultry, and fish supply protein, B vitamins, iron, and zinc. The other foods in this group provide protein and most vitamins and minerals.	Two to three servings	2 to 3 ounces of cooked lean meat, poultry, or fish 1/2 cup of dry beans or 1 egg counts as 1 ounce of lean meat. 2 tbsp. of peanut butter or 1/3 cup of nuts counts as 1 ounce of meat.
Fats, oils, and sweets	Fats, oils, and sweets provide calories. but little else nutritionally	Use sparingly	1 tsp. butter or margarine 1 tbsp. mayonnaise or salad dressing 1 oz. cream cheese

Do a nutrient check

You've no doubt heard the expression, "You are what you eat." Eating a variety of healthy foods is never more important than when you're planning a pregnancy. Don't wait until your pregnancy is confirmed before you start eating for two; begin the moment you start trying to conceive. That means ensuring that your diet includes adequate amounts of folic acid, iron, and calcium — three nutrients that have a critically important role to play during pregnancy. You don't, of course, have to up your caloric intake at this point, unless, of course, you're seriously underweight and in weight-gain mode. That part of the "eating for two" program can wait until you get the official word that there's a baby on the way.

FACTS AND FIGURES

Large doses of certain types of vitamins — particularly vitamin A — are believed to be harmful to the developing baby. That's why it's important to stick with a vitamin that's been formulated for use during pregnancy when you're trying to conceive.

Folic acid

There's a solid body of evidence to prove that consuming an adequate amount of folic acid each day can significantly reduce your chances of giving birth to a baby with a neural tube defect, such as spina bifida or anencephaly. Studies have shown that when folic acid is taken daily for at least three months prior to pregnancy, it can prevent up to 70% of neural tube defects from occurring. Note: It's particularly important to take folic acid prior to pregnancy because the neural tube — the brain and spinal column in the developing embryo — develop very early in pregnancy, around 26 to 28 days after conception.

The American College of Obstetricians and Gynecologists recommends that all women who are planning a pregnancy consume a minimum of 0.4 mg of folic acid per day (the amount found in a standard prenatal vitamin) prior to conception and throughout the first 10 to 12 weeks of pregnancy — the point at which the brain and spinal column are finished forming. Women who've previously had a baby with a neural tube defect should take 4 mg of folic acid daily. Women considered to be at moderate risk of giving birth to a baby with a neural tube defect — women who have a close relative with a neural tube defect, who have insulin-dependent diabetes, or who are epileptic and take the drugs valproric acid or carbamazepine, for example — should take 1 to 4 mg of folic acid daily. Your doctor or midwife will be able to tell you what quantity of folic acid is recommended in your case.

Here's another good reason for taking folic acid: Some new research from the Netherlands indicates that women who consume adequate quantities of folic acid prior to pregnancy are less likely to experience early miscarriages.

 FACTS AND FIGURES

According to the American Academy of Pediatrics, fewer than one in three American women consume the amount of folic acid recommended by the U.S. Public Health Service.

Iron

Folic acid isn't the only nutrient that a woman planning a pregnancy needs to be concerned about. Iron also plays an important role during pregnancy, helping the body to create the additional red blood cells needed to carry oxygen from your lungs to various parts of your body as well as to your growing baby. If you have a severe case of anemia, your baby faces an increased risk of intrauterine growth restriction and fetal hypoxia during labor, and you'll be less able to handle the blood loss associated with a typical vaginal or cesarean delivery.

Unfortunately, many women of childbearing age don't get enough iron in their diet. As a result, they may already be iron-deficient (anemic) by the time they become pregnant. Because it's important to ensure that a pregnant woman has adequate iron reserves, your doctor will likely check your hemoglobin level at your preconception health checkup and throughout your pregnancy. If it's below normal, he or she may recommend an iron supplement and suggest that you make an effort to increase your intake of iron-rich foods (see Chapter 6). You should plan to include these foods in your diet regularly, however, even if your hemoglobin result comes back as normal, since your iron requirements double during pregnancy. That way, you'll have some iron reserves to draw upon if first-trimester morning sickness has you turning your nose up at anything more exotic than unsalted soda crackers!

Even if you do make a point of consuming iron-rich foods prior to pregnancy — which I hope you will, once I climb down off my soapbox — you may still become iron-deficient toward the end of pregnancy or after giving birth. If you find yourself feeling tired and draggy during pregnancy or after you've had your baby, it could be because your iron stores are low, in which case you'll want to talk to your doctor or midwife about taking an iron supplement.

Just a quick word to the wise: Some iron supplements cause constipation and/or gastrointestinal upsets. While the side effects usually die down after a few days, some women find they have to switch to a slow-release iron supplement or a pediatric iron supplement. Your doctor, midwife, or pharmacist will be able to help you to choose the iron supplement that's right for you.

You can also combat some of the constipating effects of iron supplements by drinking more fluids and increasing the amount of fiber in your diet. Here are a few tips:

- Choose whole-grain foods such as whole-wheat bread and brown rice.

- Eat breakfast cereals that are high in fiber. (You can give your bowl of breakfast cereal an added fiber boost by topping it with fresh fruit such as bananas, blueberries, strawberries, or raisins.)

- Look for ways to increase your intake of vegetables. Eat them raw or add them to soups and casseroles.

- Find creative ways to work legumes into your diet, like adding beans to soups, chili, and pasta dishes.

FACTS AND FIGURES

Be careful about the type of beverage you use to wash down that iron supplement. Orange juice and other beverages that are high in vitamin C are thought to make it easier for your body to absorb iron, while milk, tea, or coffee at meals can interfere with iron absorption.

Calcium

We all know that calcium plays an important role during pregnancy, but many women don't realize why it's so important to go into pregnancy with adequate stores of this crucial mineral. Here's what you need to know. A woman who is calcium-deficient prior to and during pregnancy may give birth to a calcium-deficient baby who is at increased risk of being born prematurely. What's more, she may find herself at increased risk of developing osteoporosis later in life.

Even though Mother Nature does her best to ensure that a pregnant woman will obtain adequate amounts of calcium from her food — a pregnant body is twice as efficient at absorbing calcium as a non-pregnant one — if the woman isn't consuming enough calcium-rich foods, her body will start to take calcium from her bones in order to meet the needs of her developing baby. (Yes, it's true: Your baby is somewhat of a parasite. Your body will automatically do whatever it can to meet your baby's needs, and if that means depleting your calcium stores in order to ensure that the baby survives, then that's what it will do. It's kind of romantic in a Robin Hood kind of way, now isn't it?)

While most women will get more than enough calcium by consuming four servings a day from the milk, yogurt, and cheese group of the Food Guide Pyramid (see Table 2.2), if you have a milk allergy, are lactose intolerant, or are a vegetarian who's chosen not to consume milk products, you may have difficulty getting enough calcium from your diet. In this case, you'll want to talk to your doctor or midwife about the advisability of taking a calcium supplement prior to and during pregnancy.

If you're taking an iron supplement to combat anemia and a calcium supplement to boost your calcium stores, you might just end up with a Battle of the Nutrients going on in your very own body. Because iron tends to reduce your body's ability to absorb calcium, you'll have to give some thought to timing your iron and calcium supplements. One solution that some dietitians swear by is to take your iron supplement at night and your calcium supplement in the morning — assuming, of course, that morning sickness isn't preventing you from stomaching any supplement anytime!

FACTS AND FIGURES

While it was once fairly routine for doctors to prescribe large doses of calcium to pregnant women who were thought to be at increased risk of developing pre-eclampsia (a serious medical condition characterized by extremely high blood pressure), that research has been disproven over the last couple of years.

FACTS AND FIGURES

Be careful not to go overboard in the calcium department. Too much calcium during pregnancy (more than 2500 mg daily from supplements and food sources combined) can put you at greater risk of developing a urinary tract infection (due to the increased amount of calcium that needs to be excreted in the urine) or kidney stones, and it can hamper your ability to absorb other nutrients such as iron, zinc, and magnesium.

Kick your smoking habit

If you're planning to get pregnant in the near future, you owe it to yourself and your baby-to-be to quit smoking now. Here's why:

- **Smoking makes you less fertile.** Here's something to consider the next time you're tempted to light up: A University of California at Berkeley study found that smoking just ten cigarettes per day cuts a woman's chances of conceiving in half.

- **Smoking interferes with the absorption of vitamin C.** Since vitamin C has an important role to play in helping you to absorb iron, smoking can indirectly contribute to iron-deficiency anemia.

- **Smoking disrupts the flow of oxygen to the baby.** Nicotine constricts the flow of blood through the blood vessels in the placenta, thereby reducing the amount of oxygen and nutrients that the baby receives.

- **Smoking can cause birth defects.** If you smoke ten cigarettes per day, you're 50% more likely to give birth to a baby with cleft palate and cleft lip. And if you smoke more than 21 cigarettes per day, you're 78% more likely to give birth to a baby with these types of problems.

- **Smoking can harm your baby's lungs.** Brand-new research shows that mothers who smoke during pregnancy risk permanently altering the structure and function of their babies' lungs, which can make their babies more susceptible to respiratory disorders and infections during early childhood.

- **Smoking increases your risk of giving birth prematurely.** Because babies who are born prematurely tend to experience more health problems than those who are carried to term, this is yet another good reason for quitting smoking before you start trying to conceive.

- **Smoking can be fatal to the developing baby.** Women who smoke during pregnancy face an increased risk of miscarriage, stillbirth, premature birth, and of losing a baby to Sudden Infant Death Syndrome (SIDS).

- **Smoking can cause certain pregnancy-related complications.** Women who smoke during pregnancy are more likely to experience placental abnormalities and bleeding.

- **Smoking is linked to childhood behavioral problems.** A recent study showed that toddlers whose mothers smoked during pregnancy are four times as likely to be impulsive and rebellious and to take risks.

- **Smoking can interfere with breastfeeding.** Smoking can decrease the quantity and quality of breastmilk, which can lead to early weaning.

- **Smoking is bad for your baby's health.** Children who are exposed to second-hand smoke are more likely to develop asthma, bronchitis, and ear infections. What's more, exposure to second-hand smoke during childhood can cause lung cancer later in life.

MOTHER WISDOM

Trying to kick your smoking habit before you start trying to conceive? Make sure your menstrual cycle isn't working against you. A study reported in a recent issue of the *Journal of Consulting and Clinical Psychology* found that women who attempt to quit smoking during the first half of their menstrual cycles (prior to ovulation) experienced less severe symptoms of tobacco withdrawal and depression than women who tried to quit during the second half of their cycles (after ovulation).

Quitting smoking is never easy, but you've now got the best possible reason for quitting: the health of your future baby. Here are some tips on kicking your habit:

- **Decide on a quitting strategy.** Quitting "cold turkey" works well for some women but not for others. If you can't make up your mind which way to go, here's a point to keep in mind: Studies have shown that withdrawal symptoms disappear more quickly for smokers who quit completely rather than for those who gradually wean themselves off their habit.

- **Expect to experience some powerful withdrawal symptoms.** Symptoms of nicotine withdrawal include a slowed heart rate, difficulty concentrating, difficulty thinking, irritability, anger, anxiety, restlessness, insomnia, tremors, headaches, dizziness, feeling "spaced out," tingling or numbness in the arms and legs, increased hunger (especially for sweets), increased coughing (as the cilia in the lungs regain their cleaning action and begin cleaning up the lungs), and an overwhelming desire for a cigarette. Fortunately, these symptoms tend to be relatively short-lived, peaking at around 96 hours after you quit lighting up and disappearing entirely before your one-month smoke-free anniversary rolls around.

- **Talk to your doctor about your plans.** If you're planning to use a nicotine patch or nicotine chewing gum to help you break your smoking habit, your doctor will advise you to quit before you become pregnant. Neither of these aids is recommended for use during pregnancy.

- **Get your partner in on the act.** You're not the only one who should be thinking about quitting smoking — your partner should plan to quit too. Not only is smoking harmful to a pregnant woman and her baby — one study showed that exposure to second-hand smoke during pregnancy increases the baby's chances of developing certain types of childhood leukemia — it lowers a man's sperm count by 20%. (So much for those manly Marlboro ads!)

Skip that glass of wine

According to the American Academy of Pediatrics, there's no safe level of alcohol consumption during pregnancy. Women who drink large amounts of alcohol on a regular basis while they're pregnant risk giving birth to a baby with Fetal Alcohol Syndrome (FAS) — a condition characterized by prenatal and postnatal growth deficiencies, facial malformations, central nervous system dysfunction, brain abnormalities, impaired motor function, neurosensory hearing loss (problems with the nerves that run from the ears to the brain), poor hand-eye co-ordination, and problems with learning, language, and behavior. Women who drink lesser amounts of alcohol risk giving birth to babies affected by fetal alcohol effect — a milder form of FAS.

While you should do your best to avoid consuming any alcoholic beverages while you're trying to conceive, don't spend your entire pregnancy beating yourself up if you drank a glass of wine or two at some point after you conceived. It's all water under the bridge now, so it's best to just forget about it and move on.

FACTS AND FIGURES

According to the American Academy of Pediatrics, approximately 20% of pregnant women consume alcohol during pregnancy.

FACTS AND FIGURES

Your partner should also plan to abstain from alcohol while you're trying to conceive. Alcohol has been proven to contribute to ejaculatory dysfunction and depressed sperm counts and testosterone levels, and some studies have indicated that babies fathered by men who consume alcohol on a regular basis tend to have a lower birthweight.

Just say no to drugs

Like alcohol, illicit drugs should be avoided when you're try-ing to conceive and after you become pregnant. The reason is obvious: Illicit drugs have been proven to cause a smorgasbord of problems in the developing baby, including cleft palate, heart murmurs, eye defects, facial deformities, central nervous system problems, damage to major organs, and low birthweight. What's more, babies who become addicted to drugs while in the womb experience painful withdrawal effects after birth. Cocaine has been linked to both miscarriage and placental abruptions (the premature separation of the placenta from the uterine wall) and maternal death from cardiac overload, while marijuana is believed to be responsible for a variety of neurobehavioral abnormalities in the newborn.

Your partner should also plan to kick his drug habit long before the two of you plan to start trying to conceive. Studies have shown that cocaine use can reduce sperm counts for up to two years and that marijuana use may affect both sperm counts and sperm's ability to fertilize an egg. And if your partner is in the habit of using anabolic steroids to boost his athletic performance, he could be jeopardizing his chances of becoming a father: Some men find that the drop in testosterone production and the shrinking of the testes that occurs when they take anabolic steroids continue long after they've discontinued steroid use.

Get your partner on the program

Smoking, alcohol, and drugs aren't the only issues that should be of concern to fathers-to-be. If the two of you are hoping to conceive in the near future, your partner should be playing an active role in safeguarding his reproductive health. That means

- avoiding injuries to the genital area, since such injuries can hamper the production of sperm, interfere with the transport of sperm, affect hormone levels, and/or lead to ejaculatory problems

---

MOTHER WISDOM

If your partner will be having cancer-related surgery to his uro-genital area in the near future, you may want to encourage him to consider making a deposit at the nearest sperm bank before he checks into the hospital. That way, he'll still be able to father any future children the two of you decide to have.

- not exposing the genitals to excessive heat, which can hamper the production of sperm

- avoiding exposure to toxic chemicals and radiation, which can destroy sperm production and/or damage a man's genetic material

- achieving a healthy weight (men who are significantly over-weight tend to have an abundance of the female sex hormone estrogen — something that can interfere with the transmission of messages between the testes and the pituitary gland)

- getting the doctor's okay about using herbal medicine prod-ucts (some products — including St. John's wort, ginkgo biloba, and echinacea — are thought to damage sperm)

- talking to his doctor about which drugs are — and aren't — safe for him to consume while the two of you are trying to conceive. A recent study showed that miscarriages and fetal abnormalities are more common in women whose partners take the drug 6-mercaptopurine to treat inflammatory bowel disease. What's more, certain antibiotics, chemotherapeutic agents, and other drugs (e.g., cimetidine, an antacid) can reduce sperm counts, and certain types of blood pressure drugs can contribute to ejaculatory dysfunction.

Kick your coffee habit

While you might find it hard to imagine starting your day without a steaming cup of coffee, most experts agree that caffeine use during pregnancy may pose some significant risks to the developing baby. Recent studies have linked caffeine to decreased fertility, an increased risk of miscarriage (in women who consume more than five cups per day), and lower birthweight.

Unfortunately, the one thing the experts can't seem to agree on is what constitutes a "safe" amount of caffeine during pregnancy. Until the jury comes back with a more definitive answer, it's probably best to err on the side of caution. If you can't kick your caffeine habit entirely, you should at least try to limit your intake to no more than one or two cups of coffee each day. (We're talking five-ounce cups here — not those bowl-sized latte mugs!)

Still not convinced? Here are some more reasons to cut back on your caffeine consumption prior to pregnancy:

• Caffeine tends to act as a diuretic, removing both fluid and calcium from your body.

• Caffeine interferes with the absorption of iron — something that can contribute to anemia.

• Caffeine is known to heighten mood swings and cause insomnia — the last thing you need when you're trying to cope with the highs and lows of trying to conceive.

Just one additional bit of fine print before we put the caffeine discussion to bed. A far greater range of products contain caffeine than you may realize. Not only can it be found in coffee, tea, cocoa, chocolate milk, and other chocolate-based products, it also shows up in a number of non-cola beverages as well. So if you're not already in the habit of reading product labels, this is as good a time as any to get hooked!

MOTHER WISDOM

While aspartame should be avoided by women with phenylketonuria (a metabolic disorder discussed at the end of this chapter), it's generally considered safe for use during pregnancy. Since it's still a relatively
new product, however, many pregnant women choose to err on the side of
caution, limiting the number of servings of aspartame they consume during
pregnancy.

Don't douche

Douching is starting to go the way of the dodo bird, but it
hasn't completely disappeared yet. If you're in the habit of
douching, you'll definitely want to give the douche bottle the
old heave-ho before you start trying to conceive. For one thing,
douching significantly reduces your fertility: One study showed
that women who douche on a regular basis are 30% less likely
to conceive in any given month than women who don't douche
at all. And as if that weren't enough, women who douche are at
increased risk of experiencing pelvic inflammatory disease (one
of the leading causes of infertility) and ectopic pregnancy (in
which the fertilized ovum implants somewhere other than inside
the uterus, most often in the fallopian tube). Finally, don't make
the mistake of assuming that it's safe to douche with water.
Studies have shown that it's the mechanics of douching rather
than what you douche with that's responsible for any resulting
gynecological problems.

Keep your stress level down

Here's one of those bits of advice that belongs in the "easier
said than done" category: You should make a concerted effort to
reduce your stress level if you're hoping to conceive in the near
future because high levels of stress can disrupt ovulation.

Now before you start feeling stressed about, well, feeling
stressed, let's do a quick reality check. We're not talking about

minor, day-to-day stress here — conflicts at work, arguments with your partner, the frustration of being caught in a traffic jam, that kind of thing. We're talking about major, life-altering events such as the death of a close family member or a marital breakdown.

Unfortunately, as much as we might like to be able to schedule life's little catastrophes, we rarely have that option. Consequently, we need to develop ways of coping with whatever curve balls life chooses to toss our way. If you find yourself faced with a crisis while you're trying to conceive or during pregnancy, you may want to seek out the services of a counselor who can help you develop healthy ways of managing stress.

Watch out for workplace hazards

If you or your partner are exposed to hazardous substances on the job, you might have to consider a job change or, at the very least, a job modification while you're trying to start a family. (Note: You'll find a detailed discussion of your rights as a pregnant employee in Chapter 7.)

Here are some of the major types of substances that should be avoided during pregnancy:

- paints

- gases

- lacquers

- industrial or household cleansers

- wood-finishing products

- solvents

- darkroom chemicals

- nuclear medicine testing procedures

- X-rays

- anesthesia

MOTHER WISDOM

Planning to conceive in the very near future? Now's the time to deal with your root problem. While the jury is still out on the dangers of dyeing your hair during pregnancy, this is one risk to your baby you can easily avoid. Either get your hair dyed before you start trying to conceive or switch to a toxin-free type of hair color. Or plan to postpone your standard dye job while you're trying to conceive and throughout the first trimester.

What to Expect from Your Preconception Checkup

You've started making some important lifestyle changes because you're determined to get your body in the best possible shape for pregnancy. Now it's time to pay a visit to your doctor to get a clean bill of health. Here's what to expect during your preconception checkup.

Your doctor will

- talk with you about your plans to start trying to conceive and answer any questions you may have about conception, pregnancy, and birth

- ask you questions about your lifestyle and recommend any necessary changes (e.g., changing your eating habits, becoming more active, quitting smoking)

- conduct a general physical examination designed to uncover any health problems and to recommend treatment, where applicable

- review the list of medications you're currently taking (both over-the-counter and prescription drugs) and let you know which medications are safe to continue taking during pregnancy and which ones should be discontinued

MOTHER WISDOM

Be sure to ask your doctor if there's a waiting period required before you start trying to conceive after you stop using a particular prescription or over-the-counter drug product. Some medications take time to clear your system — something you'll definitely need to factor into your babymaking plans.

- answer your questions about how any chronic health conditions may affect your ability to conceive or give birth to a healthy baby (see Table 2.3 for a list of questions to ask and Table 2.4 for a summary of the effects of certain chronic health conditions on pregnancy).

TABLE 2.3

QUESTIONS TO ASK YOUR DOCTOR ABOUT ANY CHRONIC MEDICAL CONDITION

How will pregnancy affect my medical condition? Can I expect my symptoms to improve, worsen, or stay the same?
How will my medical condition affect my pregnancy? Am I at increased risk of experiencing any pregnancy-related problems as a result of my medical condition? Will my pregnancy automatically be classified as high-risk? Will I need to make any significant lifestyle modifications (e.g., will I be put on bedrest)?
Will my medications need to be changed before I become pregnant? If so, how long should I wait after changing medications before I start trying to conceive?
Will additional testing be required during my pregnancy as a result of my medical condition? If so, which types of tests will be ordered and why?

TABLE 2.4

CHRONIC HEALTH CONDITIONS AND PREGNANCY

Condition	Effect During Pregnancy
Adrenal Gland Disorders	
Addison's disease (inadequate adrenal production)	May experience life-threatening infections and other health complications during pregnancy.
Cushing's syndrome (too much cortisone)	Increased risk of stillbirth and premature birth.
Autoimmune disorders	
Lupus (an autoimmune disease that primarily affects the skin and joints, but that can also affect the heart, kidneys, and nervous system)	You face a 25% chance of experiencing a miscarriage or stillbirth, 25% chance of going into premature labor, 20% chance of developing pre-eclampsia, and a 3% chance of giving birth to a baby with neonatal lupus (a form of lupus that lasts for the first six months of life and that can leave an affected baby with a permanent heart abnormality). Women with heart, kidney, or other internal organ involvement are generally advised to avoid pregnancy.
Myasthenia gravis (an autoimmune disease that causes the skeletal muscles to weaken and that contributes to fatigue)	There's a 40% chance that your condition will worsen during pregnancy, 25% risk of giving birth to a preterm baby, and a 10 to 20% chance that baby will be born with a temporary form of myasthenia gravis.
Scleroderma (a progressive connective tissue disorder that can cause lung, heart, kidney, and other organ damage, and that's characterized by joint inflammation and decreased mobility)	There is a 40% chance that your condition will worsen during pregnancy.

Blood Disorders	
Anemia (iron deficiency)	May experience fatigue, weakness, shortness of breath, and dizziness; tingling in the hands and feet; a lack of balance and co-ordination; a loss of color in the skin, gums, and fingernails; jaundice of the skin and eyes; and — in severe cases — heart failure.
Sickle-cell anemia	There is a 25% chance of miscarriage, 8 to 10% chance of stillbirth, 15% chance of neonatal death (death during the first 30 days after birth), and a 33% chance of developing high blood pressure problems and toxemia. May experience urinary tract infections, pneumonia, and lung tissue damage. More susceptible to sickle-cell crises during pregnancy. Can pass disease along to baby if your partner also carries the gene for the disease.
Thalassemia	May develop severe anemia and congestive heart failure requiring transfusion. If you have thalassemia minor (a less severe form of thalassemia) you may require blood transfusions during pregnancy, and run the risk of passing the disease along to the baby if your partner also carries the gene for thalassemia.
Thrombocytopenia (a blood platelet deficiency)	Increased risk of cesarean section. Babies born to mothers with severe forms of this condition may have increased platelet counts and problems with hemorrhaging — especially around the brain.

continued

Condition	Effect During Pregnancy (Continued)
Blood Disorders	
Von Willebrand's disease (an inherited bleeding disorder)	May need to be treated with intravenous clotting factors to prevent severe blood loss during the delivery.
Brain Disorders	
History of strokes, hemorrhages, or blood clots	Pregnancy may not be advisable, depending on the severity of your condition.
Cancer	
Cancer (malignant diseases)	Avoid conceiving until you and your doctor feel confident that the condition won't recur while you're pregnant. Otherwise, you could find yourself faced with the heart-wrenching decision to terminate your pregnancy in order to save your own life. Radiation used in the diagnosis and treatment of cancer can be harmful — even fatal — to the developing fetus. Chemotherapy can also be harmful to the developing baby. Surgery is the least hazardous option for cancer treatment during pregnancy.
Diabetes	
Diabetes	Increased risk of miscarriage, stillbirth, birth-related trauma, cesarean section, neonatal death, of giving birth to a very large baby, and of giving birth to a baby with heart, kidney, or spinal defects. These risks can be reduced by consuming large quantities of folic acid prior to pregnancy and by keeping your blood sugar levels down in the 70 to 140 milligrams/deciliter range prior to pregnancy and averaging 80 to 87 milligrams/deciliter during pregnancy.

Gastrointestinal Disorders

Crohn's disease (inflammatory bowel disease)	50% chance of miscarriage if your condition is active when you conceive.
Peptic ulcers (chronic sores that protrude through the lining of the gastrointestinal tract and that can penetrate the muscle tissue of the duodenum, stomach, or esophagus)	12% chance that your symptoms will worsen during pregnancy.
Ulcerative colitis (inflammatory disease of colon and rectum)	Small chance that emergency surgery may be required if your disease is active during pregnancy — something that could increase your chances of requiring a premature delivery or a cesarean section.

Heart Disease

Congenital heart problems (heart defects that are present at birth)	No significant risks to you or your baby if you have a minor congenital heart condition (e.g., mitral valve prolapse), but you could face some significant risks if you have a serious congenital heart problem (such as Eisenmenger's syndrome). You may wish to have your baby screened for heart problems prenatally since certain types of congenital heart problems are genetic. There's a 4% risk of congenital heart disease in children of affected mothers, although the incidence for certain types of congenital heart disease can be even higher. Note: If you have a mitral valve prolapse, your doctor will likely order a dose of antibiotics during delivery to minimize the risk of infection.

continued

Condition	Effect During Pregnancy (Continued)
Heart Disease	
Coronary artery disease (angina, heart attacks)	Significant risk of heart attack and death during pregnancy if your disease is unstable, since pregnancy increases the workload on the heart. There's also a significant risk that you might not live long enough to see your child reach adulthood.
Rheumatic heart disease (an autoimmune response to an infection that results in damage to the heart valve)	Intensive monitoring will be required during pregnancy and multiple cardiac drugs will be required during labor. There's a high maternal mortality rate for pregnant women with this condition. The risks are much greater for women who have sustained a lot of damage to their heart.
High Blood Pressure	
High blood pressure (hypertension)	Your doctor may want to assess the functioning of your heart and kidneys throughout your pregnancy. It may be necessary to change your blood pressure medications before you start trying to conceive. Most women with mild high blood pressure deliver healthy babies, but they still require more frequent prenatal checkups and face an increased risk of premature delivery. If your condition is severe (your blood pressure is over 160/105 or your condition is complicated by either heart or kidney disease), you face a 50% chance of developing pre-eclampsia or of requiring a cesarean section and 10% chance of experiencing a placental abruption (premature separation of the placenta from the uterine wall). You also face an increased risk that your baby will develop intrauterine growth restriction. Other risk factors include age (if you're under 16 or over 40), a long

High Blood Pressure	
High blood pressure (hypertension)	history of blood pressure problems (for more than 15 years), previous clot-related problems, and if you've experienced pre-eclampsia early on in a previous pregnancy or a placental abruption in a previous pregnancy.
Kidney Disease	
Kidney disease	One-third of women with kidney disease find that their disease worsens during pregnancy. Your doctor will want to monitor you carefully for urinary tract infections, as they frequently progress into kidney infections. Women with severe kidney disease often experience fertility problems, since ovulation is frequently disrupted. Those who become pregnant face a higher-than-average risk of developing pyelonephritis (an acute kidney infection that can result in permanent damage), of experiencing a premature delivery, and/or of having the baby experience intrauterine growth restriction if they've got a severe form of kidney disease. There's a 50% chance of developing severe hypertension during pregnancy if you've got both chronic kidney disease and high blood pressure. If you were already on dialysis treatments prior to pregnancy, you'll require them more frequently during pregnancy. If you've had a kidney transplant and are on anti-rejection medications you'll need to continue taking your medications during pregnancy. (Note: Most doctors recommend that you wait for two to five years after a transplant before attempting a pregnancy.)

continued

Condition	Effect During Pregnancy (Continued)
Liver Disorders	
Hepatitis B (a virus transmitted via blood and other body fluids that can lead to cirrhosis and liver cancer)	You have a 10 to 20% chance of passing the hepatitis B virus on to your baby if you don't receive any preventative treatment. Women who become infected with hepatitis B during the third trimester have a 90% chance of passing the disease on to their babies if no preventative treatment is provided.
Hepatitis C (a virus transmitted via blood products that result in cirrhosis and liver cancer)	Approximately 7% of women carrying the hepatitis C virus transmit it to their babies during pregnancy or at the time of birth. There is no known way of preventing transmittal of the virus from mother to baby. The risk of transmittal is higher if the mother also has AIDS.
Lung Disease	
Asthma	There's a 25% chance that your symptoms will improve, a 50% chance that your condition will stabilize, and a 25% chance that it will worsen during pregnancy. You should try to avoid exposing yourself to the types of substances that tend to trigger your asthma; avoid colds, flus, and respiratory infections; consider having a flu shot; continue taking your allergy shots; continue to use your asthma medications (with your doctor's approval); and be sure to treat asthma attacks immediately to avoid depriving your baby of oxygen. Note: 1% of women who've never had trouble with asthma before will develop the disease as a complication of pregnancy.

Lung Disease

Sarcoidosis (a lung disease caused by non-cancerous tumors called tubercles)	No special monitoring required during pregnancy. Pregnancy is risky only if your lungs are badly scarred, resulting in right-sided heart failure.
Tuberculosis (a bacterial disease that attacks the lungs)	No special monitoring required during pregnancy. Some drugs used to treat this disorder, however, are not safe for use during pregnancy.

Metabolic Disorders

Phenylketonuria (PKU) (a genetically transmitted metabolic disorder that results in elevated levels of the amino acid phenylalanine in your blood)	Increased risk of miscarriage and of giving birth to a baby with microcephaly or congenital heart defects, who is mentally retarded, or who suffers from intrauterine growth restriction and/or low birthweight. Decreasing your intake of foods that are high in phenylalanine content (such as red meats and soya products) both prior to conception and during the first trimester of pregnancy can help to reduce these risks.

Neurological Disorders

Epilepsy and other seizure disorders	1/30 odds of giving birth to a baby with a seizure disorder. Many of the drugs used to treat seizure disorders have been linked to problems in the developing baby such as facial, skull, and limb abnormalities; fatal hemorrhages in newborns; unusual childhood cancers; cleft palate or cleft lip; congenital heart ease; spina bifida; intrauterine growth restriction; and fetal death.

continued

Condition	Effect During Pregnancy (Continued)
Neurological Disorders	
Epilepsy and other seizure disorders	Studies have shown, however, that you can dramatically increase your chances of giving birth to a healthy baby by taking your medications as directed by your doctor. Note: Your seizures must be well under control before you start trying to conceive. Your pregnancy will also have to be carefully monitored because you'll face a high risk of seizuring if you develop pre-eclampsia (a potentially life-threatening condition characterized by high blood pressure).
Multiple sclerosis	There's a small risk (1 to 5%) that your baby will be born with multiple sclerosis. If you don't have any sensation in your lower body, you'll need to be monitored carefully during the final weeks of pregnancy in case you're unable to detect the onset of labor. Since multiple sclerosis can affect your ability to push, you may require a forceps or vacuum-assisted delivery or a cesarean section. Note: You should contemplate a pregnancy only if you haven't had any recent relapses.
Parathyroid Disorders	
Hyperparathyroidism (too much parathyroid)	Increased risk of stillbirth, neonatal death, or of giving birth to a baby with tetany (severe muscle spasms and paralysis caused by inadequate levels of calcium).
Hypoparathyroidism (too little parathyroid)	Your doctor will likely prescribe calcium and vitamin D to reduce the likelihood that your baby will develop a bone-weakening disorder.

Pituitary Disorders

Diabetes insipidus (a rare condition caused by a deficiency of an antidiuretic hormone manufactured by the pituitary gland)	Special monitoring or treatment may be required during pregnancy.
Pituitary insufficiency	Special monitoring or treatment may be required during pregnancy.
Pituitary tumors	Special monitoring or treatment may be required during pregnancy.

Sexually Transmitted Diseases and Other Infections

Bacterial vaginosis (a vaginal infection sometimes associated with a thin, milky discharge and fishy odor)	Increased risk of preterm labor, premature rupture of membranes, and/or a preterm delivery.
Chlamydia (sexually transmitted disease that can result in pelvic inflammatory disease; often symptomless)	Increased risk of ectopic pregnancy and infertility.
Gonorrhea (sexually transmitted disease that can result in pelvic inflammatory disease)	Increased risk of ectopic pregnancy and infertility.
Hepatitis B	Treatment is required to reduce the chances that you will transmit the hepatitis B virus to your baby. (Your baby will be given the hepatitis B vaccine and then again at 1 month and 6 months of age.)

continued

Condition	Effect During Pregnancy (Continued)
Sexually Transmitted Diseases and Other Infections	
Herpes	Treatment is required to prevent the disease from being transmitted from mother to baby. Herpes can be fatal to the developing baby. A cesarean delivery will be required if the disease is active at the time of delivery or rear term.
HIV-positive	Treatment with AZT is required to reduce your chances of passing on HIV to your baby. (The risk without treatment is 20 to 32%. The risk with treatment is less than 1%.) Note: The risk of transmission is further reduced if the baby is delivered by cesarean section and you do not breastfeed.
Syphilis	Untreated syphilis can cause birth defects in the developing baby.
Thyroid Disorders	
Graves' disease (an immunological form of thyroid disease)	Can affect the fetal thyroid even if maternal thyroid levels have been brought under control.
Hyperthyroidism (overactive thyroid)	Hyperthyroidism can interfere with ovulation, making it difficult to conceive. Pregnant women with hyperthyroidism are at risk of developing thyroid storm — a severe form of hyperthyroidism that is associated with an increased risk of premature delivery and low birthweight and that can put the mother's life at risk.
Hypothyroidism (underactive thyroid)	No special risks during pregnancy as long as you continue to take your prescribed thyroid medication. Women with untreated hypothyroidism are at increased risk of experiencing infertility, miscarriage, and of giving birth to a baby with growth or developmental abnormalities.

Mental Illness	
Depression	It's important to meet with your doctor to talk about the risks/benefits of discontinuing medication use prior to trying to conceive. If this is not possible, your doctor may wish to switch you to one of the newest generation of anti-depressants since these drugs are thought to be less dangerous to the developing baby than their predecessors.
Bipolar disorder	Your doctor may suggest that you switch to anti-depressants or anti-psychotics rather than taking lithium, but that isn't necessarily an option for every woman. Lithium poses some risks to your developing baby (e.g. a risk of malformation of the heart if lithium is taken during the first three months of pregnancy, and a higher-than-average risk of stillbirth and infant death). If you stop taking lithium on the advice of your doctor, you will need to gradually wean yourself off the drug over a six- to eight-week period and then wait a few more weeks before you start trying to conceive to ensure that you don't get any recurrence of your bipolar symptoms. Because women with a history of bipolar face a high risk of experiencing postpartum psychosis in the weeks after the birth, your doctor may recommend that you start taking lithium again within a few days of the birth. Note: Women who are taking lithium should not breastfeed their babies as lithium can enter the breastmilk in sufficient amounts to be dangerous to the baby.

- examine your breasts for any unusual lumps (pregnancy can change the shape and feel of your breasts, making it harder for you to detect the early signs of breast cancer during your monthly breast self-examination, so it's best to have a breast exam prior to pregnancy)

- do a pelvic exam and Pap smear to check for symptomless infections, ovarian cysts, and any gynecological conditions that could be difficult and/or risky to treat during pregnancy

- discuss your gynecological and/or obstetrical history (e.g., how sexually transmitted diseases or venereal infections as well as any previous miscarriages, abortions, stillbirths, and infant deaths that may affect your ability to conceive or to carry a baby to term — see Chapter 4 for a detailed discussion of the effects of sexually transmitted diseases and venereal infections on fertility and Chapter 11 for a detailed discussion of the causes of miscarriage, stillbirth, and infant death)

- talk about whether or not any pregnancy-related complications that you experienced in previous pregnancies are likely to recur this time around (see Chapter 11 for a discussion of many common pregnancy-related complications)

- find out if your mother took a drug called diethylstilbestrol (DES) when she was pregnant with you (90% of so-called DES daughters have experienced abnormalities of the cervix, vagina, and uterus that make it difficult for them to conceive and carry a baby to term)

FACTS AND FIGURES

It's not just DES daughters who may experience fertility problems. The sons of women who took DES back in the 1950s and 1960s also have genital abnormalities, including smaller-than-average testicles and penis, undescended testicles, low sperm counts, poor motility of sperm, cysts, and possibly even testicular and prostate cancer.

- do a blood test to determine whether you're anemic and whether you've been infected with any sexually transmitted diseases (undiagnosed genital herpes can be harmful — even fatal — to your baby; gonorrhea and chlamydia can scar your fallopian tubes and make it difficult to conceive or increase your chances of experiencing an ectopic pregnancy; syphilis, if uncured, can cause birth defects; and your pregnancy will have to be carefully managed to reduce the risk of infecting your baby if you're HIV positive or have full-blown AIDS)

- do a urine test to screen for such conditions as diabetes, urinary tract infections, and kidney infections

- do a rubella test (German measles test) to determine whether you're immune to the disease (if you're not, you'll need to postpone your plans to start trying to conceive until three months after your vaccination — a baby who's exposed to rubella during the first three months of pregnancy will likely die or have severe malformations)

- check that your immunizations are up to date and screen for hepatitis B (a disease that can be passed on to the developing baby and that can result in liver disease and cancer during adulthood)

FACTS AND FIGURES

According to the American College of Obstetricians and Gynecologists, there's no need to postpone becoming pregnant just because you've had one of the following types of vaccines: the tetanus-diptheria booster, the hepatitis A vaccine, the hepatitis B vaccine, the influenza vaccine, or the pneumococcal vaccine.

- ask you whether you've ever had chicken pox and, if you haven't, discuss the benefits of vaccination (you'd have to delay becoming pregnant for at least one month after the vaccine, but you'd reduce the risks of pneumonia and other complications should you develop chicken pox during pregnancy — see Chapter 6 for additional information about the effects of chicken pox on both mother and baby)

- assess whether a flu shot is advisable (they're generally recommended for pregnant women with serious health problems that would place them at risk for flu-related complications)

- talk about whether you're a good candidate for genetic counseling (something that's generally recommended if you have a family history of mental retardation, cerebral palsy, muscular dystrophy, cystic fibrosis, hemophilia, or spina bidifa; if your ethnic background puts you at increased risk of giving birth to a baby with Tay-Sachs disease, thalassemia, or sickle-cell anemia; if you're over 35; or if you feel quite strongly that you'd like to know ahead of time what your risks may be of giving birth to a baby with a genetic problem) (see Table 2.5)

TABLE 2.5

GENETIC COUNSELING: WHAT TO EXPECT

If you and your partner decide to go for genetic counseling, the genetic counselor that you meet with will

explain how diseases and conditions are passed from one generation to the next and what this may mean to you and your partner

assess your odds of passing on a serious medical condition to your child

let you know whether there are any carrier identification tests that might be helpful to you and your partner, given your family history and/or ethnic background

tell you whether preimplantation diagnosis is available for any disorder that you and your partner are at risk of passing on to your child

put you in touch with families who are raising a child with this
disorder so that you can get a realistic idea of what would be
involved in caring for a child with this type of medical problem

connect you with health-care practitioners who will be able to
answer any specific questions you may have about the prognosis
and/or treatment options for a particular disease or disorder

warn you about any hazards you may face on the job that should
be avoided during pregnancy (e.g., exposure to X-rays, toxins
such as paints and solvents, and other substances like gases
that could be harmful to the developing baby) as well as any job
modifications that may be necessary (e.g., no heavy lifting)

provide your partner with information on his role in giving your
future baby the healthiest possible start in life (e.g., not drinking
when you're trying to conceive, quitting smoking so that you and
the baby won't be exposed to second-hand smoke, and avoiding
exposure to teratogens that may be harmful to sperm)

As you can see, there's a lot to think about before you start
trying to conceive: your overall health, your gynecological history, your current lifestyle, and much more. And, as you've seen
from our discussion, preparing for pregnancy isn't just a
"woman's problem." Fathers-to-be also need to take steps to
ensure that the sperm they contribute to Project Baby is every
bit as healthy as possible.

Now that I've armed you with the facts you need to know
about preconception health, let's get to the main event: the business of babymaking!

FROM HERE TO MATERNITY

Thanks to some dramatic breakthroughs in the world of genetic testing, it is now possible to take a blood test that will tell you whether you are a carrier for certain types of genetic disorders and that will help you to determine what your odds are of conceiving a baby with that particular condition — information that may prove to be invaluable when you and your partner are discussing the pros and cons of starting a family.

While carrier testing isn't available for all types of genetic problems, it's now possible to find out ahead of time what your odds are of giving birth to a baby with cystic fibrosis (a disease that causes thick secretions that can lead to chronic lung disease, gastrointestinal tract problems, and other complications); Fragile X syndrome (a condition that causes moderate-to-severe mental retardation in males and borderline-to-mild retardation in females); Tay-Sachs disease (a disorder that causes brain cells to die, leading to severe retardation, seizures, and blindness starting when a baby is 4 to 6 months of age); Canavan disease (a condition that is similar to Tay-Sachs disease and that typicaly leads to death by age 10); Niemann-Pick disease — Type A (a condition that results in severe feeding problems that leads to both developmental problems and death); Gaucher disease (a condition that causes anemia, bone pain, and enlargement of the spleen and the liver); sickle-cell disease (a condition that causes severe anemia, bone pain, organ damage, and susceptibility to infection); and thalassemia (a condition characterized by severe anemia, the need for frequent blood transfusions, and organ damage). Note: You'll find a detailed discussion of the pros and cons of carrier testing in *The Unofficial Guide to Having A Baby* (Hungry Minds, 1999), a book which I co-authored with John R. Sussman, M.D.

Sperm, Meet Egg

After years of panicking about missed birth control pills and broken condoms, it can feel more than a little strange to be consciously trying to arrange a meeting between sperm and egg. On the one hand, it can be tremendously liberating: You don't have to pause at the most passionate point in a romantic interlude in order to go find the appropriate birth control paraphernalia. On the other hand, it can be a little bit intimidating: You may find it hard to relax when you know that the next hour or two of passion could very well result in the birth of another human being!

In this chapter, we're going to talk about what's involved in conceiving a baby. We'll start out with the science of reproduction: what has to happen, biologically speaking, in order for a pregnancy to occur. Then we'll look at the art behind the science — in other words, what you can do to boost your chances of conceiving quickly. (Despite what those scary tenth-grade health films like to claim, you might not automatically get pregnant the very first time you "do it" without birth control.) We'll conclude by pondering that age-old dilemma: whether or not there's anything you can do to increase your chances of conceiving a baby of a particular sex.

The Numbers Game

While many couples naively assume that getting pregnant is simply a matter of losing the birth control for a month, many find out the hard way that it's not always quite that simple. Because even couples at their peak of fertility have, at best, a one-in-four chance of conceiving during any given cycle (see Table 3.1), it's hardly surprising that the vast majority of couples don't end up winning at baby roulette the first time around.

 MOTHER WISDOM

Wondering why conception doesn't happen each and every time a woman has sex? Because a typical woman would end up with 3,000 children, that's why! According to Robin Baker and Elizabeth Oram, authors of *Baby Wars*, that's how often a typical woman has sex over her lifetime. And since that size of family would put even the Old Woman Who Lived in a Shoe to shame, in humans, the female reproductive system is designed for just a few hits and a whole lot of misses.

A female honeybee's reproductive system works in an entirely different fashion, however. Instead of having sex far more often than is necessary to achieve a pregnancy, as is the case with humans, she can conceive millions of offspring over a period of years from a single episode of intercourse. Her secret? She stores the sperm in her body so that it'll be there whenever she's ready to get pregnant again.

While the odds that you'll end up conceiving this month may be discouragingly low, it's important to take a look at the big picture. As Table 3.1 indicates, a couple in their late 20s has an 86 to 93% chance of conceiving within one year of actively trying (e.g., having intercourse daily or every other day during the woman's most fertile period). That's not to say you have to aim to have intercourse every day, of course; most fertility experts agree that every other day is plenty.

TABLE 3.1

THE ODDS OF CONCEIVING IN ANY GIVEN CYCLE OR YEAR FOR WOMEN OF VARIOUS AGES

Age	Odds That You'll Conceive in Any Given Month	Average Number of Months It Takes to Conceive	Probability That You'll Be Pregnant Within One Year
Early 20s	20 to 25%	4 to 5 months	93 to 97%
Late 20s	15 to 20%	5 to 6.7 months	86 to 93%
Early 30s	10 to 15%	6.7 to 10 months	72 to 86%
Late 30s	8.3 to 10%	10 to 12 months	65 to 72%

Adapted from a similar chart in How to Get Pregnant by Sherman J. Silber, M.D. (New York: Warner Books, 1980). Note: The data reported by Silber is supported by more recent data from the National Center for Health Statistics, which reports that a couple under the age of 25 has a 96% of conceiving within one year; a couple between the ages of 25 and 34 has an 86% chance of conceiving within a year; and a couple between the ages of 35 and 44 has a 78% chance of conceiving within one year.

The Science of Conception

While you might think you paid enough attention in tenth-grade health class to pick up the necessary facts about human reproduction, chances are you acquired at least a few pieces of misinformation along the way. (Think about it: Maybe some cute guy in your class asked to borrow a pen at the most critical point in the lecture on conception and birth!) Studies have shown that there's still a phenomenal amount of guff out there about the science of conception. Consider these facts:

- Researchers have found that many couples wrongly assume they can become pregnant by timing intercourse to occur during the day or two following ovulation, when quite the opposite is true. It's only possible to conceive during the five days leading up to the time of ovulation (the point in a woman's menstrual cycle when the egg is released from the ovary). Once ovulation has occurred, the window of opportunity for conceiving during that cycle slams shut within about 12 hours.

- Other studies have indicated that many couples who show up for an infertility assessment don't have fertility problems, they have timing problems. There's a common misconception that a woman ovulates two weeks after the first day of her last period when, in fact, she actually ovulates 14 days before the first day of her next period. It's a moot point if you have a textbook 28-day menstrual cycle, but it can throw your babymaking efforts off by an entire week if your cycles tend to be 35 days long. After all, even the hardiest and most determined of sperm can't camp out indefinitely in the fallopian tube, hoping that some egg will come strolling by. The life cycle of a sperm cell is, after all, short and sweet: Even grade A sperm can't live for much longer than five days.

Because it's so important to have your facts straight when you're trying to conceive, we're going to take a few more minutes to talk about how the whole reproductive process works — and clear up a lot of conception misconceptions along the way. Here goes.

 MOTHER WISDOM

A recent study conducted at the University of Liverpool in England indicates that taller men tend to have more children than shorter men. The researchers decided to study this phenomenon after noting that men were willing to mention their height in personal ads only if they happened to be particularly tall. "You don't see advertisements saying, 'I'm five-foot-three, give me a call,'" one of the researchers told the Reuters news service.

MOTHER WISDOM

Wondering why you sometimes feel like two different people — Dr. Jekyll and Ms. Hyde? It's because, for all intents and purposes, you are two entirely different people, depending on which phase of your menstrual cycle you're in! You see, the hormonal cocktail that affects how you feel changes dramatically over the course of your menstrual cycle. During the first half of your cycle (the so-called follicular or proliferative phase), your hormones are focusing on preparing for ovulation; during the second half of your cycle (the so-called luteal or secretory phase), your hormones are hard at work trying to prepare your uterus to sustain any pregnancy that may have occurred. Since the recipes for these two cocktails — the follicular cocktail and the luteal cocktail — are dramatically different, you may experience some powerful physical and emotional changes over the course of your menstrual cycle.

A tale of two phases

A woman's menstrual cycle is divided into two distinct phases: the follicular (or proliferative) phase, which precedes ovulation; and the luteal (or secretory) phrase, which follows it.

During the follicular phase, your body has one mission and one mission only — to prepare itself for ovulation. Inside your ovaries, approximately 1,000 eggs begin to mature. Of these, just 20 eggs (or ova) respond to the release of follicle stimulating hormone (FSH) by the pituitary gland in the brain and begin to ripen and to occupy fluid-filled sacs known as follicles.

Since you couldn't possibly conceive and carry 20 babies to term (nor would you want to — just think of the stretch marks!), your body is just hedging its bets. It hopes that by entering 20 candidates in the Ms. Follicle contest, at least one will end up making that glorious trip down that runway known as the fallopian tube. (To qualify for the fallopian runway stroll, the follicle doesn't need a slinky ballgown or a flashy tiara à la Miss America: It simply needs to be the dominant follicle — the one that gets chosen to rupture. Yes, ladies, this is one contest where the skinnier contestants get left behind: For once, bigger is better!) Sometimes, two or more follicles will end up rupturing in the same cycle, in which case a multiple pregnancy may result; at other times, none of the 20 follicles manage to mature enough to rupture, in which case an anovulatory cycle (a cycle without ovulation) is said to have occurred. (Believe it or not, even the most fertile women in the world have anovulatory cycles on a regular basis — another one of those all-important details that they failed to teach you in health class!)

A lot of people believe that the two ovaries share egg-releasing duties on some predetermined schedule — that they alternate from month to month. This is simply not the case. Researchers have discovered that it's purely a matter of chance which ovary ends up releasing the egg — although, of course, if you have only one functioning ovary, it'll win the draw by default. This is Mother Nature's way of maximizing your childbearing potential: equipping you with a "spare" ovary.

MOTHER WISDOM

The old expression "waste not, want not" seems to go out the window as far as the female reproductive system is concerned. While the ovaries of a female fetus contain 6 to 7 million eggs by the time she reaches 20 weeks gestation, at birth, her supply will have dwindled to just 2 to 3 million eggs. And by the time she reaches puberty, just 400,000 of those eggs will be left. During her reproductive years, she'll use less than 500 of them and, in the end, she may end up giving birth to, at most, a handful of children. (Not exactly a model of efficiency, now is it?)

At the same time, the level of estrogen in your body begins to rise. This causes the endometrial lining of your uterus to thicken significantly (from 1/25" to 1/6") and prepares it for the possible implantation of a fertilized egg. The rising levels of estrogen also change the quantity and quality of your cervical mucus. Scant and sticky during the early part of your cycle, as ovulation approaches, the mucus becomes increasingly abundant and slippery — like egg white. This "egg white" cervical mucus is designed to help transport the sperm into the uterus and to protect it from the harsh vaginal environment. (Believe it or not, a healthy vagina has the same acidity level as a glass of red wine.)

The hormonal changes that occur as ovulation approaches also trigger some noteworthy behavioral changes. You may find yourself feeling increasingly interested in sex and more susceptible to the charms of the male species. Here's why:

- Studies have shown that a woman's vision and sense of smell become more acute around the time of ovulation. Scientists theorize that this may be Mother Nature's way of encouraging her to give more notice to members of the opposite sex. After all, if the man in your life starts looking more appealing and starts smelling irresistible, you're more likely to hop in the sack with him, now aren't you? There's just one disturbing footnote to this research: Apparently the one scent that we find truly irresistible as ovulation approaches is — are you ready? — the smell of male armpit sweat. I don't know about you, but I'd take a truckload of Old Spice in place of Eau de Sweat any day. (Or at least I think I would. Perhaps my subconscious mind doesn't agree. . . .)

MOTHER WISDOM

Here's another interesting finding related to the science of attraction. Researchers in Switzerland have discovered that women tend to be most attracted to those men who smell the least like themselves. There's just one small but noteworthy exception: Women who are taking birth control pills tend to experience the opposite effect. They gravitate toward those men who smell the *most* like themselves.

We're programmed to act more provocatively as ovulation approaches. Researchers have found that the skimpier the clothing

a woman wears to a nightclub, the more likely she is to be ovulating! (Bet that bit of news would encourage more than a few
would-be Romeos to turn off the charm.)

Our criteria for the ideal man changes as ovulation
approaches. While we generally tend to prefer men with slightly
more feminine facial features (we tend to link these features with
more positive personality traits, apparently), according to
researchers at the University of St. Andrews in Scotland, we're
more drawn to men with more masculine features during the
days when we're most likely to conceive. So next time you find
yourself loading up on Eastwood and Schwarzenegger flicks at
the local video outlet, reach for your calendar. Perhaps the
moment of truth has arrived again!

Hormonal changes are also responsible for triggering the big
event around which the entire female menstrual cycle is centered:
ovulation. Just prior to ovulation, rising levels of estrogen
prompt the pituitary gland to trigger a brief but intense surge of
luteinizing hormone (LH). This causes the dominant follicle to
rupture and release its egg 36 to 42 hours later. Some women
experience pain in the lower abdomen as ovulation occurs — a
sensation that the Germans call mittelschmerz or "pain in the
middle." Some scientists theorize that mittelschmerz may be
caused by the irritation of the lining of the body cavity by blood
or other fluid that escapes from the ovary at the time of ovulation.

Once the egg has been released, it needs to find its way to the
fallopian tube. (Contrary to what most people believe, the
ovaries aren't directly attached to the fallopian tubes. They just
happen to live in the same neighborhood.) Fortunately, Mother
Nature — amazing designer that she is — put some thought
into this whole process as well. Cilia (tiny hairs that line the
inside of the fallopian tubes) create a suction-like effect that's
designed to draw the egg into the fallopian tube. Once the egg
gets inside, the cilia move the egg in conveyer-belt fashion to the
inner portion of the fallopian tube (the isthmus) — the zone
where the egg can be fertilized. (There's only about a six- to

eight-hour window when fertilization can occur or else the egg shall become overripe and die, so time is of the essence.) Once the egg has been fertilized, it spends the next 80 hours making its way through the tube at a speed of about one millimeter/hour before finally reaching the uterus. (Timing is critical here. If the egg arrives too soon, the uterine lining won't yet be thick enough to promote a healthy implantation. If it takes too long to pass through the tube, the egg will implant in the tube instead, which can result in an ectopic pregnancy. See Chapter 11.)

Having accomplished Mission Ovulation, your body now switches gears, focusing its energies on creating an egg-friendly uterine environment. The ruptured ovarian follicle (now known as the corpus luteum, or "yellow body," because of its color) begins manufacturing progesterone. The progesterone causes the uterine lining to thicken so that it can receive a fertilized egg. It also causes your cervical mucus to become sticky and impermeable to sperm. (Hey, at this stage of the game, any sperm showing up would be just crashing the party. If a pregnancy is going to be achieved, it's already happened, thanks to some earlier recruits to the Sperm Battalion.)

If conception has occurred, the corpeus luteum continues to produce progesterone until the placenta takes over the manufacturing duties approximately three months down the road. If conception has not occurred, the corpus luteum begins to deteriorate, progesterone levels drop, your uterus begins to shed the endometrial layer it has built up, and your menstrual period begins.

The sperm connection

Up until now, we've been ignoring the role that sperm has to play in the whole reproductive equation. Well, ladies, it's time to right that wrong!

MOTHER WISDOM

When sperm cells were first viewed under the microscope 300 years ago, scientists thought they could see miniature human beings in each cell. Consequently, they named these cells "spermatozoa," which means "seed animals."

We've already talked about how wasteful the female reproductive system is: 1,000 follicles begin to ripen each month, but usually only one ends up rupturing. Well, the female reproductive system looks like a model of conservation compared to the male reproductive system. Here's why. When a man ejaculates, he deposits approximately 200 million sperm in his partner's vagina. Of these, just 200,000 will make it beyond the vagina (one out of every thousand) and just 400 will make it into the fallopian tube. It isn't hard to figure out what's responsible for the loss of so many sperm. Despite the fact that the semen that carries the sperm is alkaline (Mother Nature's way of providing a barrier between the sperm and the harsh vaginal environment), the vast majority of sperm are unable to survive in the acidic vaginal environment. (Remember, the poor little sperm are being asked to swim through the pH equivalent of a glass of red wine.)

Those sperm that do end up surviving are the ones that manage to make their way into the cervical mucus as quickly as possible. (Like the semen, the cervical mucus is alkaline and designed to help to protect the sperm.) Once they've reached this safe haven, they start making their way to the fallopian tube.

While we may have visions of all the sperm setting course for the fallopian tube in flotilla-like formation, medical science has proven that theory wrong. As it turns out, only a few sperm actually set out for their destination right away, arriving within an hour of ejaculation. Some choose to make a stopover at the lower end of the fallopian tube, below the fertilization zone, while others remain in storage sites within the cervix, gradually heading northward over the next five days. Consequently, rather than arriving all at once, there's a steady migration of sperm through the fertilization zone over a five-day period. Since sperm remain fertile for up to five days, this helps to maximize the chance that some sperm will be on hand whenever the egg decides to show up for a fallopian rendezvous.

While it technically takes just one sperm to fertilize the egg, it takes many more than that to ensure conception will take place. Scientists have discovered that it takes hundreds of sperm working as a team in order to penetrate the membrane of the egg — something that may help to explain, I suppose, why men are so big on team sports. Once the first sperm has managed to penetrate the egg membrane, no other sperm can pass through. (As Robin Baker puts it in *Sperm Wars,* "If you are a human sperm, there is no prize for second place.")

Now that we've completed this refresher course in human reproduction, let's get down to the real nitty-gritty: what you can do to increase your odds of conceiving quickly.

MOTHER WISDOM

Worried that the wet spot on the bed means that all the sperm have dripped out? Relax! Mother Nature's got you covered. The coagulation that occurs after ejaculation helps to minimize the amount of ejaculate that is lost. The ejaculate thickens and sticks to the area where it's been deposited — ideally the upper vagina and cervical area, if you're trying for a baby. The fluid that drips out of your vagina after intercourse tends to be made up of cervical mucus, seminal fluid, and sperm that are too old or too damaged to penetrate the cervical mucus. In other words, what you're losing are the waste products of intercourse — not the sperm itself.

MOTHER WISDOM

A study at the University of Manchester in Britain has revealed that high levels of testosterone are associated with improved verbal abilities. So the next time some guy tries to sweet-talk you into going to bed with him, you'll know what's powering all those compliments!

What You Can Do to Increase Your Odds of Conceiving Quickly

Some couples like to take a completely relaxed approach to conception, simply abandoning the birth control and deciding to let nature take its course. Others, however, are more eager to get on with the show. Having made up their minds that they want a baby, they want to conceive sooner rather than later.

Which camp you end up falling into will be determined by a number of factors, including

- your age (if the alarm of your biological clock is about to go off, you'll be eager to get down to business right away)

- your eagerness to start a family (if it's important to you to conceive this month rather than next year, you may want to ensure that you're maximizing your chances of conceiving)

- your personality (if you're a card-carrying Type A, like me, who likes to be in control of everything, you may find it impossible to take the more laid-back Type B approach to babymaking)

- the likelihood that you or your partner might have an underlying fertility problem (if there's any reason to suspect that you might have trouble conceiving, you'll want to do whatever you can to help Mother Nature along)

While there's no magic set of instructions I can give you to ensure this will be your lucky month — the month in which you conceive little Brad or Jennifer — there are some things you can do to increase your odds of winning at baby roulette. Here's what you need to know.

Know thy cycle

One of the best things you can do to increase your chances of conceiving is to get to know your menstrual cycle so that you can begin to pinpoint your most fertile days.

FACTS AND FIGURES

If your menstrual cycle is overly short (fewer than 21 days) or overly long (more than 35 days), it's possible that you have a fertility problem. Overly short or overly long menstrual cycles can be indicative of a hormonal problem that may be interfering with your efforts to conceive. Fortunately, these types of problems can often be resolved through treatment.

FROM HERE TO MATERNITY

You can find detailed advice on monitoring your fertility signals in Toni Weschler's excellent book, *Taking Charge of Your Fertility: The Definitive Guide to Natural Birth Control and Pregnancy Achievement* (New York: HarperCollins, 1995).

The first thing you need to do, of course, is to determine the length of your menstrual cycles — something that's easier said than done if your cycles tend to be a bit irregular. You may find it helpful to keep a menstrual calendar, noting the day on which your period starts, the day when it ends, any pre-ovulatory symptoms you notice, and so on. This can be helpful in deciding when it's time to start trying to get pregnant, and can be a useful diagnostic tool for your doctor if you end up having any difficulty conceiving.

While it's common knowledge that there's no such thing as a "one size fits all" menstrual cycle, what some women forget is how this simple fact can affect the timing of ovulation. While women who have 28-day cycles tend to ovulate on or around day 14, women who have shorter or longer cycles ovulate earlier or later than that. There's also no absolute guarantee, by the way, that you'll automatically ovulate on day 14 if you have a 28-day cycle. Every woman's cycle is individual in this regard. What's more, things like stress or illness can delay ovulation or cause you to experience an anovulatory cycle (a cycle in which ovulation does not occur).

In addition to paying attention to the length of your menstrual cycles, you'll also want to learn how to predict your most fertile days. That means learning how to monitor your three key fertility signals: the quantity and quality of your cervical mucus, the position and feel of your cervix, and fluctuations in your basal body temperature.

The quality and quantity of your cervical mucus: As I noted earlier, the quality and quantity of your cervical mucus changes dramatically over the course of your menstrual cycle. During the early part of your cycle the mucus tends to be sticky and opaque. (Its job at this stage is, after all, to plug the cervix and make it difficult for sperm to enter your uterus and fallopian tubes.) Then, as ovulation approaches, your mucus becomes increasingly wet, slippery, and abundant, and — on your most fertile days — it may actually resemble egg white. (The function of this sperm-friendly "egg white" mucus is to help transport the sperm through the uterus and into the fallopian tubes.) Once ovulation has occurred, your cervical mucus changes again, going back to its usual sticky and opaque texture. (It's not needed to transport sperm anymore, so it reverts to its non-fertile state.) Monitoring this particular fertility sign is relatively easy: You simply keep track of the quantity and quality of the cervical mucus that you find on the toilet tissue each time you go to the bathroom. (If you're really obsessive, you can insert your fingers into your vagina to obtain a sample of cervical mucus, but this really isn't necessary.) You can then record your results on the following chart (see Table 3.2).

The position and feel of your cervix: Your cervical mucus isn't the only thing that changes over the course of your menstrual cycle; the position and feel of your cervix changes as well.

At the beginning of your cycle, your cervix is firm and dipping slightly downward into your vagina. Then, as ovulation approaches, it rises up slightly into your vagina and becomes soft and fleshy. (This doesn't just happen by chance. It's designed to make it easier for sperm to make their way through the cervix.) At the same time, the os (opening of the cervix) dilates slightly, making it even easier for the sperm. You can monitor the changes in your cervix by checking it at the same time of day and noting its position, its feel, and the size of the os (e.g., can you insert the tip of your finger into it?). While it's challenging to monitor changes in your cervix — some obstetricians swear that even they can't get the knack of it — basically you're trying to decide whether your cervix feels soft and mushy (like your lips) or firm (like the tip of your nose). If it's soft and mushy, you're probably fertile right now — information that you can record on the chart.

Fluctuations in your basal body temperature: The term "basal body temperature" refers to the temperature of your body first thing in the morning, before you even have a chance to get out of bed. It can be used to predict your most fertile periods because it will show a distinct shift after ovulation occurs. (If there's no such shift, chances are you're not ovulating.) This shift occurs when the corpus luteum starts producing large quantities of progesterone, a hormone that causes your temperature to shoot up. Typically, right before ovulation, your temperature will dip slightly, dropping below its usual pre-ovulatory range of 97.0°F to 97.5°F and then shooting up to the post-ovulatory 97.6°F to 97.8°F. (Don't panic if you don't experience the brief temperature dip. Not everyone does.) You can monitor this fertility signal by taking your temperature before you get out of bed each morning and then plotting your results on the temperature graph in this chapter (see Table 3.2). Here are some basic instructions for using this chart:

TABLE 3.2

BASAL BODY TEMPERATURE (BBT) CHART

Date															
Time															
Intercourse															
Cervical mucus/ cervical position															
Menstruation															
Cycle day	1	2	3	4	5	6	7	8	9	10	11	12	13	14	15
99.0															
98.9															
98.8															
98.7															
98.6															
98.5															
98.4															
98.3															
98.2															
98.1															
98.0															
97.9															
97.8															
97.7															
97.6															
97.5															
97.4															
97.3															
97.2															
97.1															
97.0															
Comments (e.g., illness, insomnia, taking your temperature earlier or later than usual)															

MOTHER WISDOM

You already know that timing is everything when it comes to conception. What you might not realize, however, is that the time of day when you make love may also determine your chances of conceiving. Researchers at the University of Modena in Italy have discovered that sperm counts are 25% higher between 5:00 and 5:30 p.m. than between 7:00 and 7:30 a.m. (Unfortunately, the researchers didn't have any advice to offer on ways to get pregnant in the middle of rush hour or while you're making dinner.)

- Make a few copies of this chart and pick up a standard digital thermometer at the drugstore. (There's no need to buy one that's labeled "basal body thermometer," by the way. They're no more accurate and they cost more.) Don't be tempted to pick up a bargain-basement mercury thermometer, however. Believe it or not, the action of shaking down a mercury thermometer can create enough body heat to throw off your temperature reading. Besides, digital thermometers are faster (you'll have your results in two minutes rather than five) and they beep (a bonus if you're likely to go back to sleep while the thermometer is still in your mouth!).

- Start a new chart on the first day of each menstrual cycle (the day on which your period starts).

- Keep the chart, the thermometer, and a pencil on the night-table beside your bed. (If you have to hop out of bed to find all this paraphernalia, your temperature reading won't be accurate.)

- Place the thermometer in your mouth each morning as soon as you wake up. Record your temperature on the chart provided in Table 3.2 by drawing a dot in the center of the appropriate box and then connecting the dot to the previous day's dot. (This will help to give you a feel for the pattern of your temperature readings.) If you had less than four hours' sleep, be sure to note this on your chart because it can affect your temperature reading.

- Note the days when you have menstrual bleeding or spotting by placing a checkmark in the boxes for those days. (If you're really into charting, you can differentiate between bleeding and spotting by writing a "B" or an "S" in the appropriate spots on the chart.)

- Record your babymaking efforts by placing a checkmark in the "intercourse" section of the chart for the appropriate days.

- If you're also monitoring your cervical mucus and your cervical position, there's room on the chart for these obser-vations, too. You'll probably want to come up with some form of shorthand for this: perhaps a "+" or "−" to indicate changes in the quantity of cervical mucus, an "s" to describe sticky mucus, a "c" to describe creamy mucus, and an "e" to describe egg-white mucus; an "h" for high and an "l" for low to describe the position of your cervix, and an "f" for firm and "m" for mushy to describe how your cervix feels. How you use this part of the chart is up to you.

- Use the "comments" section at the bottom of the chart to note anything else that may have thrown your temperature reading off (e.g., illness, insomnia, or the fact that you consumed a lot of alcohol the night before).

Just a few quick words about what a temperature chart can — and can't — do for you, before we move on. The one thing a temperature chart can't do is the one thing that you probably want it to do — tell you when to have intercourse. The reason is obvious: By the time your temperature graph picks up the shift in your temperature, the window of opportunity for babymaking has already slammed shut. (Remember, you have to have intercourse in the five days leading up to ovulation if you hope to conceive.)

But despite the fact that it's not exactly the fertility world's equivalent of a crystal ball, temperature charting can still provide you with a lot of valuable information about your reproductive system:

MOM'S THE WORD

"When I sometimes consider how small a window exists for conditions to be ripe for conception, it's a miracle that the world is as populated as it is."

— *Rosa, 34, mother of two young children*

• It may be able to tell you whether or not you're ovulating. If you don't experience that classic temperature shift at ovulation, you're probably not ovulating. (Five percent of women who ovulate don't experience this classic temperature shift.)

• It can tell you whether your luteal phase (the last half of your menstrual cycle) is long enough to allow for implantation and the early development of the fertilized egg.

• It can tell you whether your progesterone levels are sufficiently high to support a pregnancy. (If your temperature levels are roughly the same both before and after ovulation, it's possible that your body isn't manufacturing sufficient quantities of progesterone, which can lead to miscarriage.)

• It can help you to figure out whether or not you're pregnant. (If your temperature remains elevated for at least 18 days after ovulation — or for at least three days longer than your longest-ever non-pregnant luteal phase — you're probably pregnant.)

• It may be able to tell you if you've miscarried. If your temperature remains elevated for at least 18 days and then begins to drop, you may have experienced a miscarriage.

- It can help you to pinpoint your most fertile days — assuming, of course, that you've been blessed with relatively regular menstrual cycles. If you go back and analyze a couple of months' worth of temperature charts, you'll likely begin to see some patterns to your cycles. This can help you to time future babymaking activities more precisely.

- It can save you time if you end up having to see a fertility specialist. One of the first things that many fertility doctors ask for is a couple of months' worth of temperature charts. If you've already gathered this information, your treatment may be able to move forward more quickly.

MOM'S THE WORD

"We tried to get pregnant for about six months before it happened. It's a joke now, but at the time whenever I suspected I was going to ovulate, David was required to perform, whether he liked it or not! The poor guy. His friends envied the amount of sex he was getting — I gave myself a 16-day window for babymaking! — but David was actually dreading each passing month. He was relieved he could abandon his rigorous sex routine when I finally got pregnant."

— *Tracy, 31, mother of one*

So is temperature charting for everyone? Well, no. Some couples find that charting creates more problems than it solves, eliminating the spontaneity from sex and making intercourse feel like some sort of clinical laboratory procedure. It can also have a rather dampening effect on the male libido. Many guys find that their urge to make love disappears the moment they're confronted by a woman who's frantically waving a temperature chart and gesturing toward the bedroom. The pressure to perform can be simply too daunting. The moral of the story? If you do decide to go the temperature chart route but you're worried about the effect that too much information will have on your guy, simply keep your lips sealed until after the deed's been done.

There's another way to predict ovulation — a method we haven't discussed up until now. What I'm talking about, of course, are ovulation predictor kits, those pricey, high-tech kits that are always conveniently situated next to the pregnancy kits on the drugstore shelves. (When I say pricey, by the way, I'm not kidding. These things cost $20 or more a pop and you may need more than one kit per cycle. Given that it takes a "typical" couple around six months to conceive, you could easily end up spending $120 or more before you manage to get pregnant.) And if you splurge for the fertility world's latest-and-greatest gadget — a computerized fertility monitor — you can expect to fork out $200 for the monitor and another $50 a month in supplies!

Just in case you haven't had occasion to use an ovulation predictor kit, let me explain how they work. Basically, they're designed to predict the LH surge that typically occurs anywhere from 24 to 36 hours before a woman ovulates — information that you can't pick up from your temperature chart alone. In most cases, that handy bulletin can help you ensure that an ample supply of sperm is waiting to greet the egg by the time it makes its way into the fallopian tube.

Sound great, don't they? And for many couples, they are. Unfortunately, they aren't necessarily the amazing crystal balls their manufacturers would have you believe. They suffer from a few key drawbacks: They can't tell you whether a particular LH surge is the real thing (some women have a couple of false starts before the real one occurs), and they can't tell you whether you're actually ovulating (it's possible to have an LH surge without ovulating). What's more, they don't work for everyone: Some women have such low levels of LH that the kit never tests positive, while others have a base level that's above the threshold, so the test results are inaccurate.

Still, despite these obvious drawbacks, some couples swear by them. Consider what Tracy, a 31-year-old mother of one, has to say: "The kit showed me that I was completely wrong about the time I thought I was ovulating. When I discovered the correct time, we were able to get pregnant that month."

Make love on the right days

This may seem like a no-brainer, but it's at the root of more fertility problems than you might think. Studies have shown that there's a fairly limited window of opportunity for conception. A woman can only conceive as a result of having had intercourse during the five days preceding ovulation. (While she has just a 5% chance of conceiving on the fifth day prior to ovulation or on the day of ovulation itself, she has 33% odds of conceiving two days before ovulation — the reproductive world's equivalent of hitting the jackpot.) So you and your partner really need to make hay during your most fertile period.

Does this mean that you should make love every day? It's up to you, but it's probably not necessary. As I mentioned earlier, sperm are capable of surviving inside the female reproductive tract for up to five days (unlike eggs, which have an incredibly short "best before" date).

Have unbelievably great sex

This is one bit of babymaking advice that shouldn't be too hard to swallow! Believe it or not, some researchers maintain that one of the keys to conceiving on your fertile days is to have unbelievably great sex.

Now no one is suggesting that you try any outlandish positions. After all, the missionary position is about the most conception-friendly position around. What the experts are saying, however, is that pleasure shouldn't be sacrificed in the name of procreation. If anything, it should be maximized.

These experts argue that there's a biological reason why having an orgasm may increase your odds of conceiving. They note that a suction effect is created when the female partner reaches orgasm, causing the cervix to dip down into the vagina, drawing sperm into the uterus. Since this can help to transport sperm out of the acidic vaginal environment as quickly as possible, it may help to ensure that a greater number of sperm make it across the great divide (a.k.a. the cervix).

MOTHER WISDOM

Looking for a way to relieve the stress of trying to conceive? An orgasm could be just what the doctor ordered. Studies have shown that a typical orgasm is 22 times as relaxing as a typical tranquilizer.

MOTHER WISDOM

You don't have to stand on your head after having sex, but it helps to remain in a horizontal position for at least five minutes after you've finished making love. The reason is obvious: Gravity is a formidable adversary to swimming sperm!

Don't get too much of a good thing

If some sex is good, more sex must be better, right? Not necessarily. Not only can attempting to make love every single day be physically and mentally exhausting (particularly if you start your monthly babymaking routine too early on in your cycle), it doesn't do much to boost your odds of conceiving. Consider the facts: Researchers at the National Institute of Environmental Health Sciences have concluded that couples who have intercourse every other day during their most fertile period are only slightly less likely to conceive in any given cycle than couples who have intercourse daily. This is one of those situations where you have to sit down and do a cost-benefit analysis!

There are some couples who should definitely plan to cancel the daily romantic rendezvous: Daily sex is not recommended when the male partner is subfertile as a result of a lower-than-average sperm count. Fertility specialists advise such couples to stick with an "every other day" babymaking regime during their most fertile period and to conserve sperm by refraining from ejaculating at all during the couple of days leading up to this period.

Abstaining from intercourse longer than that isn't a good strategy, however. Studies have shown that sperm counts begin to decline if a man doesn't ejaculate for more than seven days. (Researchers have found that any gain in sperm count resulting from this temporary abstinence is more than offset by the buildup of aged sperm cells that have lower fertilization potential.) Even worse, if you accidentally miscalculate the timing of your fertile period, you could drastically reduce your chances of conceiving in any given cycle: Studies have shown that couples who have intercourse only once during their fertile period have just a 10% chance of conceiving.

Create a "sperm-friendly" vaginal environment

We've already talked about the importance of not douching. What you might not realize is that other personal hygiene habits are also decidedly unfriendly to sperm. While you're trying to conceive, you should make a point to avoid

- vaginal sprays and scented tampons, both of which can cause a pH imbalance in your vagina

- artificial lubricants, vegetable oils, glycerin, and natural lubricants such as saliva, all of which kill off sperm

If you need some help in the lubrication department, try using egg whites that have been warmed to room temperature. They mimic the consistency of fertile cervical mucus and aren't considered harmful to sperm. (Obviously, anyone with an egg allergy should avoid using egg whites as a lubricant.)

Get your partner on board

Make sure your partner is doing his bit to maximize his own fertility. This means not exposing his genitals to excessive heat (e.g., hot tubs, hot baths, or jobs that require a lot of sitting); avoiding exposure to toxic chemicals and radiation; not using anabolic steroids or recreational drugs; avoiding medications (e.g., 6-mercaptopurine for inflammatory bowel disease) and herbal products (e.g., St. John's wort, ginkgo biloba, and echinacea) that are thought to be harmful to sperm; not smoking; not consuming large amounts of alcohol; avoiding injuries to the genital area; limiting the amount of time he spends on his bike (one study showed that cycling more than 100 miles per week can cause damage to the arteries and nerves in the genital area); postponing surgery to the urogenital area (wherever possible); and maintaining a healthy body weight.

Can You Choose Your Baby's Sex?

You've no doubt heard whispers about all the things you should and shouldn't do to increase your odds of giving birth to a baby of a particular sex. Just in case you haven't tapped into the buzz around the water cooler lately, allow me to bring you up to speed on the latest theories about sex selection:

- According to the Shettles Method, if you want to conceive a baby boy, you should time intercourse so that it occurs as close to ovulation as possible. (Shettles makes the case that sperm cells resulting in the conception of a male move more quickly but don't last as long.)

- According to the Whelan Method, if you want to conceive a male baby, you should have sex as early in your fertile period as possible — four to five days prior to ovulation. (Whelan argues that biochemical conditions in a woman's body become less favorable to male sperm as ovulation approaches.)

- According to an article in the British journal *Nature,* the age of your mate may help to determine the sex of your child. A recent study showed that women with partners at least five years older than they were twice as likely to give birth to sons, while women who married younger men produced twice as many daughters as sons.

- Another study indicates that climate has an effect on the sex of your baby. Researchers at the University of Malta Medical School found that warmer countries record higher numbers of male births than do colder and more northerly countries.

- Researchers in North Carolina have uncovered a link between the length of the follicular (pre-ovulatory) phase of a woman's menstrual cycle and the sex of the baby subsequently conceived. The researchers found that conception cycles with short follicular phases and early ovulation are more likely to produce boys, while cycles with long follicular phases and later ovulation tend to produce girls.

While it's fun to think you can determine the sex of a baby by taking these factors into account, most medical experts will pooh-pooh your chances of succeeding. A 1995 study conducted by the National Institute of Environmental Health Sciences, for example, concluded in no uncertain terms that there's no connection between the timing of intercourse and the ability to conceive a baby of a particular sex. (Hey, even the best sperm separation clinics aren't able to offer couples much better than 75-25 odds.)

Bottom line? Go ahead and have fun with these sex selection theories, but don't take any of them too seriously. And hold off painting the nursery pink or blue until you're sure about the sex of your baby.

CHAPTER 4

Missed Conceptions

While the vast majority of couples manage to conceive relatively quickly, others aren't quite so lucky. According to the American Society for Reproductive Medicine, infertility affects approximately 6.1 million Americans — roughly 10% of couples of reproductive age.

In her book, *Missed Conceptions: Overcoming Infertility,* Anne Mullens describes what it's like to struggle with infertility: "The odd thing about infertility . . . is that it is completely based on a state of mind, a want. If you did not want to be pregnant, if you did not want to have children, it would not be a problem. . . . But the act of wanting children changes all of that. Infertility takes what could be a choice and turns it into no choice."

In this chapter, we're going to talk about the challenges of coping with infertility: how to tell if you have a fertility problem, what you can expect from the infertility workup, what types of treatments are available to you and your partner, and what the two of you can do to stay sane while you're on board the fertility treatment roller coaster.

FACTS AND FIGURES

According to the American College of Obstetricians and Gynecologists, at least 14% of American couples who are actively trying to become pregnant will still not have managed to conceive after one year.

Do You Have a Fertility Problem?

Your odds of conceiving in any given cycle are at best 25%, so there's no need to hit the panic button if you're not pregnant after a few months of active trying. If, however, an entire year has gone by and you still haven't managed to conceive, you and your partner should at least consider the possibility that one or both of you may have a fertility problem.

As with anything else in the weird and wonderful world of reproduction, there are a few bits of fine print that are helpful in deciding when to schedule that initial infertility appointment. Most experts agree that you should seek treatment before the one-year mark if

- you're over 35

- you have an underlying medical problem that might be making it difficult for you to conceive (e.g., a history of endometriosis, fibroids, irregular periods, or past exposure to a sexually transmitted disease such as chlamydia; if your mother took DES when she was pregnant with you; or if you have a medical condition that's known to contribute to infertility — a topic we discussed back in Chapter 2)

- your partner has some underlying problem that could be making it difficult for you to conceive (e.g., varicoceles, undescended testicles, previous surgery to the urogenital area, a sports injury or other injury to the genital area)

- you're likely to face a lengthy wait before you can get in to see a specialist

If you and your partner decide to seek help for a suspected fertility problem, you can expect to be treated by one or more of the following types of doctors: your family doctor, an obstetrician/gynecologist who regularly treats couples with fertility problems, a reproductive endocrinologist (a gynecologist who's completed additional training in the treatment of reproductive disorders), or a urologist (a doctor who specializes in the treatment of urogenital problems, including male reproductive disorders).

FACTS AND FIGURES

While you may not want to rush to the doctor's office immediately if you're having trouble conceiving, it doesn't make sense to postpone treatment indefinitely if you're committed to having a child. Not only does the dreaded biological clock keep on ticking, but studies have shown that couples who haven't conceived after two years of trying have just a one in four chance of conceiving on their own without medical assistance.

FACTS AND FIGURES

According to a survey conducted by the World Congress on Fertility and Sterility, 20 percent of couples who seek treatment for infertility are found to have a timing problem rather than a fertility problem: They're simply not having sex at the right times of the month.

The infertility workup

The term "infertility workup" is used to describe the fact-finding mission that your doctor initiates when you show up in his office with a fertility problem. It is designed to answer four basic questions:

- Is the female partner ovulating regularly?

- Is the male partner producing healthy, viable sperm?

- Are the egg and sperm able to unite?

- Is there some other type of problem?

It may not be possible for the doctor to gather all the necessary information from you and your partner during a single visit, particularly if a number of investigative tests are required, so don't be surprised if you end up going for multiple appointments without receiving any sort of definitive diagnosis. (Note: You should also prepare yourself for the possibility that your doctor might not be able to determine the cause of your fertility problem, even after conducting a thorough investigation: Approximately 10% of infertility cases remain unexplained.) Table 4.1 describes what types of tests may be ordered for you and your partner as the investigation progresses. Just one quick word of warning before you look at the chart: Don't make the mistake of assuming that you'll need all the tests. Those in the shaded boxes are ordered only if a more thorough investigation is deemed necessary. Many fertility problems are diagnosed and treated without the need for all these tests, some of which can be unpleasant or even painful.

The Major Causes of Infertility

In generations past, men tended to blame their wives for any fertility problems the couple was experiencing. After all, wasn't it her wifely duty to give him a male heir?

We now know that men have just as many fertility problems as women. In fact, most fertility experts now agree that one-third of fertility problems are caused by the male, one-third are caused by the female, and one-third are due to some sort of unexplained or combined problem (e.g., the inability of the man's sperm to penetrate the woman's cervical mucus). (Some experts peg the numbers at 40%, 40%, and 20%, respectively, percentages that are in roughly the same ballpark.)

Regardless of the cause, there are three basic treatments for male and female infertility: drug and hormone therapy, surgery, and artificial insemination (the introduction of sperm into the female reproductive tract by means other than sexual intercourse). (See Table 4.2 for a more detailed breakdown of the most common types of fertility problems and how they're treated.) In some cases, the only way to address a particular fertility problem is to use a high-tech treatment such as in vitro fertilization. (Table 4.3 describes the more common high-tech fertility treatments and their usual success rates.)

 FACTS AND FIGURES

To ensure that the semen analysis results are as accurate as possible, a man should refrain from ejaculating during the two to three days prior to providing the sperm sample; collect the sperm sample in a clean container (one that hasn't been contaminated with dish detergent residue or other substances); keep the sample at body temperature (in the winter months, he should keep the sample next to his body while he's transporting it to the lab); and deliver the sample to the designated lab within one hour of collection. (Hey, it's a tall order, but these precautions are necessary to prevent the sperm sample from becoming damaged.)

Table 4.1

THE INFERTILITY INVESTIGATION: WHAT TO EXPECT

Infertility Workup on the Female Partner

Type of Information Gathered	How It May Help in Diagnosing Your Problem
Menstrual history (e.g., the age at which you started menstruating, the length of your cycles, your bleeding patterns, whether you experience any pain when you're menstruating, whether you have any other symptoms such as breast tenderness and bloating either prior to or during your period, whether you have a history of endometriosis or pelvic inflammatory disease, whether you've had any previous pregnancies — including any that resulted in miscarriages, stillbirths, or abortions)	May help to identify hormonal problems or gynecological diseases or infections that may be contributing to your fertility problems.
Sexual history (e.g., type of contraceptive you were using prior to trying to conceive, how long you've been trying, how you've been timing intercourse, whether you've had a large number	May help to identify some possible causes of your fertility problems — complications resulting from a past birth control method (e.g., a pelvic infection caused by an IUD or a delay in the resumption of normal menstrual functioning after using

Type of Information Gathered	How It May Help in Diagnosing Your Problem
of partners in the past, whether you use lubricants during sex, whether you douche, whether you and your partner have experienced any sexual problems) Note: Both you and your partner should also expect to answer questions about the frequency and timing of intercourse, your preferred positions, and so on, all of which can provide clues to any possible fertility problems.	Depo-Provera as a method of birth control), whether you're timing intercourse to coincide with your most fertile days, whether you may have contracted a sexually transmitted disease from a previous sexual partner, whether the lubricants or douching products you use could be altering the vaginal environment and/or killing sperm, and whether sexual problems such as premature ejaculation or inadequate penetration may be hampering your efforts to conceive.
Lifestyle (e.g., smoking, drinking, drug use, eating disorders)	May help to identify any unhealthy lifestyle habits that may be contributing to your fertility problems.
General health history (e.g., overall health, chronic health conditions, medication usage, whether you've lost or gained a significant amount of weight recently, whether you've experienced appendicitis at some point)	May help to identify whether a particular health problem (diagnosed or undiagnosed) or the use of a certain type of medication may be preventing you from becoming pregnant. Your doctor will want to know, for example, if you've experienced appendicitis, in case you ended up developing some sort of pelvic infection that could be contributing to your fertility problems.

continued

Infertility Workup on the Female Partner (Continued)

Type of Information Gathered	How It May Help in Diagnosing Your Problem
Your family history (e.g., how long it took your mother to conceive her first child; whether she had any miscarriages, and if so, how many; whether she ever experienced an ectopic pregnancy; whether she experienced menstrual irregularities and cramping; at what age she started menstruating and at what age she entered menopause; whether she ever took DES to prevent miscarriage)	May help to identify any reproductive health problems that may run in your family (e.g., premature menopause) and to highlight areas requiring further investigation (e.g., ordering an ultrasound to detect possible uterine abnormalities in a DES daughter). Note: Don't panic if your mother experienced a number of miscarriages or ectopic pregnancies, since it doesn't mean that you necessarily will.
Physical examination (e.g., height/weight, blood pressure, urinalysis, blood test, general physical examination, breast examination, abdominal examination, pelvic examination, Pap smear)	May help to reveal underlying health problems (e.g., an undiagnosed diabetes or thyroid problem that may be making it difficult for you to conceive); to diagnose gynecological problems (e.g., fibroids, infections, sores, growths, sexually transmitted diseases, cancers, or other abnormalities); to detect hormonal imbalances (possible symptoms include inadequate breast development, unusual fat distribution, a milky discharge from the nipples, and hair growth around your nipples and on your face and abdomen); and to uncover abnormalities of the reproductive organs (e.g., problems with the size, shape, or position of your uterus; signs of any unusual lumps or enlargements of your reproductive organs).

Type of Information Gathered	How It May Help in Diagnosing Your Problem
Hysterososalpingogram (hSG) (a test that involves shooting X-ray dye into your reproductive tract through a tube placed in your cervix, and then taking X-rays)	Can help to reveal obstructions in your fallopian tubes, uterine fibroids, scarring, and so on Note: There is some anecdotal evidence that hSGs that use oil-based dyes can enhance your fertility in the months following the procedure, but this has yet to be substantiated in any official research study. Note: Some women find hystersosalpingograms to be quite painful, so your caregiver will probably advise you to take some sort of pain medication prior to the procedure.
Serum progesterone test (a blood test performed midway through your luteal phase — around day 21 of a 28-day cycle)	Helps to confirm that you're ovulating.
Prolactin blood test (a blood test that measures levels of prolactin — a hormone that inhibits ovulation in nursing mothers)	Elevated levels of prolactin can indicate the presence of a benign pituitary tumor that can cause fertility problems.

continued

Infertility Workup on the Female Partner (Continued)

Type of Information Gathered	How It May Help in Diagnosing Your Problem
Thyroid hormone blood test (a blood test that measures thyroid levels)	Can aid in the diagnosis of such thyroid problems as hyperthyroidism (overactive thyroid) and hypothyroidism (underactive thyroid), both of which can be associated with menstrual and ovulatory disorders.
Blood tests for other reproductive hormones	Can help to uncover a variety of hormonal problems. Note: Some of these tests have to be conducted at a specific point in your menstrual cycle.
Endometrial biopsy (a sample of tissue from the lining of your uterus is removed through a combination of suction and gentle scraping) Note: This test is taken a few days before your period is due.	Can confirm whether or not you're ovulating and indicate if your endometrial tissue is healthy and substantial enough to allow a fertilized egg to implant. (Basically, the purpose of the test is to see if the menstrual lining is as thick as it should be at this point in your menstrual cycle.) Note: The odds of this procedure causing a miscarriage are extremely small, but if you're concerned about this possibility you might want to consider using birth control during the cycle in which the endometrial biopsy is scheduled or having a sensitive blood pregnancy test performed the day before the biopsy.

Type of Information Gathered	May Help in Diagnosing Your Problem
Laparoscopy (a surgical technique that allows your doctor to look inside your pelvis using a tiny fiber-optic scope inserted into your abdomen while you're under general anesthetic)	Aids in the detection of fallopian tube obstructions and damage caused by endometriosis, pelvic inflammatory disease, or adhesions from pelvic surgery. It can also be used to detect uterine fibroids and ovarian cysts and to look for evidence that you are, in fact, ovulating.
Hysteroscopy (a fiber-optic scope is inserted into the uterus through the cervix)	Can be used to detect abnormal growths or uterine abnormalities.
Post-coital test (two or more samples of cervical mucus are removed two to 16 hours after you and your partner have had intercourse; it's timed to occur midcycle, just prior to when ovulation is expected)	Can be used to assess whether your mucus is inhospitable to your partner's sperm; whether there are antibodies in your body or your partner's body that are killing sperm; and whether the sperm is being deposited close enough to the cervix to allow conception to occur (something that can be a problem if your partner experiences premature ejaculation).Note: The post-coital test is generally considered to be less reliable than other types of infertility tests. Some doctors don't do them at all, preferring to move right to sperm washes and intrauterine insemination instead.
Ultrasound	Can reveal problems with the size or shape of the uterus and ovaries.

continued

Infertility Workup on the Male Partner

Type of Information Gathered	How It May Help in Diagnosing Your Problem
Sexual history (e.g., questions about his sexual and developmental background, such as whether both of his testicles were descended when he was born, at what age he went through puberty, how many partners he's had, whether he has any problem with impotence or ejaculation, whether he's ever fathered a child with someone other than you, whether he's ever been treated for a sexually transmitted disease) Note: Both you and your partner should also expect to answer questions about the frequency and timing of intercourse, your preferred positions, and so on, all of which can provide clues to any possible fertility problems.	May help to uncover problems that could be contributing to your fertility problems: undescended testicles, hormonal problems, sexually transmitted diseases, sexual dysfunction a history of fertility problems, etc.
Lifestyle (e.g., caffeine consumption, smoking, drinking, drug use, type of occupation, hot tub use)	May help to identify lifestyle habits that could be making it difficult for the two of you to conceive: heavy caffeine consumption, smoking, alcohol use, illicit drug use, exposure to chemicals or radiation on the job, exposing the genitals to heat for prolonged periods of time (a possibility if he's a long-distance trucker who sits for extended periods or if he's in the habit of hitting the hot tub at the health club).

Type of Information Gathered	How It May Help in Diagnosing Your Problem
General health history (e.g., whether he's been sick or had a fever during the past three months, whether he's ever had the mumps, whether he's had surgery to the urogenital area, whether he's taking any medications)	May help to determine if an illness may have caused temporary or permanent infertility (mumps in adulthood can cause sterility); if surgery to the urogenital area may have resulted in a buildup of scar tissue or other complications that may be hampering your efforts to conceive; or if he's taking any medications that are known to be harmful to sperm, etc.
Physical examination (height/weight; blood pressure; heart and lung checks; urinalysis; blood tests; examination of penis, testes, and prostate gland; observation of secondary sex characteristics such as hair growth, deepness of voice, and physical build; checks to ensure that he has full sensation throughout his external genital area, etc.)	May help to reveal underlying health problems (e.g., severe obesity or thyroid problems) or reproductive problems (e.g., undescended testicles and other structural problems with the male reproductive organs, hormonal disorders, undiagnosed sexually transmitted diseases, varicoceles — varicose veins of the testicles) that may be contributing to your fertility problems.
Semenalysis (analysis of a sample of semen; more than one sample will be required if the initial sample comes back with abnormal results or if the fertility specialist routinely requests at least two semen samples collected on two	The sample will be subjected to the following tests in the laboratory: **Coagulation:** If the semen doesn't coagulate at the time of ejaculation, there could be a problem with the seminal vesicles.

continued

Infertility Workup on the Male Partner (Continued)

Type of Information Gathered	How It May Help in Diagnosing Your Problem
Semenalysis separate days as the American Society for Reproductive Medicine recommends) Note: Most doctors will allow the male partner to collect the sample at home — either through masturbation or by having intercourse using a special lubricant-free and spermicide-free condom — and then bring the sample to the lab, rather than requiring that the man masturbate on the premises, which many men feel uncomfortable about. If the sample is collected at home, however, it must be brought to the lab promptly: In most cases the sample must be analyzed within one hour of collection.	**Liquification:** If the semen doesn't turn back into liquid form within 30 minutes of ejaculation, there could be a problem with the man's prostate. **Color:** A yellowish hue can indicate infection and a reddish or brownish tinge may indicate the presence of blood. Healthy semen is whitish-grey upon ejaculation and translucent once it's had the chance to reliquify **Odor:** An unpleasant odor may indicate an infection while an absence of odor may indicate a prostate problem. **Volume:** If there's too little semen (less than one half to one teaspoonful), some of the semen may have been ejaculated backward into the bladder (retrograde ejaculation), the seminal vesicles may be missing, there may be an obstruction in a duct, or there may be a problem with semen production. If there's too much semen, the seminal or prostate glands may be overactive, which can affect the quality and motility (ability to move) of the sperm.

Type of Information Gathered	How It May Help in Diagnosing Your Problem
Semenalysis	**pH:** A pH level that's too high or too low may indicate an infection in the seminal vesicles or prostate.
	Sperm concentration: A healthy sperm count is considered to be 20 million/mL or more.
	Motility: The sample will be assessed for both percentage of sperm that are moving and the quality of that movement (e.g., lethargic vs. healthy amounts of movement). More than 50% of the sperm should be moving forward.
	Morphology: If more than half of the sperm in the sample are abnormal (e.g., unusual shape or appearance), fertility may be affected.
	Culture: The sample will be checked for the presence of bacteria and sexually transmitted diseases.
	White blood cells: Too many white blood cells may indicate an inflammation such as prostatitis.
Semenalysis (Less standard tests)	**Sperm antibodies:** If the sperm tend to clump together, the semen may contain sperm antibodies or some sort of infection. In some cases, a man's body produces antibodies to his own sperm.

continued

Infertility Workup on the Male Partner (Continued)

Type of Information Gathered	How It May Help in Diagnosing Your Problem
Semenalysis (Less standard tests)	**Fructose test:** This test can help to determine whether the seminal vesicles are adding fructose to the semen as they should be. **Mucus penetration:** The sperm's ability to penetrate cervical mucus will be tested using a sample of cervical mucus from a cow. Note: Other related tests (the crossover sperm invasion test or the hamster egg penetration test, for example) may be ordered in some cases where a mucus penetration problem is suspected.
Further investigations (if two or more semen analyses yield consistently abnormal results, the doctor may order blood tests or a testicular biopsy)	Blood tests can be used to measure the levels of male and female hormones in the male partner's body; a biopsy may reveal a lack of sperm-generating cells in his testicles, in which case he'll be considered permanently sterile; a vasography can locate any obstructions in the ducts of the male reproductive system.

Note: The shaded boxes indicate tests that are not routinely part of the standard infertility workup.

TABLE 4.2

CAUSES AND TREATMENT OF THE MOST COMMON FERTILITY PROBLEMS

Problems with the Male Partner

Type of Problem	Treatment Options
Environmental factors (smoking, drinking, illicit drug use, exposure to toxins/radiation on the job)	Lifestyle changes and/or work modifications
Use of medications that can affect libido, reduce sperm production, destroy normal DNA production, and alter the hormonal balance	Discontinue medication use or switch to another medication without these undesirable side effects. Note: Unfortunately, some medical conditions require drugs that contribute to fertility-related problems, and there may not be any alternative medications available. Obviously, this is something your partner will need to discuss with his doctor.
Infection of prostate and seminal vesicles	Drug therapy (antibiotics)
Marginal sperm count or mucus penetration problems	Artificial insemination (with male partner's sperm, if possible)

continued

Problems with the Male Partner (Continued)

Type of Problem	Treatment Options
Sexual problems (e.g., impotence, premature ejaculation, ejaculatory dysfunction, retrograde ejaculation — a neurological problem that causes ejaculation into the bladder rather than out through the urethra)	Artificial insemination (with male partner's sperm, if possible). Retrograde ejaculation can sometimes be treated with medication
Hypospadias (a congenital anomaly in which the opening of the urethra is found on the underside rather than tip of the penis, causing semen to be deposited too low in the vagina)	Artificial insemination (with male partner's sperm, if possible)
Hormonal imbalances such as hypogonadotropic hypogonadism (a condition in which levels of FSH and LH result in a lack of normal testicular function and a lack of masculine characteristics), congenital adrenal hyperplasia (the lack of an enzyme required for the production of male hormones), and hyperprolactinemia (a condition in which there is too much prolactin in the blood)	Hormone therapy
Immunological problems (when a man's antibodies attack his own sperm)	Sperm washing, intracyto-plasmic sperm injection (ICSI) (see below), or artificial insemination with donor sperm

Type of Problem	Treatment Options
Testicular failure due to a blow to the testes, exposure to the mumps, or a birth defect	Artificial insemination with donor sperm
Undescended testes (a congenital abnormality which, if uncorrected by age 2, results in sterility)	Artificial insemination with donor sperm
Varicocele (a varicose vein in the spermatic cord that can kill off sperm)	Surgery
Blockages in the ejaculatory ducts	Sometimes sperm can be aspirated above the blockage. If that doesn't work, then surgery is another option.
Obstructions in the epidiymis	Sometimes sperm can be aspirated above the blockage. If that doesn't work, then surgery is another option.
Unexplained infertility	Artificial insemination (with male partner's sperm, if possible) Note: Some doctors will simultaneously treat the female partner with fertility drugs.

Problems with the Female Partner

Type of Problem	Treatment Options
Tubal and pelvic problems (e.g., scarring of or damage to the fallopian tubes caused	Surgery can help to correct certain types of structural problems (e.g., congenital uterine abnormalities such as a double uterus,

continued

Problems with the Male Partner (Continued)

Type of Problem	Treatment Options
Tubal and pelvic problems by an ectopic pregnancy, endometriosis, pelvic inflammatory disease, gonorrhea, chlamydia, or an intrauterine device; congenital abnormalities of the reproductive organs; fertility problems caused by uterine growths such as polyps and fibroids, and other conditions such as Asherman's Syndrome, in which bands of scar tissue in a woman's uterus cement its walls together)	bicornate uterus (surgery isn't always required), or separate uterus; congenital defects caused by your mother's use of DES when she was pregnant with you; and damage to the female reproductive system caused by such conditions as pelvic inflammatory disease and endometriosis'. Surgery is not without its own risks, however, and may result in the formation of adhesions that can add to your fertility problems. Lifestyle changes such as quitting smoking may also be recommended (smoking has been linked to an increased incidence of pelvic inflammatory disease and other fertility problems). Note: If tubal problems are severe, in vitro fertilization is generally considered a better option than surgery.
Ovulatory dysfunction (irregular ovulation) Common causes include polycystic ovarian syndrome (where the ovaries develop small cysts that interfere with ovulation and hormone production); hyperprolactinemia (where the secretion of an excessive amount of the hormone prolactin interferes with ovulation); deficiencies in gonadotropin-releasing hormone (the hormone responsible for triggering the release	Depending on the cause and nature of the ovulatory disorder, ovulation may be induced using such drugs as clomiphene citrate (Clomid or Serophene) — a pill that stimulates ovulation; human menopausal gonadotropin (hMG) (Pergonal) or follicle stimulating hormone (FSH) (Fertinorm HP or Gonal-F) — medications that are injected to stimulate the development of multiple eggs within the ovaries; human

Type of Problem	Treatment Options
of FSH and LH from the pituitary gland); a luteal phase deficiency (when inadequate levels of progesterone prevent the fertilized egg from implanting properly); other hormonal imbalances (caused by pituitary failure, glandular disorders, premature menopause, and so on); an excess of adrenal androgens (male sex hormones); amenorrhea (lack of menstruation); anovulation (lack of ovulation); and oligo-ovulation/menorrhea (infrequent ovulation/menstruation)	chorionic gonadotropin (hCG) (Profast HP) — a medication injected to encourage the developing eggs to mature and to trigger ovulation; and gonadotropin-releasing hormone — (GnRH) — a rarely used fertility hormone administered by infusion pump every 90 minutes and used to stimulate ovulation. Other drugs used to treat hormonal problems include bromocriptine (Parlodel), which suppresses the pituitary gland's production of prolactin; gonadotropin-releasing hormone (GnRH), which induces ovulation (rarely used); and Lupron, a drug used to treat endometriosis and to enhance the response to Pergonal in selected patients. Lifestyle changes may also be recommended, as excessive stress, dieting, and exercise are known to interfere with ovulation.
Immunological problems, thyroid problems, and other unusual causes	Varies depending on the underlying disorder. May include drug treatment, immunization.
Unexplained infertility	Some couples with unexplained infertility will be treated with a combination of drug therapy and artificial insemination. Note: Approximately half of those couples with unexplained infertility will manage to conceive without treatment during a three-year period.

TABLE 4.3

HIGH-TECH FERTILITY METHODS: YOUR ODDS OF SUCCESS

Type of Procedure	Success Rate per Attempt (Percentage of treatment cycles resulting in live births)	What It Involves
Donor Eggs	42.2% per retrieval	Eggs from a donor female are fertilized with sperm from the male partner and then implanted in the female partner's uterus through in vitro fertilization (when an egg that has been fertilized outside the womb is implanted into the woman's uterus).
Zygote Intrafallopian Transfer (ZIFT)	27.7%	Fertilized eggs are transferred to the fallopian tube.
Gamete Intrafallopian Transfer (GIFT)	26.8%	Eggs and sperm are inserted into a healthy fallopian tube using a laparoscope.
Intracyto-Plasmic Sperm Injection (ICSI)	24%	Ovulation is induced, eggs are retrieved, a single sperm is injected into an egg, and any resulting embryos are transferred to the woman's uterus two to five days later. Note: Spare embryos not needed for this treatment cycle can be stored and later transferred without the need for subsequent ovulation induction or egg retrieval.

In Vitro Fertilization (IVF)	22.3%	An egg (either from the female partner or from a donor) that has been fertilized outside the womb is implanted in the woman's uterus. Basically, ovulation is induced, eggs are retrieved, the eggs are inseminated in the laboratory, and then any resulting embryos are transferred two to five days later. Note: Spare embryos not needed for this treatment cycle can be stored and later transferred without the need for subsequent ovulation induction or egg retrieval.
Frozen Embryo Transfer (FET)	15.4%	Embryos left over from an IVF cycle are frozen and stored for implantation in the uterus at some future date.
Intrauterine Insemination (IUI)	15–20%	A sperm sample is washed to remove abnormal or dead sperm and then injected into the uterus via a catheter. Either fresh or frozen sperm can be used. The sperm can be from a woman's partner or from a donor. Frequently used to treat unexplained infertility and in cases where mild to moderate abnormalities or abnormal mucus production are hampering a couple's chances of conceiving, or in cases where there may be problems in the male partner. This is also a popular method of conceiving for lesbian couples.

continued

Type of Procedure	Success Rate per Attempt (Percentage of treatment cycles resulting in live births)	What It Involves (Continued)
In Vitro Maturation (IVM)	Not available (still an experimental treatment)	Ovulation is induced, eggs from the female partner or a donor are retrieved, the eggs are ripened for a day or two in the laboratory before being inseminated, and then any resulting embryos are transferred to the uterus two to five days later.

Sources: "Patient's Fact Sheet — Infertility." Birmingham: American Society for Reproductive Medicine, 1997. Available from American Society for Reproductive Medicine Web site: www.asrm.com

1998 Assisted Reproductive Technology Success Rates: National Summary and Fertility Clinic Reports. Atlanta: Centers for Disease Control and Prevention, 2001. Available online at www.cdc.gov/nccdphp/drh/art.htm.

Journal articles cited in "IUI FAQ" at www.fertilityplus.org

FACTS AND FIGURES

A fallopian tube measures just 1/7th of an inch at its widest point, while at its narrowest point it's just 1/100th of an inch.

FACTS AND FIGURES

Approximately one in four women over the age of 30 has uterine fibroids. In most cases, fibroids do not require treatment. If, however, you have a large number of fibroids, your fibroids are exceptionally large (e.g., the size of a grapefruit), your fibroids are causing you pain and bleeding, or they are interfering with your ability to conceive or to carry a pregnancy to term, your doctor may recommend surgery.

The Brave New World of Assisted Reproduction

It's hard enough to decide whether to proceed with treatment for infertility when you're considering more traditional, low-tech approaches such as drug therapy and surgery. It can be that much more difficult if you're venturing into the brave new world of assisted reproduction.

For one thing, depending on the nature of your treatment, you may have to grapple with issues that don't arise with low-tech methods:

- how you or your partner may feel about conceiving a child that may not be genetically your own (e.g., if you use donor eggs and/or sperm)

- whether you or your partner may feel jealous or inadequate if a donor was able to conceive a child with one of you, but the other partner wasn't

- whether you intend to tell any child that you conceive the details surrounding his or her conception (you'll find some sensible advice on handling this situation at the American Infertility Association Web site: www.americaninfertility.org)

- what you intend to tell family members, friends, co-workers, and others in your life about your fertility treatments

- how many attempts you and your partner are prepared to make (for physical, psychological, and financial reasons)

- what you'll do with any frozen sperm, eggs, or embyros you don't end up using (e.g., donate them, allow them to be used for genetic research, or have them destroyed) and what you'd do with them if you and your partner separated or if one of you died

- how you'd cope if you were to conceive multiples (and how you'd cope if one or more of the babies died or if your doctor suggested selective reduction — the termination of one or more of the fetuses in the hope of increasing the odds of survival of the others)

FACTS AND FIGURES

According to the **Centers for Disease Control and Prevention,** more than 28,000 babies were born in 1998 as the result of assisted reproductive technology (ART).

And if that isn't enough to wrap your head around, you've also got to be prepared to play detective when sizing up the merits of a particular fertility clinic. That means cutting through the marketing hype and looking for hard evidence about the so-called "take home" baby rate for various fertility clinics. Fortunately, uncovering this type of information isn't nearly as difficult as it was ten years ago. In 1992, the United States Congress passed a law mandating the Centers for Disease Control and Prevention to publish a report detailing clinic-by-clinic live birth rates for U.S. fertility clinics. Reports for U.S. fertility clinics for 1995, 1996, 1997, and 1998 can be downloaded free of charge from the Centers for Disease Control Web site: www.cdc.gov/nccdphp/drh/art.htm.

Damned lies and statistics

Most fertility experts agree that the most meaningful statistic is the "live birth per treatment cycle" for both the clinic and the specialist who will be performing the procedure — the so-called "take home" baby rate. (Some clinics like to cite the live birth rate per egg retrieval rate — a statistic that conveniently omits women whose treatment cycles were cancelled because their eggs didn't mature according to plan — and the live birth rate per egg transfer rate — a statistic that doesn't acknowledge the number of women whose cycles were cancelled or whose eggs failed to survive the three- to five-day incubation period in the laboratory.) But unfortunately, even the "live birth per treatment cycle" statistic can be misleading if you're not considered a particularly good candidate for the procedure because of your age or some other factor.

MOTHER WISDOM

If a fertility clinic quotes you data on its success rates, be sure to find out what period of time those statistics cover. It's possible that the data is no longer current or that it reflects a very good month or quarter that isn't particularly representative of the clinic's long-term track record. As a rule, you shouldn't put much faith in statistics that cover less than a one-year period.

FACTS AND FIGURES

The American Society for Reproductive Medicine urges couples who are considering intracytoplasmic sperm injection to proceed with caution because long-term risks to the offspring have not been clearly identified. While some studies have shown that ICSI may be associated with a higher-than-average incidence of congenital defects and lower than average performance scores on a standard measure of infant development at age 1 year, other studies have contradicted those findings.

Reading between the lines

As well as a particular treatment's likelihood of success, when you're trying to decide whether to proceed you'll want to consider some other important criteria:

- how frequently this particular procedure is performed at the clinic you're considering (since practice makes perfect, you want to ensure that you're being treated by someone who's both competent and highly experienced)

- the rate of multiple births for the procedure you're considering

- under what circumstances fetal reduction is recommended (the term *fetal reduction* refers to the process of selectively aborting one or more developing fetuses in the hope that this will increase the odds of one or more babies surviving)

- the potential side effects of the procedure

- the number of treatment cycles that are recommended (to assess whether you're willing or able to make the necessary commitment of time, money, and other resources)

You'll also need to find out as much as possible about the clinic itself:

- how long the clinic has been in operation

- whether it meets the American Society for Reproductive Medicine's (ASRM) guidelines

- whether the program reports its results to the Society for Assisted Reproductive Technology (SART) and the Centers for Disease Control and Prevention (CDC) for inclusion in its annual fertility clinic report

- the types of counseling and support services it provides

- how many doctors will be involved in your care and whether one or more of the doctors who will be treating you is board certified in reproductive endocrinology

- whether there's an age limit in place to determine which women are and aren't accepted into the program

- if someone is available to take your call after hours if you have questions or concerns about your treatment

- whether the clinic has access to donor eggs and/or donor sperm

- whether the clinic freezes and stores embryos

- the range of services that are offered by the clinic

 FACTS AND FIGURES

According to the Centers for Disease Control, the overall success rate for the 809 gestational carrier arrangements (surrogate motherhood) reported to the Centers in 1998 was 29.2%.

Money talk

And then there's the whole business of financing your baby-making plans. Unless you have a particularly comprehensive private health insurance plan, you're likely to be picking up much of the tab for these high-tech fertility treatments yourself. And with the cost of a single cycle of IVF treatment averaging $7,800, according to the American Society for Reproductive

Medicine, those costs can quickly add up. (See Table 4.4 for details on the costs of other types of ART procedures.)

TABLE 4.4

THE COST OF CERTAIN TYPES OF ASSISTIVE REPRODUCTIVE TECHNOLOGY TREATMENTS

Type of Treatment	What You Can Expect to Pay
In-Vitro Fertilization (IVF)	$6,000 to $10,000 per attempt
Gamete Intrafallopian Transfer (GIFT)	$6,000 to $10,000 per attempt
Zygote Intrafallopian Transfer (ZIFT)	$8,000 to $10,000 per attempt
Frozen Embryo Transfer (FET)	$500 to $1,500 per cycle
Intracyto-Plasmic Sperm Injection (ICSI)	$10,000 to $12,000 per cycle
Donor eggs	$9,000 per cycle
Intrauterine Insemination (IUI)	$300

Source: The Unofficial Guide to Having a Baby by Ann Douglas and John R. Sussman, M.D. (Hungry Minds, 1999).

Of course, these types of statistics don't even begin to factor in the hidden costs of fertility treatments, including the costs of taking time off work during and after treatment; traveling to appointments with specialists; freezing, storing, and transferring embryos; and canceling cycles because an egg has failed to mature.

Before you embark on any sort of infertility treatment program, it's important to find out upfront exactly what your health insurance plan will — and will not — cover. That means

- finding out if insurance companies in your state are mandated to cover some or all of the costs of infertility diagnosis or treatment (see the American Society for Reproductive Medicine Web site for details: www.asrm.org)

- inquiring about the type of treatment and drug coverage you or your partner have through your health plans at work (something that may require a couple of phone calls or a meeting with your company benefits administrator or an insurance company representative)

- developing a detailed understanding of which types of infertility treatments are and are not covered under your insurance plan, whether or not there's a cap on the amount of money that can be paid on any individual claim or a limit to the number of cycles of assisted reproduction you can attempt, and so on

- getting in touch with RESOLVE, an infertility patient advocacy and information organization, for guidance on dealing with your insurance company (Note: You'll find the contact information for RESOLVE in Appendix D.)

- asking your doctor to advocate on your behalf with the insurance company to ensure that as much of your infertility treatment program as possible is covered by your insurance plan

- filing a complaint with your state insurance regulator if you feel that your claim for coverage has been unfairly denied by your insurance company (You can find links to the various state insurance regulators on the National Association of Insurance Commissioners Web site: www.naic.org/1regulator/ usamap.htm.)

You'll also want to find out as much as possible upfront about the payment policies of the clinic you're intending to deal with (e.g., when you're expected to pay and what modes of payment are accepted; how much you should expect to pay if your treatment cycle is canceled before egg recovery or embryo transfer; what fees are charged for such services as embryo freezing, storage, and transfer — costs that can easily be overlooked initially). In most cases, you'll find that you are expected to pay in advance for any portion of your treatment that is not covered by your insurance plan. And even if your treatment is supposed to be fully covered by your insurance company, you may be asked to provide a signed credit card authorization form prior to the start of treatment so that the clinic will be able to collect any fees for your treatment that the insurance company refuses to cover unexpectedly.

How to Stay Sane

Regardless of the type of infertility treatment you and your partner choose to pursue, you're likely to find yourself hitched to a roller coaster that follows the pattern of your menstrual cycle. Early in your cycle, you may be filled with hope that this will be your lucky go. Around ovulation, you may be obsessed with timing intercourse to maximize your chances of conceiving. Then you'll find yourself in a 14-day holding pattern in which you second-guess each symptom, wondering if you could actually be pregnant this time. If your period then shows up, you may feel crushed with disappointment and angry because what seems to come so naturally to so many couples has proven to be so difficult for you.

While nothing short of conceiving a child can make the pain of infertility go away entirely, there's plenty you can do to minimize the toll it's taking on you and your partner:

MOM'S THE WORD

"Trying to conceive puts a major stress on a relationship. It's hard when one has to 'perform' on a schedule. There's anger, frustration, resentment, sadness, hope, and fear. There are so many ups and downs. I've found that unless someone has had trouble conceiving, they really have no idea what you are going through."

— *Kimberley, 37, mother of three*

- Don't allow yourself to forget the other areas of your life. Turning down job opportunities, postponing holidays, and otherwise putting your entire life on hold until you become pregnant will only add to your stress level.

- Try to keep your sex life separate from your reproductive life. If all the fun has disappeared from sex, consider taking a brief vacation from your fertility treatment so that you can keep your relationship with your partner on track. You might even wish to consider using birth control during these cycles to avoid falling into the familiar trap of spending the second half of your cycle wondering if you actually managed to conceive.

- Keep yourself healthy and find outlets for your stress. You'll feel worse, not better, if you drink too much, don't eat properly, and fail to get the exercise your body needs.

- Talk about how you're feeling with someone who truly understands. If you don't want to lean on your partner too much, seek out the services of a counselor or hook up with a fertility support group in your community or online. (Note: You can find leads on these types of resources in the appendices at the back of the book.)

- Encourage your partner to seek treatment if he's suffering from depression. Not only is it bad for his mental health, it could also be affecting his fertility. A study at the Clinical Institute of Psychiatry in Munich revealed that men who suffer from major depressive illnesses have lower concentrations of testosterone and higher levels of stress hormones.

- Make sure you're working with the right doctor. If you aren't happy with the treatment you're receiving or if you're put off by his or her less-than-compassionate bedside manner, consider making a change.

- Consider other routes to parenthood, even if you don't feel ready to abandon your dream of giving birth to a biological child. Read up on both domestic and international adoption and think about whether either one would be acceptable to you and your partner. (Note: You'll find the contact information for a number of adoption-related agencies in Appendix D.)

• Remind yourself that the odds of conceiving are in your favor. Studies have shown that 65% of people with persistent infertility problems ultimately conceive.

FACTS AND FIGURES

Here's another good reason for getting your feelings out if you're dealing with the stress of infertility. A study at the Harvard University Medical School showed that 42% of female fertility patients who participated in group therapy sessions aimed at stress reduction conceived without medical treatment, as compared to 20% of women who didn't participate in such sessions.

Up until now, we've been talking about the business of baby-making. Now let's move on and talk about what happens once the pregnancy test comes back positive.

CHAPTER 5

Winning at Baby Roulette

The two weeks after ovulation are the reproductive world's equivalent of purgatory. You're desperate to find out whether you've actually managed to conceive, but it's still too early to dash out to the drugstore and load up on home pregnancy tests. So instead you spend hours obsessing over every little symptom and twinge, trying to decide if the bloating you're feeling in your belly means you're actually pregnant or if it's signaling the impending arrival of that most unwelcome of visitors — your next menstrual period.

In this chapter, we're going to talk about the heady days of early pregnancy: finding out you're pregnant, shouting your news to the world, and hooking up with Dr. Right. (Of course, you may want to consider using the services of a midwife — something else we'll be talking about in this chapter.) Finally, we'll talk about what your due date really means and how your baby will develop during the exciting months ahead.

MOTHER WISDOM

The more things change, the more they stay the same. Four thousand years ago, a woman who was wondering if she was in the family way mixed barley seed into her urine to test for pregnancy. If the barley grew more quickly than normal, thanks to the high levels of estrogen in her urine, chances are she was pregnant.

A Little Bit Pregnant

You can always tell when a soap opera character is pregnant. She loses the impeccable makeup, her picture-perfect coiffure becomes a thing of the past, and the mere mention of food has her dashing for the nearest bathroom.

In real life, however, pregnancy symptoms aren't always quite this obvious. While most women experience a suspicious symptom or two, other women don't experience anything out of the ordinary until they've missed a period or two.

You see, despite what certain best-selling pregnancy books would have you believe, there's no such thing as a one-size-fits-all pregnancy. Not every woman ends up experiencing tender, swollen breasts within a few days of conception, nor does every woman happen to notice any implantation bleeding about a week before her period is due.

To make things even more tricky, some of the most common pregnancy symptoms — things like tender breasts, bloating, and cramping — can also double as symptoms of premenstrual syndrome (PMS). As a result, it can be hard to tell whether there's a baby on order or if you're simply about to get your next period.

I've provided a list of the most common symptoms of early pregnancy in Table 5.1. But before I set you loose on the chart, I want you to promise me that you'll take the information with a grain of salt. (Actually, make that at least a shakerful.) You may be experiencing all the symptoms listed on the chart, or you might not be experiencing any at all. Bottom line? If you wait for each and every possible pregnancy symptom to show up, you could be on your way to labor and delivery before you accept the fact that you're really and truly pregnant!

MOTHER WISDOM

Finding it hard to believe that you're actually pregnant? Stop second-guessing that pregnancy test! Studies have shown that the latest generation of tests is extremely accurate — over 97% accurate, in fact. When errors do occur, they tend to be false negatives (the test says you aren't pregnant, even though you are) rather than false positives. Inaccurate test results tend to occur for one of the following reasons: The urine was incorrectly collected or stored; the urine and the home pregnancy test weren't at room temperature when the test was conducted; or the woman had traces of blood or protein in her urine, had an active urinary tract infection, or is premenopausal.

Testing, testing . . .

There's no denying it: Whoever develops a test that diagnoses pregnancy at the time of conception is going to make a killing in the marketplace. But until that happens, the impatient women of the world will have to make do with the current generation of pregnancy tests, which are accurate approximately two weeks after ovulation.

While some women are able to get away with using these tests a few days early (I know women who've been able to confirm their pregnancies just 10 to 12 days after ovulation), it generally takes the full two weeks to get accurate results. That's because your body needs time to produce enough human chorionic gonadotropin (hCG) for the test to confirm your pregnancy.

TABLE 5.1
EARLY PREGNANCY SYMPTOMS

Symptom	What Causes It to Occur During Pregnancy	Other Possible Causes
Menstrual Changes		
A missed period	Rising levels of progesterone fully suppress your menstrual period.	Jet lag, extreme weight loss or gain, a change in climate, a chronic disease such as diabetes or tuberculosis, severe illness, surgery, shock, bereavement, or other sources of stress Note: Taking birth control pills can also cause you to miss a period.
A lighter-than-average period	Your progesterone levels are rising, but not enough to fully suppress your menstrual period. Note: This can make it difficult for your doctor or midwife to pin down your due date.	Can be experienced by users of birth control pills
A small amount of spotting	May occur when the fertilized egg implants in the uterine wall — about a week after conception has occurred	Can be experienced by users of birth control pills and women with fibroids or infections. What's more, some women routinely

Menstrual Changes

| | experience some mid-cycle spotting. Spotting may also be the earliest sign of an impending miscarriage. (See Chapter 11.) | |

Breast Changes

| Breast tenderness and enlargement | Hormonal changes of early pregnancy. Note: You may also notice some related physical changes. The areola (the flat area around the nipple) may begin to darken, and the tiny glands on the areola may begin to enlarge. | Premenstrual syndrome (PMS), excessive caffeine intake, or fibrocystic breast disease |

Cramping and/or Nausea

| Abdominal cramping (period-like cramping in the lower abdomen and pelvis and/or bloating and gassiness) | Hormonal changes of early pregnancy | PMS, constipation, irritable bowel syndrome |
| Morning sickness (a catch-all term used to describe everything from mild nausea to vomiting to the point of dehydration) | High levels of progesterone and human chorionic gonadotropin (hCG). Note: Can occur at any time of day, but tends to be worse first thing in | Flu, food poisoning, or other illnesses |

continued

Symptom	What Causes It to Occur During Pregnancy	Other Possible Causes (Continued)
Cramping and/or Nausea		
Morning sickness	the morning, when your blood sugar is at its lowest.	
Increased Need to Urinate and/or Constipation		
Increased need to urinate	Increased blood flow to the pelvic area, triggered by the production of human chorionic gonadotropin (hCG) during early pregnancy	A urinary tract infection, uterine fibroids, or excessive caffeine intake
Constipation	Progesterone relaxes the intestinal muscles, resulting in varying degrees of constipation	Inadequate intake of high-fiber foods or inadequate consumption of fluids
Food Aversions and Cravings and/or Heightened Sense of Smell		
Food aversions and cravings (e.g., a metallic taste in the mouth and/or a craving for certain foods)	Hormonal changes of early pregnancy	Poor diet, stress, or PMS

Food Aversions and Cravings and/or Heightened Sense of Smell

Heightened sense of smell (e.g., sudden dislike of the smell of coffee, perfume, strong-smelling foods like onions, and/or cigarette smoke)	Hormonal changes of early pregnancy	Illness

Decreased Energy Level

Fatigue	Increased production of progesterone (which acts as a natural sedative) and an increase in your metabolic rate (your body's way of ensuring it will be able to support the needs of you and your developing baby)	Not getting enough sleep, not eating properly, flu, illness, or some other medical condition

Changes to the Reproductive Organs

Changes to the cervix and the uterus (The cervix will take on a slightly purplish hue, and both the cervix and uterus will begin to soften.)	Hormonal changes of early pregnancy. Note: These types of changes can be detected by your doctor or midwife during a pelvic examination.	A delayed menstrual period

Some women find that their bodies still aren't manufacturing enough hCG even two weeks after ovulation. Consequently, they end up spending a small fortune on pregnancy tests waiting for their hCG levels to rise to a detectable level. If you find yourself in this frustrating situation and you've been charting your temperature, your chart may be able to save you enough money on pregnancy tests to treat yourself to dinner out! All you have to do is to count the number of days your temperature has remained elevated since ovulation. If you've had 18 consecutive high temperatures (or at least three more high temperatures than you've experienced in any previous luteal phase to date), it's probably time to crack open the non-alcoholic champagne.

Here are some other things you need to know about home pregnancy tests:

- It's important to use your first morning urine when you're conducting the test. The concentration of hCG will be highest at that time of day.

- You should check that the test hasn't passed its expiration date. Most have a clearly marked "best before" date.

- Make a point of following the testing instructions to the letter. Pay particular attention to how long you have to wait before you read the test results and at what point the results are no longer valid. (Some tests will eventually turn positive, even if they originally came back with a negative result. This doesn't mean you're pregnant; it means it's time to toss out the test!)

- If you initially test positive on a pregnancy test, but retest a week later and get a negative result, chances are you've experienced an early miscarriage. Contact your doctor or midwife right away. He or she may want to order an hCG test to confirm you were pregnant and to verify that your hCG level is returning to normal. (You'll find a detailed discussion of miscarriage in Chapter 11.)

How you may feel about being pregnant

While the television commercials would have you believe that there's only one way to react when the pregnancy test comes back positive — apparently, you're supposed to jump with joy and then run into the arms of your drop-dead-gorgeous husband — those of us who've been around the block a few times know that the scene you've been scripting in your head doesn't always play out that way. You may find yourself feeling one or more of the following ways during the first few hours and days:

MOM'S THE WORD

"I felt a whole flurry of emotions: excitement, nervousness, anxiety, fear, every emotion you can imagine. My husband was thrilled and excited as well. We were both giddy like little kids."

— Jennifer, a 29-year-old mother of one

- Elated. You may feel as if you're going to burst with excitement and that you've got to tell somebody — anybody! — about your pregnancy. Jane, a 33-year-old mother of two, remembers how she felt when she found out she was expecting her first baby: "I was elated! It was a snowy day, and I actually called into work and said I couldn't make it in. I then spent the day celebrating being pregnant. I stopped by my husband's office on the way home from my doctor's appointment to tell him. We hugged in the falling snow."

- Awestruck. It's one thing to want to be pregnant, and quite another to discover that the deed has actually been done! Some women find themselves feeling positively wonderstruck at the realization that there's a baby growing inside their bodies. In fact, it may be all they can think about at first. Jennifer, 26, who is midway through her first pregnancy, describes how she continues to feel about being pregnant: "I still sometimes just sit back and shake my head at how overwhelmed I feel about carrying a child that's half me and half this man that I love more than anything in the world. I hope every day that the baby is happy and cozy inside of me, and that he or she is growing strong and healthy. I'm still very emotional about this awesome adventure."

- Proud. If becoming pregnant has been a goal of yours for some time, you may feel a tremendous sense of accomplishment when you discover you've actually managed to conceive. "I remember feeling as if I'd made this momentous step forward — that an entirely new chapter had opened in my life," says Marie, a 36-year-old mother of three. "And, in fact, it had."

- Shocked. Finding out that you're really and truly 100% pregnant can be unnerving, even if you've been consciously trying to have a baby. "I was initially quite shocked and somewhat panicked," recalls 32-year-old Janet, who recently gave birth to her first baby. "I had expected it to take much longer. My husband was asleep when I did the test, and I woke him up to tell him the news. I don't think either of us got very much sleep that night. It took us both a few weeks to get used to the idea, and then we were both very happy about it."

- Overwhelmed. It's not unusual to feel completely overwhelmed and possibly even slightly panicked when you realize that you're going to become a mother. "Up until that point, it had all seemed like a game," recalls Maria, a 31-year-old mother of two young children. "Then I was thinking, 'What have we done?'"

- Worried. If you've been pregnant in the past, but had that pregnancy end in miscarriage, stillbirth, or infant death, you may feel extremely anxious about being pregnant again. You may wonder if something will go wrong this time, too — whether you'll actually end up with a healthy baby in your arms nine months down the road or if your hopes and dreams will be shattered again. (Note: You'll find a detailed discussion of the challenges of pregnancy after a loss in Chapter 11.)

- Unenthused. Some women find that the symptoms of early pregnancy leave them feeling less than thrilled about the situation. (Hey, it's hard to feel like celebrating when you're constantly dashing to the bathroom!) That was certainly the case for 31-year-old Debbie, who is currently pregnant with her first child: "I've found that people expect me to always be in a state of ecstasy. Even throughout the morning sickness and weeks of physical exhaustion, it felt like I was disappointing people if I wasn't skipping around talking about baby names, etc. It made me wonder how many women cover up their real feelings, especially in early pregnancy."

- Dismayed. If your pregnancy was unplanned, you may need a little time to get used to the idea of having a baby. "I conceived in the blink of an eye — or perhaps even faster than that!" admits LeeAnne, a 29-year-old mother of three. "This made for a bit of a mental adjustment with each pregnancy, as we weren't really planning and trying to conceive."

By the way, if you're expecting your partner to react like all the men in the television commercials — he's supposed to pick you up and swing you in circles while declaring his undying love for you and the baby — you could be in for a bit of a disappointment. Not all guys react with quite that much enthusiasm: "My husband said, 'Oh, that's good' and kept watching the hockey game because he was in shock," recalls Darci, a 29-year-old mother of one. "Darin was a little more cautious than me," said Julie, 29, who is currently pregnant with her second child. "He looked at the pregnancy test and said, 'The line's not very dark.' I wanted to hit him!"

Of course, some women find that the men in their lives are even more excited than they are. This was certainly the case for Marinda, a 30-year-old mother of two, who was initially shocked to discover she was unexpectedly pregnant with baby number two. "It took me about two weeks to come to terms with being pregnant and to start looking forward to having another baby. My husband, on the other hand, was happy right away."

Sharing your news with the world

One of the first decisions you and your partner will face as a newly pregnant couple is when to share your exciting news with the rest of the world. You may decide to tell the entire world all at once, or to be a bit more selective about whom you tell and when.

Marguerite, a 36-year-old mother of two, took the first approach: "I phoned everyone right away — as soon as I found out I was pregnant. I couldn't contain myself." Although she knew that spreading her news early on meant she might have to share some sad news if she ended up miscarrying, Marguerite felt that it made more sense to announce her pregnancy right away. "David and I decided not to wait until the pregnancy was further along because as soon as the pregnancy was confirmed, we were strongly attached to the presence of the baby in our lives. We felt that if any unforeseen problems arose it would affect us significantly and we'd therefore want and need the support of the people around us."

Anne, a 29-year-old mother of one, decided to wait before sharing the news with everyone until she'd passed the peak risk period for miscarriage (the first trimester): "We told our parents early on but we held off telling other family members and friends until we were about three months along. I felt that our parents would be there to help us through a miscarriage, but I couldn't cope with having to tell all our family members and friends if we were to miscarry."

Sometimes special circumstances force you to spill the beans about your pregnancy a little sooner than you might normally have planned. Jenna, a 25-year-old mother of one, had a particular reason for choosing to announce her pregnancy sooner rather than later: "My grandfather was very sick and I wanted him to know about his great-grandchild," she explains.

Just one quick word of caution: Once you decide to share the news with one member of your extended family, you'd better plan to get on the phone to the rest of the clan as soon as possible. The family grapevine is never more effective than when there's news of a pregnancy to spread, and you don't want the grandparents-to-be (particularly first-time grandparents-to-be!) to hear your exciting news from someone else.

MOM'S THE WORD

"I told my dad about my pregnancy over the phone because I didn't want to confront him in person. To my surprise, I heard a choke in his words and I thought he might be crying. I just didn't know if it was for joy or because he was upset that I was pregnant but not yet married. About an hour later, an absolutely huge bouquet of flowers arrived at my office door. It was from my dad. My question was answered and I was happy."

— *Tracey, 31, mother of one*

Sharing your news at work

You kicked your coffee habit weeks ago, but for some reason your boss still hasn't clued into the fact that you're pregnant. Now you're wondering how — and when — to announce your pregnancy at work. While there's no single "right time" to make your big announcement, you're more likely to meet with a positive reaction if you plan that announcement carefully. Here are a few tips:

- Respect the power of the office grapevine. Share your news with your boss before he or she hears it from someone else. If you feel an overwhelming need to confide in a co-worker before you're ready to fully come out of the pregnancy closet, make sure he or she realizes that they're the only one who knows. That way, he or she will be less likely to spill the beans in the middle of a staff meeting.

- Time your announcement carefully. If you're expecting a performance review or a raise in the near future, keep your pregnancy to yourself for now. That way, if the news is less than what you'd hoped for, you won't have to wonder whether your poor review or less-than-spectacular raise is due to your performance or your pregnancy. It's also a good idea to time your announcement to coincide with a major achievement at work: That way, you can reassure your boss with actions as well as words that you're still as productive and committed to your job as ever.

MOM'S THE WORD

"I was in the process of receiving a promotion so I didn't tell my employer until after we'd hammered out my new compensation package. They were surprised, but for the most part everyone took the news well."

— *Jenny, 31, mother of one*

FACTS AND FIGURES

The federal Pregnancy Discrimination Act of 1978 is designed to protect the rights of pregnant workers who are employed by companies that have 15 or more employees. (Note: Most women who work for smaller companies are covered by similar legislation at the state level.) The Act:

- prevents employers from refusing to hire a woman solely because she is pregnant, provided that she is capable of fulfilling the major requirements of the position
- prohibits employers from introducing any special procedures that would in any way discriminate against pregnant employees (e.g., treating pregnant employees who are on medical leave differently

than employees who are on medical leave for other health reasons, or treating health insurance expenses for pregnancy-related conditions differently than those for other types of medical conditions)

• guarantees a pregnant woman's right to continue working as long as she is able.

If you feel that you have been the victim of pregnancy discrimination at work, you should keep detailed notes on everything that has happened (e.g., print out copies of e-mail messages that may be helpful in making your case), ask to review the contents of your personnel file and make copies of anything that may prove to be relevant (e.g., copies of particularly glowing performance reviews), and discuss your concerns with your company's human resources manager. You might also want to obtain advice and information from the U.S. Equal Employment Opportunity Commission (1-800-669-4000; www.eeoc.gov).

• Don't neglect safety concerns. If you work in a hazardous type of environment — in an X-ray laboratory or a chemical manufacturing plant, for example — you may need to announce your pregnancy sooner rather than later so that you can be reassigned to a different type of work for the duration of your pregnancy. To find out about laws concerning safety at work and your rights as a pregnant employee, get in touch with your state or county health department.

• Keep the news under your hat if you can. If your job doesn't pose any immediate risks to your developing baby, you might want to consider keeping the news to yourself until you've passed through the highest-risk period for pregnancy loss. Of course, if you're experiencing severe morning sickness or other pregnancy-related complications, you may have little choice but to share your news right away.

• Think seriously about postponing your announcement if your boss is having a particularly bad day. You're less likely to be met with a positive reaction if your boss is in the middle of dealing with a major computer problem or if he's spent the entire morning trying to placate the Customer from You-Know-Where.

- Be prepared for a lukewarm reaction — and try not to take your boss's lack of enthusiasm personally. As happy as your employer may be for you, you've just dropped a major staffing challenge in her lap! If this is the first time she's ever had to deal with a pregnant employee, she may be particularly apprehensive about what your pregnancy may mean for both her and the company.

- Don't make promises you may not be able to keep. Rather than trying to reassure your boss that you'll work right until the bitter end of your pregnancy and that you'll return to work as soon as possible after your baby is born — commitments you might not be willing or able to honor in the end — simply agree to discuss your plans when your pregnancy is further along.

MOM'S THE WORD

"I told my employer shortly after I reached the three-month mark because I knew he'd need considerable time to find and train a replacement for me."

— *Anne, 29, mother of one*

Finding Dr. Right

Decisions, decisions. Who would have thought pregnancy could be this complicated? Well, believe it or not, you've got yet another important decision to make — assuming, of course, that you didn't already resolve this back at your preconception checkup. What I'm talking about is the need to choose a doctor or midwife to care for you during your pregnancy and to be present at the birth of your baby.

If you decide to go the doctor route, your baby will be delivered by either a family physician (a medical doctor who has had several years of specialized training in all aspects of family medicine, including obstetrics) or an obstetrician (a medical doctor who has received specialized training in obstetrics).

If you choose to work with a midwife instead, you'll have the option of working with whatever type(s) of midwives are in practice in your particular state:

- certified nurse-midwives (CNMs) (registered nurses who have taken additional training in midwifery and who have been certified by the American College of Nurse-Midwives Certification Council)

- certified midwives (CMs) (midwives with training in a health-care field other than nursing who have received specialized training through a midwifery education program accredited by the American College of Nurse-Midwives Division of Accreditation)

- independent midwives (also known as direct entry midwives or lay midwives) (midwives who have apprenticed with other midwives, but who have not received any formal training in midwifery)

- certified professional midwives (CPMs) (an independent midwife who has met the certification standards as set by the North American Registry of Midwives)

While certified nurse-midwives are able to practice legally in all 50 states and the District of Columbia, the legal status of certified midwives, independent midwives, and certified professional midwives varies from state to state. You can get up-to-date information on the status of midwifery in various states by visiting the Web sites of the American College of Nurse-Midwives and the Midwives Alliance of North America. (See Appendix D for Web site addresses and other contact information for these two organizations.)

FACTS AND FIGURES

According to the American College of Nurse-Midwives, 9% of vaginal births in 1998 were attended by certified nurse-midwives.

MOM'S THE WORD

"Our midwives were wonderful. We had a standard doctor-assisted delivery the first two times and, in comparison, our experience with our midwives was incredible. I think of the experiences as night and day, with the midwives providing a consistent level of care and expertise that, in our view, cannot be matched."

— *LeeAnne, 29, mother of three*

Once you've decided whether you would like to have your birth attended by a doctor or a midwife, your next step is to find the caregiver who's right for you. Here are some things you'll want to look for when you're meeting prospective caregivers:

- Someone who's capable of providing the type of care you're likely to require during your pregnancy. If you know from the outset that your pregnancy is likely to be high-risk (e.g., you have a pre-existing health condition such as diabetes or high blood pressure), an obstetrician may be your best choice. But if your pregnancy is likely to be low-risk, there's no reason why a family physician or midwife shouldn't be able to provide you with equally good care during your pregnancy. If, for some reason, you unexpectedly develop some sort of pregnancy-related complication that causes your pregnancy to be classified as high-risk, your family physician or midwife will either transfer you to an obstetrician or ask him or her to consult on your case. So you needn't fear that you won't have access to the care of a specialist if you need it. The door is still open to make a change down the road.

- Someone with whom you have a good rapport. If you get along famously with your family physician, you may prefer to turn to him or her for your prenatal care. If you don't get along, however, you'll definitely want to give serious thought to finding someone else to care for you during your pregnancy. There are so many important issues to discuss during pregnancy, and you want to be sure that you feel comfortable with the person who'll be caring for you and your baby.

• Someone whose philosophies are compatible with your own. When you're shopping around for a caregiver, it's important to look for someone who shares your outlook on pregnancy and birth — for example, your views on important issues like pain relief during labor, episiotomy, breastfeeding, and so on. That's not to say you'll necessarily end up with "the perfect birth," of course! No one in the baby business can offer that sort of guarantee.

• Someone who can provide you with consistent care. Studies have shown that women and babies are better off being cared for by the same caregiver or by one of a small group of caregivers who share the same basic philosophies about pregnancy and birth. If your caregiver works in a group, you'll want to make sure that you feel comfortable with the other members of the medical or midwifery practice. After all, there's always the possibility that one of them could end up attending your baby's birth instead of your primary caregiver.

• Someone who meets any other special criteria you may have. You may have some other criteria that need to be considered when you're shopping around for a caregiver. If, for example, you're a survivor of sexual abuse or a member of a religious group that would consider it inappropriate for any male other than your husband to be present at the birth of your baby, it may be very important to you to find a female caregiver. If you're in a large urban area with plenty of caregivers to choose from, you may be in luck. Otherwise, you could find yourself forced to compromise on this point.

🔊 MOM'S THE WORD

"My feeling about caregivers is that they should provide the services I can't do for myself and not interfere with my decisions about the birth. I don't need someone to teach me about pregnancy and birth, as I've taught myself through experience and books. I just need someone to do the routine stuff like making sure I'm not sick and the baby's not sick."

— *Elvi, 32, currently expecting her third child*

Here are some specific questions you may want to ask when you're trying to determine whether a particular caregiver is right for you:

About the practice

- How long have you been practicing? How many births have you attended? What percentage of your patients' babies do you end up delivering yourself?

- Other than you, who might be present at the birth of my baby? Will I have the opportunity to meet some or all of these backup caregivers at some point during my pregnancy?

- How should I go about reaching you in the event of an emergency? Are there times when you may be unavailable to take my call? In that case, whom would I call instead?

- How often are you on call? Do you expect to be on call around the time that my baby is due?

- Do you involve residents, interns, or student midwives in your practice? If so, what role would they play in my care?

- What hospitals and/or birth centers are you affiliated with?

- Do you attend home births? (While many midwives attend home births, only a handful of doctors are willing to do so.)

Pregnancy-related policies and procedures

- What's your standard schedule for prenatal appointments? (According to the American College of Obstetricians and

Gynecologists, a typical woman with a low-risk pregnancy is seen monthly until the 28th week of pregnancy, every two weeks between weeks 28 and 36, and weekly from 36 weeks until she gives birth — something that typically happens around the 40-week mark.)

- Under what circumstances would you decide to see me more often than this? (Note: If you've previously experienced the death of a baby through miscarriage, stillbirth, or neonatal death, you might want to ask whether the caregiver would be willing to schedule additional appointments if you required added reassurance between appointments or, at the very least, if he/she would agree to see you on an as-needed basis if your anxiety level suddenly shot sky-high.)

- How much time do you set aside for each appointment? (Doctors tend to schedule about 10 minutes for prenatal appointments, while midwives typically spend 45 minutes to an hour with each client.)

- What types of tests are you likely to recommend over the course of my pregnancy (e.g., ultrasound, maternal-serum screening, amniocentesis, gestational diabetes, group B strep)?

- Under what circumstances, if any, would you need to transfer me into the care of another health-care provider? Under what circumstances would it be possible for you to coordinate shared care with a specialist?

Approaches to birth and postpartum care

- What percentage of your patients write birth plans? What advice would you offer if I decided to write one? (Note: You'll find a sample birth plan in Appendix B.)

- Under what circumstances do you induce labor?

- How much time will you be able to spend with me while I'm in labor?

- Do the majority of women who you care for have medicated or non-medicated births? Which methods of pharmacological and non-pharmacological pain relief do they tend to use the most often (e.g., epidurals vs. laboring in water)?

- Do you encourage couples to attempt unmedicated deliveries?

- How would you feel if I were to decide to use the services of a doula (a professional labor support person) or some other labor support person?

- Do you routinely use electronic fetal monitoring during labor?

- What percentage of women in your care receive episiotomies?

- How often do the women in your care end up delivering through cesarean section? (Note: A doctor who specializes in high-risk pregnancies may have a higher-than-average cesarean rate just by virtue of the nature of his or her practice.)

- What percentage of the women in your care who are attempting a vaginal birth after cesarean (VBAC) are able to deliver vaginally?

- Will my baby be able to remain with me after the birth?

- Do you provide breastfeeding support?

- How often will I see you during the postpartum period? Should my baby be checked by another health-care provider during this period?

While you'll want to spend some time making sure that a particular caregiver is right for you, don't wait too long to make up your mind or you could find out that his or her practice is full. Jane, a 33-year-old mother of two, encountered this frustrating situation: "When I was nine weeks pregnant with my first child, I phoned the nearest midwifery practice to inquire. I was already too late to secure the services of a midwife! The second time around, I phoned the practice as soon as I knew I was pregnant."

Hospital or home birth?

Something else to keep in mind when you're shopping around for a caregiver is where you intend to give birth. If you're hoping to give birth at home, you'll probably need to use the services of a midwife. If you're hoping to give birth in a hospital, a doctor will likely handle your delivery (unless, of course, you're fortunate enough to live in a part of the country where midwives have hospital privileges).

While 99 percent of babies are born in hospitals, some women choose to deliver their babies at home, preferring to welcome their newborns in a setting in which they feel comfortable and relaxed. "My biggest fears were that once I was at a hospital, I'd be lost among the other expectant mothers and treated as though I were part of a babymaking assembly line rather than a person partaking in the making of a miracle," explains Bevin, 27, who recently gave birth to her first child. (See Table 5.2 for a summary of the pros and cons of hospital and home birth.)

While the American College of Obstetricians and Gynecologists (ACOG) is firmly opposed to home births (ACOG argues that giving birth poses potential hazards to both mother and baby and that it simply isn't possible to make the home setting as safe as a hospital setting), some health-care providers consider home birth to be a reasonably safe alternative to hospital birth for women with low-risk pregnancies. You should, however, consider a home birth only if

- you are in good medical condition and your pregnancy is considered low-risk (e.g., you aren't experiencing gestational diabetes, pre-eclampsia, or other complications)

- there aren't any obstetrical red flags to indicate that home birth might be a poor choice for you (e.g., you have a history of difficult deliveries)

- you have a qualified caregiver lined up to attend the birth, and this person has all the necessary emergency medical supplies (e.g., oxygen, resuscitation equipment, and so on)

- you're willing to take responsibility for having all the necessary birth-related supplies on hand (see Table 5.3) and are prepared to abandon your plans for a home birth immediately if any sort of complication arises

- your home is reasonably close to a hospital (say within 10 minutes)

- your partner and/or children are supportive of home birth and you have some additional support people available to help you before, during, and after the birth.

TABLE 5.2

THE PROS AND CONS OF HOSPITAL BIRTH VS. HOME BIRTH

Pros	
Hospital Birth	*Home Birth*
All the high-tech medical equipment is on hand in case you or your baby need them.	You're able to give birth in the privacy of your own home, surrounded by people you care about.
You can be prepped for an emergency cesarean in a matter of minutes.	You don't need to head for the hospital when you're in labor.
You have more options for pain relief.	You have greater control over your birthing experience (e.g., you can eat and drink according to your own appetite, rather than adhering to any strict hospital policies).
	You may be more relaxed, which can help reduce your need for pain medications during labor.
	There's less chance of picking up a postpartum infection.
	You're less likely to be subjected to unwanted medical interventions.

Cons

Hospital Birth	**Home Birth**

Hospital Birth

Despite an effort to create more home-like birthing environments, many hospital birthing centers still feel sterile and clinical.

You may find yourself having to hop in the car and head for the hospital when you're in the heat of labor, which can be painful and upsetting.

Rigid hospital policies may interfere with your plans for the birth.

There's a greater risk of infection in a hospital setting than at home.

You may find it difficult to relax in the hospital environment, which can increase your need for pain relief medications during labor.

You may be needlessly subjected to certain interventions (e.g., electronic fetal monitoring, artificial rupture of membranes, augmentation of labor, or a cesarean delivery) simply because the technology is available. (Some studies have shown that women giving birth in a hospital setting are sometimes subjected to these types of interventions without any specific medical reason.)

Home Birth

If an acute emergency were to arise during labor (e.g., if the placenta were to suddenly separate from the uterine wall), you and your baby could be at risk. It might not be possible to obtain the necessary medical attention in time to prevent a tragedy, even if the hospital were within minutes of your home.

You don't have access to the same range of pain relief options that would be available to you in a hospital.

TABLE 5.3

HOME BIRTH SUPPLIES

If you decide to plan a home birth, your midwife will likely advise you to have the following types of supplies on hand:

Two or more sets of clean sheets (a set for use during the delivery and a set for use after the birth)
A waterproof pad, shower curtain, or large plastic tablecloth to prevent the mattress of your bed from being damaged
Disposable absorbent pads or large diapers to absorb amniotic fluid and blood during labor and the birth
Clean towels and washcloths
Sterile gauze pads
A dozen or more pairs of disposable gloves
Umbilical cord clamps
A three-ounce bulb syringe for suctioning mucus from the baby's mouth and nose
A large bowl to catch the placenta
Receiving blankets for the baby
Sanitary napkins

Note: If you're planning a water birth, you'll also need to round up some additional supplies: a portable birthing tub (unless you intend to use your existing bathtub, Jacuzzi, or hot tub), a water thermometer (to ensure that the temperature remains around 100°F/37°C), a flashlight that works underwater (so that the caregiver can view the birth), an inflatable plastic pillow (to keep you comfortable), a fishnet (to scoop out placental fragments and other remnants from the birth), and plenty of clean towels. There is still a great deal of controversy about the safety of water birth, so this is an issue you'll want to discuss with your caregiver early in your pregnancy.

Some women feel quite strongly that giving birth at home is the right choice for them. Bevin, 27, who recently gave birth to her first child, was immediately sold on the idea of having a home birth. It just took a bit longer to sell her partner, Ben, on the whole idea: "I knew right away that I didn't want to give birth in a hospital — I have a fear of doctors and hospitals — but trying to convince Ben that there were other options was almost like trying to pull a semi-truck with dental floss.

"In the end, Ben listened to my arguments in favor of a home birth. I did a ton of research and presented my case to him. I also pointed out that we're just six minutes away from the closest hospital and 15 minutes from the biggest hospital, should anything go wrong. He finally agreed reluctantly, and our doctor recommended a very experienced midwife. By our second visit with her, Ben was actually convinced that having a home birth was probably better than going to the hospital!"

Marinda, 30, was similarly determined to deliver her second baby at home. She'd gone with a hospital birth the first time around, but wanted to have baby number two somewhere other than in the clinical hospital setting. "I had my second child at home in our bedroom, which was cozy and dimly lit and extremely relaxing," she recalls. "Three hours after the birth, everyone in the house was trying to sleep and the midwives were gone."

LeeAnne and her partner had planned to deliver their child at home, but ended up having to abandon those plans. "Unfortunately, because I tested positive for group B strep, we had to be at the hospital," she explains.

Home birth isn't necessarily for everyone. Some women prefer to give birth in a setting where all the medical bells and whistles are close at hand. That was certainly the case for Marie, a mother of three. "I don't think I'd be able to forgive myself if I decided to give birth at home and something happened to the baby that could have been prevented if I'd given birth in the hospital. I simply felt safer giving birth knowing that the necessary medical equipment and specialists were nearby if I needed them."

Your First Prenatal Checkup

Regardless of whether you intend to give birth at home or in hospital, and to be cared for by a midwife, family physician, or obstetrician, you'll want to get in to see your caregiver as soon as possible after you find out that you're pregnant. This is particularly important if your pregnancy was unplanned and you weren't able to schedule a preconception checkup.

MOTHER WISDOM

Your prenatal checkup will fly by in a flash, so you'll want to get in the habit of bringing a written list of questions to ask your doctor or midwife. That way, you won't realize half an hour after your appointment ends that you forgot to ask an important question.

During your initial prenatal checkup, your caregiver will

- confirm your pregnancy by doing a urine or blood test or by conducting a physical examination to look for changes in your uterus and cervix that would indicate you're pregnant

- estimate your due date by considering such factors as the date of your last menstrual period, the types of pregnancy symptoms you've been experiencing, physical changes to your uterus and cervix, and any information you can provide concerning the possible date of conception. (You may have this information if you've been using ovulation predictor kits or charting your fertility signals — see Chapter 3.)

- perform a blood test to check for anemia, hepatitis B, HIV, syphilis, antibodies to rubella (German measles), and — depending on your ethnic background and family history — certain genetic diseases

- take a vaginal culture to check for infection. (Some caregivers do this routinely; others do it only if there's a specific reason.)

- do a Pap smear to check for cervical cancer or pre-cancerous cells. (If you've had this test within the past year, your doctor or midwife is unlikely to repeat it. Some doctors and midwives try to avoid performing Pap smears during pregnancy because they can result in a small amount of spotting, which isn't harmful to the pregnancy, but can be quite alarming to the pregnant woman nonetheless.)

- check your urine for signs of infection, blood sugar problems, and excess protein

- weigh you to establish a baseline so that your weight gain during pregnancy can be monitored

- take your blood pressure

- talk to you about how you and your partner feel about the pregnancy and ask you whether you have any questions or concerns

If you didn't have a preconception checkup, your doctor or midwife will want to ask you about your medical and reproductive history. He or she will ask you questions about

- any chronic health problems or conditions you may have

- any medications you're taking (both prescription and over-the-counter)

- the state of your general health

- your gynecological and obstetrical history

- your family medical history

- your general nutrition and lifestyle habits (e.g., whether you smoke, drink, or use drugs, and whether you exercise regularly)

- whether you'll be working during your pregnancy (and, if so, whether you'll require any work modifications for safety reasons)

- whether there are any special circumstances that he/she should know about in order to care for you during your pregnancy and birth (e.g., whether you have a history of sexual abuse that might lead to heightened anxiety about the birth; whether there are any ethnic or religious traditions that might affect your pregnancy and birth)

- whether or not your pregnancy was planned (and, if not, how you and/or your partner are adjusting to the news)

Note: Your doctor or midwife will record details about your pregnancy on your prenatal record. He or she may also provide you with a patient version of this record so that you can keep your own pregnancy records as well. If you aren't given such a record during your initial prenatal appointment, you may want to use the one at the back of the book. (See Appendix G.)

What your due date really means

One of the most important bits of information you'll walk away with at the end of your first prenatal checkup is your doctor's or midwife's best guess about when your baby will be born — your so-called "estimated date of confinement," or due date.

To calculate this all-important date, your caregiver will consult a due-date chart (see Table 5.4) or due-date wheel or will either

- add 266 days or 38 weeks to the date you ovulated, or

- add 280 days or 40 weeks to the date of the first day of your last menstrual period (assuming, of course, that you have a textbook 28-day cycle)

TABLE 5.4

YOUR ESTIMATED DATE OF DELIVERY

The row of boldface numbers indicates the date of the first day of your last menstrual period. The date underneath indicates your approximate due date (assuming, of course, that you have a 28-day menstrual cycle). If your cycle is anything other than 28 days in length, your doctor or midwife will likely adjust your due date by adding or subtracting the appropriate number of days.

January	**1**	**2**	**3**	**4**	**5**	**6**	**7**	**8**	**9**	**10**	**11**	**12**	**13**	**14**	**15**	**16**	**17**	**18**	**19**	**20**	**21**	**22**	**23**	**24**	**25**	**26**	**27**	**28**	**29**	**30**	**31**
October	8	9	10	11	12	13	14	15	16	17	18	19	20	21	22	23	24	25	26	27	28	29	30	31	1	2	3	4	5	6	7
February	**1**	**2**	**3**	**4**	**5**	**6**	**7**	**8**	**9**	**10**	**11**	**12**	**13**	**14**	**15**	**16**	**17**	**18**	**19**	**20**	**21**	**22**	**23**	**24**	**25**	**26**	**27**	**28**			
November	8	9	10	11	12	13	14	15	16	17	18	19	20	21	22	23	24	25	26	27	28	29	30	1	2	3	4	5			
March	**1**	**2**	**3**	**4**	**5**	**6**	**7**	**8**	**9**	**10**	**11**	**12**	**13**	**14**	**15**	**16**	**17**	**18**	**19**	**20**	**21**	**22**	**23**	**24**	**25**	**26**	**27**	**28**	**29**	**30**	**31**
December	6	7	8	9	10	11	12	13	14	15	16	17	18	19	20	21	22	23	24	25	26	27	28	29	30	31	1	2	3	4	5
April	**1**	**2**	**3**	**4**	**5**	**6**	**7**	**8**	**9**	**10**	**11**	**12**	**13**	**14**	**15**	**16**	**17**	**18**	**19**	**20**	**21**	**22**	**23**	**24**	**25**	**26**	**27**	**28**	**29**	**30**	
January	6	7	8	9	10	11	12	13	14	15	16	17	18	19	20	21	22	23	24	25	26	27	28	29	30	31	1	2	3	4	
May	**1**	**2**	**3**	**4**	**5**	**6**	**7**	**8**	**9**	**10**	**11**	**12**	**13**	**14**	**15**	**16**	**17**	**18**	**19**	**20**	**21**	**22**	**23**	**24**	**25**	**26**	**27**	**28**	**29**	**30**	**31**
February	5	6	7	8	9	10	11	12	13	14	15	16	17	18	19	20	21	22	23	24	25	26	27	28	1	2	3	4	5	6	7
June	**1**	**2**	**3**	**4**	**5**	**6**	**7**	**8**	**9**	**10**	**11**	**12**	**13**	**14**	**15**	**16**	**17**	**18**	**19**	**20**	**21**	**22**	**23**	**24**	**25**	**26**	**27**	**28**	**29**	**30**	
March	8	9	10	11	12	13	14	15	16	17	18	19	20	21	22	23	24	25	26	27	28	29	30	31	1	2	3	4	5	6	
July	**1**	**2**	**3**	**4**	**5**	**6**	**7**	**8**	**9**	**10**	**11**	**12**	**13**	**14**	**15**	**16**	**17**	**18**	**19**	**20**	**21**	**22**	**23**	**24**	**25**	**26**	**27**	**28**	**29**	**30**	**31**
April	7	8	9	10	11	12	13	14	15	16	17	18	19	20	21	22	23	24	25	26	27	28	29	30	1	2	3	4	5	6	7
August	**1**	**2**	**3**	**4**	**5**	**6**	**7**	**8**	**9**	**10**	**11**	**12**	**13**	**14**	**15**	**16**	**17**	**18**	**19**	**20**	**21**	**22**	**23**	**24**	**25**	**26**	**27**	**28**	**29**	**30**	**31**
May	8	9	10	11	12	13	14	15	16	17	18	19	20	21	22	23	24	25	26	27	28	29	30	31	1	2	3	4	5	6	7
September	**1**	**2**	**3**	**4**	**5**	**6**	**7**	**8**	**9**	**10**	**11**	**12**	**13**	**14**	**15**	**16**	**17**	**18**	**19**	**20**	**21**	**22**	**23**	**24**	**25**	**26**	**27**	**28**	**29**	**30**	
June	8	9	10	11	12	13	14	15	16	17	18	19	20	21	22	23	24	25	26	27	28	29	30	1	2	3	4	5	6	7	
October	**1**	**2**	**3**	**4**	**5**	**6**	**7**	**8**	**9**	**10**	**11**	**12**	**13**	**14**	**15**	**16**	**17**	**18**	**19**	**20**	**21**	**22**	**23**	**24**	**25**	**26**	**27**	**28**	**29**	**30**	**31**
July	8	9	10	11	12	13	14	15	16	17	18	19	20	21	22	23	24	25	26	27	28	29	30	31	1	2	3	4	5	6	7
November	**1**	**2**	**3**	**4**	**5**	**6**	**7**	**8**	**9**	**10**	**11**	**12**	**13**	**14**	**15**	**16**	**17**	**18**	**19**	**20**	**21**	**22**	**23**	**24**	**25**	**26**	**27**	**28**	**29**	**30**	
August	8	9	10	11	12	13	14	15	16	17	18	19	20	21	22	23	24	25	26	27	28	29	30	31	1	2	3	4	5	6	
December	**1**	**2**	**3**	**4**	**5**	**6**	**7**	**8**	**9**	**10**	**11**	**12**	**13**	**14**	**15**	**16**	**17**	**18**	**19**	**20**	**21**	**22**	**23**	**24**	**25**	**26**	**27**	**28**	**29**	**30**	**31**
September	7	8	9	10	11	12	13	14	15	16	17	18	19	20	21	22	23	24	25	26	27	28	29	30	1	2	3	4	5	6	7

Because these calculations tend to be more accurate if they're based on the timing of conception rather than the date of your last menstrual cycle, it's important to let your doctor or midwife know if you have a temperature chart or ovulation predictor kit result that could help to pinpoint the timing of ovulation. If your due date is calculated based on the date of your last menstrual period, it's important to let your caregiver know if your cycles tend to be longer or shorter than normal.

Now, before you reach for your calendar and scrawl "have baby" in the appropriate square, allow me to reveal the plain, unvarnished truth about due dates: Babies don't have a whole lot of respect for them. Studies have shown that just 5% of babies bother to show up on schedule — although, to be fair, 85% do manage to make their grand entrance within a week of their due date.

Multiple pregnancy

While 40 weeks tends to be the typical duration of a singleton pregnancy, women who are carrying more than one baby typically deliver a few weeks ahead of that. Twins usually make their debut at 36 weeks, triplets at 32 weeks, and quadruplets at 30 weeks. Some multiples arrive considerably earlier than that, of course, just as some singletons make an early appearance. (See Table 5.5.)

TABLE 5.5

PERCENTAGE OF SINGLETONS AND MULTIPLES BORN BEFORE 35 WEEKS AND 31 WEEKS

Number of Babies	Percentage Born Before 35 Weeks	Percentage Born Before 31 Weeks
Singletons	5%	1%
Twins	35%	10%
Triplets	80%	30%

Source: Based on statistics in When You're Expecting Twins, Triplets, or Quads *by Barbara Luke and Tamara Eberlein (HarperCollins, 1999).*

Here are the three main reasons why multiple pregnancies are likely to result in an earlier delivery:

- One of the ways your body determines when it's time to go into labor is by tracking your baby's growth. When growth begins to slow down, your body concludes that it's time for the baby to be born. Because this tends to happen earlier in multiple pregnancies, these babies tend to be born earlier.

- The placentas of multiples tend to age more quickly and to function less efficiently, which is thought to directly or indirectly lead to a shorter gestation.

- The uterus has its limits. Even though it's capable of expanding tremendously during pregnancy, it can only stretch so far. As Barbara Luke and Tamara Eberlein note in their book, *When You're Expecting Twins, Triplets, or Quads,* "The combined weight of several babies, several placentas, and a whole lot of amniotic fluid eventually signals to the body that it's time for labor to start, no matter now much longer the calendar says pregnancy should continue. By the time she reaches 32 weeks, the uterus of a woman carrying twins is already as large as that of a singleton mom at the full 40 weeks. For the mother of triplets, the uterus is stretched to full-term size by 28 weeks. And with quadruplets on board, a woman's uterus reaches full-term size as early as 24 weeks." Note: You'll find a detailed discussion of the joys and challenges of a multiple pregnancy in Chapter 11.

 FACTS AND FIGURES

By the 36th week of pregnancy, the volume of your uterus is 1,000 times greater than it was before you conceived.

The Incredible Growing Baby

Approximately 30 hours after the sperm fertilizes the egg, the process of cell division that will ultimately lead to the creation of a human being begins. What happens during the remaining weeks of pregnancy is nothing short of miraculous. That tiny bundle of cells is slowly but surely transformed into a newborn infant. (See Table 5.6.)

TABLE 5.6

HOW YOUR BABY GROWS AND DEVELOPS DURING PREGNANCY

Here's the inside scoop on your baby's growth and development during the 40 weeks of pregnancy. Of course, there's nothing much to report during the first two weeks, since you haven't actually managed to conceive yet! But once conception occurs — approximately two weeks after the start of your last menstrual period — the fertilized egg rapidly begins to develop into a tiny human being.

Week of Pregnancy	Highlights of Fetal Development
Week 1	Your period starts and your menstrual cycle begins.
Week 2	The endometrium (lining of the uterus) begins to build up in order to prepare for the implantation of a fertilized egg in the event that you're able to conceive. Your cervical mucus develops an egg white–like consistency, and ovulation occurs.
Conception Occurs — Embryonic Period Begins — First Trimester of Pregnancy Begins	
Week 3	The egg is fertilized by sperm cells that have been camping out in your fallopian tubes, waiting for this very opportunity. At the end of this week, the fertilized egg embeds itself in the lining of your uterus and then divides itself into two parts: the future placenta and the future embryo.
Week 4	Amniotic fluid is now being produced and the fetus's eyes have started to develop. By the end of this week, the umbilical cord — the developing

Week of Pregnancy	Highlights of Fetal Development
Week 4	baby's lifeline for the next eight months — will have started to form.
Week 5	The hands have started to appear and major organs are now being formed. The embryo is now the size of an apple seed.
Week 6	The embryo's heart has begun to beat, and other major organs such as the kidneys and the liver have begun to develop. The neural tube — the structure that connects the brain to the spinal cord — closes over.
Week 7	The embryo's eyes continue to develop and begin to develop pigment. Fingers, toes, and outer ears begin to take shape. The embryo is now approximately 1 inch long.
Week 8	The embryo has parchment-like skin. You can see its veins right through the skin. The teeth, palate, and larynx are beginning to take shape. The embryo is now approximately 1 1/4 inches long — the size of a large grape.
Week 9	The embryo's organs, muscles, and nerves begin to function, and it begins to make its first spontaneous movements — movements that are far too tiny for you to detect at this stage of your pregnancy.
Week 10	The amniotic sac has formed around the embryo. The sac, which is filled with amniotic fluid, helps to protect the embryo from harm and assists with proper temperature control. If the embryo is a boy, this is the week when his scrotum forms. All the embryo's major organs have been formed by now. From this point forward the embryo is referred to as a fetus.

continued

Week of Pregnancy	Highlights of Fetal Development (Continued)
First Trimester of Pregnancy — Fetal Period Begins	
Week 11	The fetus's head now makes up approximately half of its length. While the ovaries and testicles are fully formed and the external genitalia are developing, it's still too early to distinguish the sex. The fetus is now about 2 inches long and weighs approximately half an ounce.
Week 12	The fetus's face is properly formed. Even its eyelids are present. Blood has started to circulate through the umbilical cord, carrying oxygen and nutrients from the placenta to the embryo and carrying away waste products. Urine produced by the kidneys is excreted into the amniotic fluid. The fetus is now approximately 2 1/2 inches long.
Week 13	This is the week when the fetus's intestines migrate from the umbilical cord into the abdomen. The eyes and ears have almost moved into their permanent position, and the fetus has already acquired some rudimentary reflexes.
Week 14	The fetus's lungs are fully functional: It can "breathe" amniotic fluid in and out. The fetus is now approximately 3 1/2 inches long and weighs roughly 2 ounces.
Beginning of the Second Trimester	
Week 15	The fetus is covered in fine, downy hair (lanugo) that usually disappears shortly after birth. It has developed a full repertoire of facial expressions.
Week 16	The fetus's joints are now fully functional. At some point over the next four weeks, you'll likely feel its kicks for the very first time. The fetus is sensitive to light.

Week of Pregnancy	*Highlights of Fetal Development*
Week 17	The fetus is now about 5 inches long and weighs approximately 6 ounces.
Week 18	The bones in the fetal skeleton continue to be very soft and pliable.
Week 19	The fetus now has as many nerve cells as an adult. Connections between the muscles and the nerve cells are now being established.
Week 20	The fetus's senses of taste and smell are fully developed. It is now approximately 6 1/2 inches long and weighs about 9 ounces.
Week 21	The fetus is acquiring a layer of fat that will help to keep it warm after birth. Its skin is covered in a layer of vernix caseosa (a slick, fatty substance designed to protect the skin while the fetus is immersed in amniotic fluid).
Week 22	The fetus's skin is sensitive to touch, and the fetus will often respond when pressure is placed on your abdomen. By this stage of pregnancy, the fingernails have been formed and the eyebrows and eyelids are fully developed. The fetus is now approximately 7 1/2 inches long and weighs approximately 3/4 of a pound.
Week 23	The fetus's lungs are starting to develop surfactant — the dish soap–like substance that keeps the lungs from sticking together and that enables them to expand easily when the baby is born. While the fetus now has similar proportions to those of a newborn baby — its head no longer takes up half of its length — it is still extremely thin, weighing in at just a pound. During the remaining weeks of pregnancy the fetus will add another 6 1/2 pounds or so to its weight.

continued

Week of Pregnancy	Highlights of Fetal Development (Continued)
Second Trimester — Fetus Is Potentially Viable	
Week 24	The fetus's vital organs have developed enough to give it a chance to survive after birth, but outcomes for babies born this prematurely tend to be extremely poor.
Week 25	The fetus regularly experiences episodes of hiccuping during the second half of pregnancy. It is now approximately 9 inches long and weighs approximately 1 1/2 pounds.
Week 26	The fetus has developed distinct periods of sleeping and waking, and its brain patterns now resemble those of a newborn baby.
Week 27	At this stage of pregnancy, the fetus is passing a pint of urine into the amniotic fluid each day — fluid that is subsequently removed from the body via the mother's kidneys.
Beginning of the Third Trimester	
Week 28	The fetus is between 12 and 15 inches long and weighs approximately 2 1/2 to 3 pounds.
Week 29	The fetus has red, wrinkly skin.
Week 30	The fetus is capable of reacting to sound.
Week 31	From this point onward, the fetus will grow more in weight than in length.
Week 32	The fetus's lungs and digestive tract are almost mature. Due to cramped conditions in the uterus, its movements may be less noticeable than they've been in recent weeks. You should still be able to detect fetal movement on a regular basis, however.

Week of Pregnancy	Highlights of Fetal Development
Week 33	The fetus's skull bones are not yet joined together — nor will they be until after birth. This provides some added flexibility during birth, just in case you happen to have a smaller-than-average pelvis and a baby with a bigger-than-average head. The fetus is now approximately 19 inches long — nearly its full length — and weighs approximately 4 1/2 pounds.
Week 34	The fetus is gaining weight at a rapid rate, depositing layers of fat under the skin so that it will have some built-in insulation to help keep itself warm after birth.
Week 35	The fetus has generally settled into a head-down position by this stage of pregnancy, but it may still make a few more flip-flops before labor begins.
Week 36	The fetus's lungs are hard at work producing surfactant.
Week 37	The fetus is now approximately 21 inches long and weighs approximately 6 1/2 pounds.
Week 38	The rapid period of weight gain continues, with the fetus gaining approximately 1% of its body weight each day. (A 150-pound woman gaining weight at the same rate would be packing on a mind-boggling 10 1/2 pounds per week!)
Week 39	The fetus's intestines are filled with a dark green, sticky substance known as meconium that will be excreted as the baby's first bowel movement. The fetus's adrenal glands are in overdrive, producing vast amounts of cortisone — a hormone that may help to trigger the start of labor.

continued

Week of Pregnancy	Highlights of Fetal Development (Continued)
Third Trimester	
Week 40	The fine, downy hair and the slippery white vernix have all but disappeared from the fetus's body, although you're still likely to find some bits of vernix in the skin creases of the groin, under the armpits, and behind the knees.

In this chapter, we focused on the early weeks of pregnancy — that exciting but overwhelming period when you're struggling to come to terms with the fact that you're really and truly pregnant. In the next few chapters, we're going to move on and talk about some of the biggest concerns you're likely to encounter during the remaining weeks and months of your pregnancy.

CHAPTER 6

Operation Healthy Baby

Thee moment the sperm and the egg hooked up in the darkest recesses of your fallopian tube, you signed on for a super-secret mission called Operation Healthy Baby — a mission so secret, in fact, that for the first few weeks of your pregnancy, you didn't even know you'd been recruited!

Super-secret spy stuff aside, your mission over the next nine months is pretty straightforward: to do everything in your power to maximize your chances of ending up with a healthy baby. That means gaining a healthy amount of weight, ensuring that your body gets an ample supply of nutrients, maintaining an active lifestyle, practicing "safe sex" during pregnancy (it's not what you think!), steering clear of hazards in the workplace, and avoiding substances that could be harmful to your baby. That, in a nutshell, is what this chapter is all about.

There's just one bit of fine print that I have to toss out, in the interests of full disclosure. Doing everything by the book doesn't necessarily guarantee that you'll end up with a picture-perfect outcome. (Remember: The reproductive world doesn't offer any guarantees!) But by doing whatever you can to give your baby the healthiest possible start in life, you're definitely putting the odds in your favor.

FROM HERE TO MATERNITY

If you've suffered from an eating disorder in the past, you may require some extra support during and after your pregnancy. According to a recent study conducted at Harvard Medical School, women with eating disorders face a higher-than-average risk of developing certain types of complications during pregnancy, giving birth to a child with a congenital problem, and experiencing postpartum depression.

The Weighting Game

Everyone knows that weight gain is part of the whole pregnancy turf. But what you might not realize is just how much weight you actually need to gain — and why. While past generations of women were told to keep their weight gain under 20 pounds, your doctor or midwife is likely to give you some very different advice today.

As you can see from Table 6.1, there's no such thing as a one-size-fits-all pregnancy "gain" plan. Some women need to gain 40 pounds, while others can get away with something in the range of 15 pounds. Either way, your body needs to gain a significant amount of weight in order to provide for your growing baby (see Table 6.2).

TABLE 6.1

**WEIGHT GAIN DURING PREGNANCY:
HOW MUCH DO YOU NEED TO GAIN?**

Weight Status	Recommended Weight Gain (pounds)
Underweight	28-40
Normal weight	25-35
Overweight	15-25
Carrying Twins	35-45

Source: The American College of Obstetricians and Gynecologists

If you're going to be giving birth to more than one baby, your doctor or midwife will likely encourage you to gain more weight than if you were carrying a single baby. According to Barbara Luke and Tamara Eberlein, co-authors of *When You're Expecting Twins, Triplets, or Quads,* you should aim for a weight gain of 40 to 50 pounds if you're carrying twins (slightly more than the 35 pounds to 45 pounds recommended by the American College of Obstetricians and Gynecologists), 50 to 60 pounds if you're carrying triplets, and 65 to 80 pounds if you're carrying quadruplets. Not all doctors get equally hung up on the number on the scale. Some feel it's more important for a woman carrying multiples to focus on eating a variety of nutrient-rich foods than to fixate on gaining a particular number of pounds.

TABLE 6.2

WHERE THE POUNDS GO

A typical newborn weighs in at just 7 pounds, but your body needs to gain considerably more than that over the course of your pregnancy. The reason is obvious: Your body needs to create an entire support system for your baby. Here's what your body does with a 30-pound pregnancy weight gain (which is typical for a normal-weight woman):

Baby	7 1/2 lbs.
Breasts	2 lbs.
Maternal stores of fat, protein, and other nutrients	7 lbs.
Placenta	1 1/2 lbs.
Uterus	2 lbs.
Amniotic fluid	2 lbs.
Blood	4 lbs.
Body fluids	4 lbs.

It's important to try to keep your weight gain within the healthy range. Women who gain too much or too little during pregnancy face a higher-than-average risk of experiencing a number of unwanted complications:

FACTS AND FIGURES

According to a study conducted by the Research Institute of Bassett Healthcare in Cooperstown, New York, overweight women are significantly more likely to gain more than the recommended amount of weight during pregnancy than normal-weight women. The researchers found that while 38 percent of normal-weight women gained more than the 25 to 35 pounds recommended for women in their weight range by the Institute of Medicine of the National Academy of Sciences, 68 percent of overweight women gained more than the recommended 15 to 25 pounds recommended for women in their weight range.

FACTS AND FIGURES

The risks associated with high gestational weight gain and high birthweight are even greater for shorter women. That's why most doctors and midwives encourage these women to aim for a weight gain that's in the lower end of the range indicated for pregnant women in their particular BMI category.

- Gaining too much weight during pregnancy doesn't merely leave you with potentially permanent souvenirs of your pregnancy on your hips and thighs. It can also boost your chances of experiencing such pregnancy-related complications as back pain, high blood pressure, pre-eclampsia, and gestational diabetes. What's more, according to a study at the Duke University Medical Center gaining too much weight also increases your odds of requiring a cesarean delivery. (This is because women who gain large amounts of weight during pregnancy are more likely to give birth to high-birthweight babies — babies who weigh in at more than 4,000 grams, or 8.8 pounds — and consequently, because of the baby's size, to experience such birth-related complications as prolonged labor and pushing stages, birth trauma, birth asphyxia, and an increased risk of infant death.)

- Gaining too little weight during pregnancy increases your odds of giving birth to a low-birthweight baby (one who weighs less than 2,500 grams, or 5.5 pounds). Low-birth-weight babies often experience health and developmental problems and are more likely to die during infancy than their heftier peers.

Just as important as how much weight you gain, of course, is when you gain that weight. Ideally, you should aim for a slow, steady weight gain. While you're not likely to gain much weight at all during the first trimester — most women tend to gain somewhere between two and eight pounds — you should expect to continue to gain weight at a more rapid rate during the second and third trimesters. Your weight gain will, however, tend to taper off during the last week or two of pregnancy, as your body begins to prepare for the birth.

Of course, not every pregnant woman manages to gain weight in this prescribed fashion. You may end up losing rather than gaining weight during the first trimester if you're experiencing a particularly nasty bout of morning sickness. And, as your pregnancy progresses into the second and third trimesters, you may find that there are some weeks when you gain two or three pounds and others when you don't manage to gain any weight at all. What matters is the overall pattern of your weight gain — that you're slowly but surely gaining weight as your belly begins to blossom.

FACTS AND FIGURES

It takes approximately 80,000 extra calories to grow a baby. To ensure that your body is getting enough food to meet your baby's needs, you should plan to increase your intake by 100 calories per day during the first trimester and 300 calories per day during the second and third trimesters. If you're planning to breastfeed, you'll need even more food after your baby arrives: an extra 450 calories per day. Of course, if you're particularly active or your metabolism is very high, this still may not be enough food for you and your baby. You may have to experiment a little until you figure out how much food your body requires to gain weight at a slow but steady pace.

MOTHER WISDOM

Don't get too hung up about the number on the scale. Most women will gain appropriate amounts of weight during pregnancy if they maintain an active lifestyle and eat a variety of healthy foods when they're genuinely hungry. (You can get a quick refresher course in the art of choosing healthy foods by flipping back to Chapter 2.)

Nutrient Check: The Sequel!

Back in Chapter 2 we talked about the nutrients your body needs in order to prepare for pregnancy. Now let's zero in on the nutrients you need in order to sustain a healthy pregnancy: calcium, vitamin D, folic acid, iron, and essential fatty acids.

FACTS AND FIGURES

Iron deficiency is quite common during pregnancy. You're likely to be low on this important nutrient if

- you're carrying more than one baby
- you're pregnant for the third or subsequent time
- your diet is low in meat, fish, poultry, and/or vitamin C
- you're in the habit of drinking tea or coffee close to mealtime — something that can interfere with the absorption of iron
- you use acetylsalicylic acid (ASA) regularly
- you have a history of heavy menstrual bleeding
- you give blood three or more times each year

As you can see from Table 6.3, each of these nutrients has an important role to play during pregnancy, as do essential fatty acids. Calcium helps to maintain your bones while providing for the development of your baby's skeletal system; vitamin D helps your body to absorb and use calcium; folic acid plays an important role in tissue growth, blood cell generation, and the prevention of open neural tube defects; iron helps to increase the quantity of red blood cells and to meet the iron needs of both the placenta and the growing baby; and essential fatty acids help to promote neural and visual development in the fetus.

It can be difficult to meet your body's demands for all these nutrients through diet alone — although that's certainly the way to go if you can swing it. If, like many of us, you aren't likely to be named an inductee to the Healthy Eating Hall of Fame any time soon, you might want to talk to your doctor or midwife about the advisability of taking a prenatal vitamin supplement.

Here are a few important points to keep in mind when it comes to vitamin supplements:

- Food tends to interfere with the absorption of both calcium and iron. That's why it's best to take your calcium and iron supplements between meals, if your stomach will let you. Unfortunately, taking any type of vitamin on an empty stomach can trigger morning sickness, so taking them between meals may not be possible. A nutritionist that I know recommends washing your iron supplement down with a glass of orange juice because vitamin C enhances iron absorption.

- Never take more than the recommended number of prenatal vitamins per day. (If you're carrying more than one baby, your caregiver may recommend that you take two vitamins per day.) As I noted back in Chapter 2, large doses of certain types of vitamins — particularly vitamin A — are believed to be harmful to the developing baby. This is one of those situations in which more is definitely not better.

TABLE 6.3

THE BIG FIVE: THE NUTRIENTS YOUR BODY NEEDS MOST DURING PREGNANCY

What You Need	How Much You Need	Where to Find It	Why You Need It During Pregnancy
Calcium	1,200 to 1,500 mg per day (depending on age)	Excellent sources (275 mg/serving or more): milk, Swiss cheese, tofu set with calcium sulphate, plain yogurt, whole sesame seeds, fortified plant-based beverages Good sources (165 mg/serving or more): cheeses such as mozzarella, cheddar, edam, brick, Parmesan or Gouda, feta, processed cheese slices, and processed cheese spread; flavored yogurt; canned sardines, canned salmon (including bones) Other foods containing calcium (55 mg/serving or more): creamed cottage cheese, ricotta cheese, cooked or canned legumes (e.g., beans), cooked bok choy, kale, turnip greens, mustard greens, broccoli, oranges, cooked scallops, cooked oysters, almonds, dried sunflower seeds	To maintain your bones while providing for the development of your baby's skeletal system

Vitamin D	200 IU (international units)	Excellent sources: evaporated milk, fortified soy beverages, margarine, and fatty fish (e.g., salmon) Good sources: egg yolks	To increase the intestine's ability to absorb calcium and the body's ability to use it efficiently
Folic acid	0.4 mg per day Note: Women with a higher-than-average risk of giving birth to a baby with a neural tube defect require more than 0.4 mg/day of folic acid. See Chapter 2 for details.	You'll have to make a conscious effort to add folic acid to your diet. A typical woman of childbearing age obtains just 0.2 mg per day from her diet. Excellent sources (more than 0.055 mg/serving): cooked fava, kidney, pinto, roman, soy, and white beans; chickpeas; lentils; cooked spinach; asparagus; romaine lettuce; orange juice; canned pineapple juice; sunflower seeds Good sources (more than 0.033 mg/serving): lima beans (cooked), corn, bean sprouts, broccoli (cooked), green peas, Brussels sprouts, beets, oranges, honeydew melons, raspberries, blackberries, avocado, roasted peanuts, wheat germ	To support your expanding blood volume, to promote the growth of both maternal and fetal tissues, and to decrease the risk of neural tube defects (NTDs)

continued

What You Need	How Much You Need	Where to Find It	Why You Need It (Continued) During Pregnancy
Folic Acid		Other foods containing folic acid (0.011 mg or more): cooked carrots, beet greens, sweet potato, snow peas, summer or winter squash, rutabaga, cabbage, cooked green beans, cashews, roasted peanuts, walnuts, egg, strawberries, banana, grapefruit, cantaloupe, whole wheat or white bread, pork kidney, breakfast cereals, milk	
Iron	First trimester: 13 mg Second and third trimesters: 18 mg	Excellent sources of iron (3.5 mg/serving or more): non-heme sources — cooked beans, white beans, soybeans, lentils, and chick peas; clams and oysters; pumpkin, sesame, and squash seeds; iron-enriched breakfast seeds Good sources of iron (2.1 mg/serving or more): heme sources — ground beef or steak, blood pudding. Non-heme sources — canned lima beans, red kidney beans, chickpeas, split peas, enriched cooked egg noodles, dried apricots Other foods containing iron (0.7 mg/serving or more): Heme sources — chicken, ham, lamb, pork, veal, halibut, haddock, perch, salmon, shrimp, canned sardines, tuna, eggs. Non-heme	

What You Need	How Much You Need	Where to Find It	Why You Need It During Pregnancy
		sources — peanuts, pecans, walnuts, pistachios, roasted almonds, roasted cashews, sunflower seeds, cooked egg noodles, bread, pumpernickel bagels, bran muffins, cooked oatmeal, wheat germ, canned beets (drained), canned pumpkin, raisins, peaches, prunes, apricots	To increase the quantity of red blood cells and to supply the placenta and growing baby. Women who consume inadequate quantities of iron during
		Note: Heme sources of iron (iron from meat, poultry, and fish) are more easily absorbed than non-heme sources. It's important not to pair foods containing non-heme types of iron with the following types of foods, all of which can interfere with iron absorption: tea, coffee, legumes, soybeans, whole grains, spinach, chard, beet greens, rhubarb, sweet potato, calcium.	pregnancy are at increased risk of premature delivery, giving birth to a low-birthweight baby, or experiencing fetal loss. They also tend to experience fatigue, reduced immunity to infection, and other problems.
		Note: An iron supplement (30 mg) is generally recommended during the second and third trimesters because many women will have depleted their pre-pregnancy iron stores by this point.	

continued

What You Need	How Much You Need	Where to Find It	Why You Need It (Continued) During Pregnancy
Essential fatty acids	Not applicable	Include sources of essential fatty acids such as soybean, canola oils, and non-hydrogenated margarines; soy-based products (tofu, vegi burgers); and salad dressings made from non-hydrogenated oils such as canola or soybean oils in your diet. Limit your intake of fried foods, higher fat commercial bakery products, and snack foods.	To promote proper fetal neural and visual development

The deprivation trap

Despite what the authors of one best-selling pregnancy book would have you believe, healthy eating during pregnancy doesn't have to be a nine-month exercise in deprivation. Sure, this is one time in your life when you might want to kick your Twinkie-for-breakfast habit. And it goes without saying that you shouldn't be trying to live on decaf coffee and diet soda alone. Each of these foods can be enjoyed in moderation, provided you're also consuming ample quantities of healthier foods. (Of course, if you're tempted to count those Twinkies as one of your servings from the grain group, you might want to flip back to Chapter 2 and review the food pyramid fundamentals!)

That's not to say this is a time for an orgy of overeating — a food-focused free-for-all. You may be eating for two, but the other person you're eating for is considerably smaller than a 250-pound trucker! While you may experience cravings for certain types of foods during your pregnancy, you do have the option of saying no to that craving. (Okay, it's not always easy, but ultimately you're the one in charge.) If you don't learn how to "just say no" to that daily fling with a Twinkie, you could find yourself toting around a lot more baby fat than baby. (Not surprisingly, studies have shown that women who gain too much weight during pregnancy are far more likely to be carrying around extra pregnancy-related weight by the time their babies' first birthdays roll around.)

FACTS AND FIGURES

Despite what your mother or grandmother may try to tell you, you don't have to lay off the salt shaker just because you're pregnant. While previous generations of women were told to restrict their salt intake during pregnancy in the name of minimizing edema (water retention), we now know that doing so can actually make edema worse. So much for that particular nutritional theory. . . .

Of course, if you're having difficulty with hypertension (high blood pressure) or water retention, or you suffer from certain kidney diseases, your caregiver may suggest that you avoid highly salted foods and refrain from adding extra salt to your foods.

FACTS AND FIGURES

There's no hard evidence to show that products with artificial sweetners are harmful to the developing baby, but some women choose to err on the side of caution by avoiding these products during pregnancy. The only women who definitely have to steer clear of products containing aspartame are women with phenylketonuria (PKU) — a metabolic disorder.

Special diets

If you're following any sort of special diet, you may wish to consult with a dietititian in order to find out what types of dietary modifications, if any, may be recommended during pregnancy. Before you pay for this type of service out of your own pocket, be sure to find out up front whether or not it's covered by your health insurance plan.

Lactose-free diets

If you're following a lactose-free diet because you have difficulty digesting the sugar in milk, you may be able to treat yourself to small servings of dairy products during the months ahead. Some studies have shown that pregnancy improves a woman's ability to digest lactose.

If, however, you continue to have difficulty digesting lactose, you'll need to focus on obtaining calcium from as many non-milk food sources as possible: tofu, calcium-fortified bread or juice, dark-green leafy vegetables, sardines, salmon, and so on.

Here are some other ways to cope with lactose-intolerance during pregnancy:

- Look for lactose-free dairy products in your grocery store.

- Try eating yogurt that contains acidophilus (active cultures that can actually aid in the digestion of lactose).

- Try drinking milk at mealtime rather than on its own — something that can help to eliminate some people's lactose-intolerance problems.

- Stick to very small servings of dairy products that are naturally low in lactose, like aged cheese. The smaller the serving, the less likely you are to run into problems.

- Take Tums. They're an inexpensive source of calcium that can be easily digested by people with lactose intolerance.

Vegetarian/vegan diets

If you're a vegetarian or vegan who doesn't eat meat, you may need to make a special effort to ensure you're obtaining adequate quantities of vitamins B12, B2, and D; calcium; iron; and zinc.

As well as maximizing your iron absorption by combining iron-rich foods (e.g., eggs, fish, and vegetables such as spinach) with foods that are rich in vitamin C and that can help with the absorption of iron (e.g., citrus fruits, strawberries, and tomatoes), you may want to ask your doctor to recommend a vitamin B12 supplement and/or to check your hemoglobin regularly to ensure that you aren't becoming anemic.

FACTS AND FIGURES

Don't avoid milk products during your pregnancy out of some mistaken belief that this will prevent your baby from developing food allergies. According to Ellen Lakusiak, R.D., author of *Eating Well When You're Pregnant*, you'd be needlessly depriving your body of some important nutrients. "There is virtually nothing that can be done during pregnancy to prevent your baby from developing allergies, if they are at risk of developing them. Eliminating total food groups from your diet, such as milk and milk products, is not a good idea for pregnant women since this food group is the major and best source of calcium. Without a calcium supplement, it is almost impossible to meet the greater calcium needs of pregnancy from non-milk foods alone."

MOTHER WISDOM

Worried that you aren't keeping enough food down to nourish a flea, let alone a growing baby? You'll find plenty of reassuring words, plus some practical tips on coping with this all-too-common rite of pregnancy, in Chapters 7 and 8.

Food safety

It's also important to pay careful attention to food safety during pregnancy. That means taking steps to prevent listeriosis (a type of food-borne illness) and avoiding certain types of fish that have high levels of methylmercury.

Preventing listeriosis

Listeria monocyotogenes is a bacterium that can cause a serious infection called listeriosis in humans. If contracted by a pregnant woman, it can lead to miscarriage, stillbirth, and premature labor, and can result in severe — even fatal — illness in the newborn (pneumonia, a bacterial blood infection known as septicemia, or meningitis). Because this bacterium can grow at refrigerator temperature and is found in ready-to-eat foods, the Food and Drug Administration (FDA) advises consumers to reduce the risk of illness by

- using a refrigerator thermometer to ensure that the refrigerator always stays at or below 40 degrees F

- cleaning the refrigerator regularly

- using perishable items (e.g., precooked or ready-to-eat foods) as soon as possible

Because their immune systems are at higher risk, pregnant women need to take some added steps to prevent listeriosis. That means avoiding

- hot dogs and luncheon meats unless they are reheated until they are steaming hot

- soft cheeses such as feta, brie, Camembert, blue-veined cheeses, and Mexican-style cheeses such as "queso blanco fresco." (It's still okay to eat hard cheeses; semi-soft cheeses such as mozzarella; pasteurized processed cheeses such as slices and spreads; cream cheese; and cottage cheese.)

- smoked seafood (unless it is contained in a cooked entrée such as a casserole)

- unpasteurized milk, and foods that contain unpasteurized milk

Preventing methylmercury poisoning

Certain types of fish contain high levels of a form of mercury called methylmercury that is known to be harmful to the nervous system of the developing baby. That's why the Food and Drug Administration (FDA) recommends that pregnant women avoid eating shark, swordfish, king mackerel, and tilefish. (Note: It's also best to avoid these types of fish while you're breastfeeding.)

Because there are smaller amounts of methylmercury in other types of fish, the FDA recommends that pregnant women limit their weekly intake of fish to 12 ounces and that they choose from a variety of different types of fish (as opposed to eating only one type of fish).

You can find out more about food safety during pregnancy by visiting the FDA's Food Safety Web site: www.cfsan.fda.gov.

Exercising During Pregnancy

Although there's nothing you can really do to "train" for labor, studies have shown that your labor is likely to be shorter and less complicated if you're in good physical condition when those first contractions hit. That's why most pregnant women are encouraged to make exercise part of their regular routine. Your goal, however, should be to maintain your current level of physical conditioning during pregnancy — not to embark on a heavy-duty training program.

You'll note that I said "most." That's because exercise is not recommended across the board to every pregnant woman. You can expect your doctor or midwife to recommend that you hang up your running shoes for a while if

- you're significantly underweight

- you're carrying multiples

- you've been diagnosed with pregnancy-induced hypertension (high blood pressure)

- your membranes (amniotic sac) have ruptured prematurely

- you're currently experiencing premature labor

- you've had problems with premature labor during a previous pregnancy

- you've been diagnosed with a condition known as incompetent cervix, in which the cervix dilates prematurely

- you have a history of second-trimester miscarriage

- you've been having persistent problems with vaginal bleeding throughout your second and/or third trimester — something that could indicate a possible placental problem

- you have been diagnosed with placenta previa or other types of placental problems

- you've become anemic over the course of your pregnancy

- you're experiencing significant pubic or lower back pain

- your baby isn't growing as quickly as expected for a baby of that gestational age (a condition known as intrauterine growth restriction)

- you have a serious medical condition such as chronic hypertension; an overactive thyroid; or cardiac, vascular, or pulmonary disease, all of which make exercise inadvisable

Assuming you do get the go-ahead from your caregiver, you've got plenty of great reasons to be physically active:

- Exercise helps to boost your energy level. If you've been feeling tired and dragged out since the moment the pregnancy test came back positive, exercise can help to re-energize you.

- Exercise makes it easier for you to keep your weight gain within the target range. Studies have shown that women who work out regularly during pregnancy are less likely to find themselves stuck with a huge amount of weight to lose after giving birth.

- Exercise leaves you feeling relaxed and positive. Since pregnancy is a time when many women report experiencing intense mood swings, this is welcome news indeed!

- Exercise helps to keep your blood glucose levels stable, which can reduce your likelihood of developing gestational diabetes.

- Exercise lowers your blood pressure, which can reduce your risk of developing pregnancy-induced hypertension (a condition that affects 12% of pregnant women).

- Exercise helps to ward off a number of pregnancy-related complaints. You're less likely to be troubled by insomnia, backache, hip soreness, leg cramps, and constipation if you're exercising regularly.

• Exercise helps to prepare your body for the rigors of labor. Studies have shown that women who are physically fit prior to labor experience faster labors and require fewer inductions, fewer forceps deliveries, and fewer cesarean deliveries than their less fit counterparts.

• Exercise helps to reduce the amount of time it takes your body to recover from the delivery. That means you'll be in the best possible shape for the next marathon you'll face — becoming a mother.

FACTS AND FIGURES

While moderate exercise is thought to be safe for both mother and baby, excessive exercise may increase a pregnant woman's risk of giving birth to a low birthweight baby. According to a study reported in the *American Journal of Obstetrics and Gynecology*, pregnant women who engage in strenuous exercise five or more times each week during the last trimester are four times as likely to give birth to a low birthweight baby as moms-to-be who engage in more moderate exercise regimes. The researchers concluded that pregnant women who exercise three or four times a week have the best chance of giving birth to a healthy weight baby.

As beneficial as prenatal exercise can be to a pregnant woman and her baby, it's still necessary to proceed with caution. Here are some important points to keep in mind when you're planning your fitness program:

• Choose your fitness activity with care. Certain forms of exercise are not recommended for pregnant women. Avoid anything that could leave you susceptible to injury — deep knee bends, full sit-ups, double-leg raises, straight-leg raises, and so on. These types of maneuvers can result in injury because a hormone called relaxin relaxes all your joints and ligaments to make it easier for your body to give birth. You can reduce the risk of injury by incorporating a warm-up and a cool-down into your workout.

MOTHER WISDOM

Put your plans for that adventure vacation on hold until after Junior arrives! Mountain climbing is out, due to the reduced oxygen content of air at high altitudes, and so is deep-sea diving, because of the harmful effects of underwater pressure on the developing baby.

MOTHER WISDOM

If you're having problems with sciatica (pain starting in the buttock and radiating down the outer thigh and into the calf), you'll probably want to avoid high-impact aerobics because this type of exercise may stress your joints and increase the amount of pain you're experiencing.

- Avoid activities that could result in abdominal trauma or other types of injuries. Remember: Your growing uterus has thrown off your sense of balance, which can make it easier for you to fall or injure yourself. Your best bets are walking, swimming, stationary cycling, and low-impact aerobics. Activities that aren't recommended include contact sports such as football, basketball, and volleyball; adventure sports such as parachuting, mountain climbing, and scuba diving; sports with a high risk of trauma, such as downhill skiing, horseback riding, waterskiing, surfing, and ice skating; and high-impact, weight-bearing sports such as running or jogging.

- Proceed with caution if you're planning to continue with your strength training program. While researchers at Queen's University in Kingston, Ontario, recently discovered that it's perfectly safe for a pregnant woman to continue with a moderate strength training program, they advise against exercising in the tilted supine (semi-reclined) position — a position that can result in decreased oxygen available to the fetus.

- Plan to include some floor exercises that can help your body prepare for the rigors of giving birth. (See Table 6.4 for a list of your four best bets.)

- Keep in mind that you'll probably tire more easily than usual since you're carrying around some additional weight. It might be a good idea to reduce the intensity of your usual workout until you're sure you'll be able to keep up your regular pace.

- Don't go crazy during the first trimester. It's not a good idea to launch a new fitness program or increase the intensity or duration of your existing program prior to the 15th week of pregnancy. Besides, you may not feel like hitting the gym at this stage of the game: "I had started exercising about a month prior to conception, but I gave it up in early pregnancy," confesses Jennifer, a 32-year-old mother of one. "I was experiencing exhaustion beyond anything I had ever felt before. It was a major accomplishment to get out of bed and get dressed. The thought of lacing up sneakers and going to the gym reduced me to tears."

- Don't overexert yourself. Otherwise, blood and oxygen may end up being diverted from your baby to your muscles.

- Don't allow your body to become overheated. An overly high body temperature can cause certain brain and spinal defects, particularly if the overheating occurs during the first trimester of pregnancy. Decrease the duration and intensity of your workout; wear lightweight clothing; avoid exercising during the hottest times of the day or on hot, humid days; and skip your workout if you have a fever.

- Consume enough liquids to keep yourself well hydrated. Remember: You're exercising and drinking for two! That means drinking before, during, and after exercise.

- Make sure that you're eating enough. If you're particularly active, the extra 300 calories a day recommended to most women during the second and third trimesters of pregnancy might not be enough for you. You may have to bump your caloric intake up further to avoid weakness, dizziness, and inadequate weight gain.

- Pay attention to your body. If you start feeling winded or shaky; if you experience vaginal bleeding or uterine contractions; or if your membranes rupture, stop exercising immediately.

- Wear a supportive bra. Your breasts are bigger and heavier than they were before you became pregnant, and the ligaments that support breast tissue can be permanently damaged if they become overstretched. This can lead to a saggy bosom and a lot of discomfort during exercise.

- Avoid exercising on your back after the 20th week of pregnancy. According to the American College of Obstetricians and Gynecologists, when you're lying in this position, your uterus rests on the vena cava — the vein responsible for returning blood from the lower body to the heart. This can disrupt the flow of blood, leaving you feeling very faint.

- Don't overdo things during the last trimester. Most prenatal fitness experts advise against increasing the intensity, duration, or frequency of your workouts at any point after the 28th week of pregnancy. Fetal demands for nutrition and oxygen are highest during this period.

- Start thinking ahead about what you will do to stay fit after the baby arrives. You'll find plenty of helpful advice in Chapter 12.

And now the most important piece of advice: Have fun! Sign up for a prenatal fitness class so that you can get to know other pregnant women in your community. Hop on your stationary bike while you're reading your favorite pregnancy magazine. And make an after-dinner stroll with your partner part of your daily routine. (Hey, that's one tradition that you can easily continue even after your baby arrives. Unfortunately, I can't necessarily say the same thing about the candlelit dinners.) Bottom line? Pregnancy is a time to enjoy and celebrate your body and the miracle that's taking place inside. It's the perfect time to be physically active.

TABLE 6.4

THE FOUR BEST PREGNANCY FLOOR EXERCISES

Type of Exercise	What It Does for You
Squatting	Stretches the legs and opens the pelvis; great preparation for birth if you intend to do some of your laboring and birthing in a squatting position
Pelvic tilting	Strengthens the muscles in your abdomen and back to improve your overall posture and help prevent or relieve backache
Abdominal curl-ups	Strengthens the abdominal muscles that support the uterus
Pelvic floor exercises	Strengthens the muscles that support the abdominal organs, helps to prevent pregnancy incontinence, and can make birth easier

 FACTS AND FIGURES

While you're exercising, your body releases a neurotransmitter called norepinephrine. It causes all the muscles in your body to contract, including the muscles of your uterus — which helps to explain why your uterus may sometimes feel rock-hard during your workout.

Sex During Pregnancy

A recent study conducted by researchers at Memorial University in Newfoundland confirmed what most doctors and midwives have known for years: More than half of couples believe that making love during pregnancy poses some sort of threat to the developing baby.

Yet quite the opposite is true. Sex during pregnancy is generally considered perfectly safe for couples who are experiencing low-risk pregnancies. Your doctor or midwife is likely to recommend that you forgo intercourse, orgasm, or both for all or part of your pregnancy only if

- you have a history of recurrent, first-trimester miscarriage or you're threatening to miscarry this time around

- if you have been diagnosed with an incompetent cervix (a condition in which the cervix opens prematurely)

- you've been diagnosed with placenta previa (a condition in which the placenta blocks all or part of the cervix) or a placental abruption (a condition in which the placenta begins to separate from the uterine wall)

- you're carrying more than one baby

- you have a history of premature labor, or you're showing signs of going into premature labor

- you or your partner have an untreated sexually transmitted disease

- your membranes have ruptured

If your doctor or midwife tells you that sex is off-limits for now, make sure that you're clear about what you can and can't do. Some couples are given the go-ahead to enjoy everything but intercourse, while others are told to avoid nipple stimulation and any form of sexual activity that could lead to orgasm. (Both activities cause the uterus to contract.)

The concept of "safe sex" takes on an entirely different meaning during pregnancy, by the way. While you still need to use a condom if you have unprotected intercourse with a new partner or if you have reason to suspect that your current partner may have a sexually transmitted disease, you also have to exercise caution if oral sex is part of your usual bedroom routine. It's okay to have oral sex (unless, of course, your doctor or midwife has forbidden any activity that could lead to orgasm), but it's not okay to allow your partner to blow air into your vagina. Believe it or not, this could cause an air embolism to travel to your brain, something that could result in stroke or even death! No sexual encounter is worth that kind of risk, so be careful.

While your doctor or midwife will probably talk to you about how the physical changes of pregnancy may affect your sex life — you're likely to find yourself with abundant vaginal secretions, super-sensitive breasts, and a belly that requires some maneuvering to get around — what they might not get around to discussing is how your feelings about sex may change over the course of your pregnancy. You may find that your interest goes through the roof, or that you couldn't care less if you ever "do it" again. And you may find that your interest rises and falls as particular pregnancy-related complaints come and go. (Hint: Morning sickness isn't exactly an aphrodisiac.)

MOTHER WISDOM

Try not to panic if you experience a small amount of bleeding after intercourse at some point during your first trimester. If your cervix — which becomes sensitive during pregnancy — happens to get bumped by your partner's penis, a small amount of bleeding can occur. Even though it can be alarming to see any type of bleeding coming from your vagina when you're pregnant, this type of bleeding doesn't pose any risk to the developing baby. Still, if it's going to cause you undue stress, it might be best to put the lovemaking on hold until you're into your second trimester and past the peak risk period for miscarriage.

Here's what some of the women interviewed for this book had to say about their interest in sex during pregnancy:

- "In the beginning, exhaustion reigned supreme. In the second trimester, my sex drive was pretty much normal. In the third trimester, I don't know if it was hormones or my newly ballooned status, but I just couldn't get enough! Not every day, but some days it was on my mind all the time. My poor husband!"

- "My husband had heard stories of women who wanted sex all the time at certain points in their pregnancies. Boy, was he disappointed. We didn't lose our closeness, however. There was always lots of snuggling, etc., because we found the whole experience of sharing the pregnancies brought us closer together as a couple. But as for the rest — it just didn't happen."

- "Throughout my pregnancy I've had very little interest in sex. I just seem to have lost my drive. It's not that I don't feel attractive. My husband thinks I've never looked better and I feel great. Perhaps it's a hormonal thing. It's been a little hard on us, but we both realize that it's not that we don't love and aren't attracted to each other. I'm sure things will eventually get back to normal — maybe even better. Who knows — they say women reach their sexual peak at 30, and I'm still three years away!"

- "I always want more sex when I'm pregnant. I'm so scared of miscarriage though that we've only had sex once since we found out I was pregnant. It's hard, though, because I really, really want to! After the first trimester is over, I'm sure I'll feel more comfortable."

- "We only had sex a few times during the first trimester. After that, we completely stopped because my husband was worried that he was hurting the baby. We compensated with lots of affection, cuddling, hugging, and kissing."

- "With my first pregnancy, I was just as interested in sex as before pregnancy — maybe even more so! — and we had sex right up until the end of my pregnancy. With the subsequent two pregnancies, however, my sex drive went through the floor and there was not much action in the bedroom. When I went to bed, all I wanted to do was sleep."

Most couples find that it helps to keep your sense of humor and — if you can swing it — your sense of adventure, too. After all, you won't always have that watermelon-sized belly to maneuver around. Why not consider it a temporary challenge and make the most of it?

FACTS AND FIGURES

A study conducted at Memorial University in Newfoundland revealed that 58% of women are less interested in sex while they're pregnant, while 42% are more interested or at least as interested as they were prior to pregnancy.

Working During Pregnancy

Gone are the days when a woman was expected to resign from her job the moment she found herself "in the family way." Pregnant women are as much a part of the modern office landscape as photocopiers and fax machines.

According to the American College of Obstetricians and Gynecologists, most women who experience low-risk pregnancies can safely continue to work outside the home.

If, however, your job is physically demanding (e.g., it requires repeated stooping and bending, repeated climbing of ladders, poles, or stairs, heavy lifting, or a lot of standing); exposes you to radiation, toxins, or other harmful substances (see Table 6.5); or involves shift work or prolonged standing, you might want to consider switching jobs or requesting a job modification for all or part of your pregnancy. Jobs such as these can modestly increase your chances of miscarrying, going into labor prematurely, or having a low-birthweight baby.

FACTS AND FIGURES

Women who work in jobs that involve a lot of physical exertion and prolonged periods of standing face an increased risk of experiencing premature rupture of the membranes, a condition that often precedes a preterm delivery. Researchers at the Medical University of South Carolina in Charleston found that women with the most fatiguing types of jobs faced a 7% chance of experiencing premature rupture of the membranes as opposed to the 2% risk faced by women who do not work outside the home.

Even if your job doesn't present any obvious threat, you'll still need to make an effort to take care of yourself while you're on the job. Here are a few tips:

- Get up and move around as often as you can — at least once every couple of hours. Sitting down for more than three hours at a stretch can lead to fluid retention in your legs and feet, reduced blood flow to your baby, muscle strain (particularly in your lower back), and tension in your back and shoulder areas.

- Find a position that's comfortable for you while you're working at your desk. Place a pillow behind the small of your back, prop your feet up on a footstool or an open desk drawer, and make sure that you take regular breaks from typing if you work at a computer all day. Pregnant women are at increased risk of developing repetitive stress disorders such as carpal tunnel syndrome.

TABLE 6.5

HAZARDS IN THE WORKPLACE

Here are a few of the more common workplace hazards that pose a risk to the pregnant worker or her baby.

Type of Risk	Potential Effect on Pregnant Worker	Potential Effect on Developing Baby
Chemical Exposure		
Anesthetics		Miscarriage, premature birth, congenital abnormalities
Carbon monoxide		Miscarriage, premature birth, congenital malformation
Solvents such as benzene, trichoroethylene, trichloroethylene, carbon tetrachloride, vinyl chloride, chloroprene, epichlorhydrine, carbon bisulfide	Increased susceptibility to poisoning (liver, kidney, blood, and central nervous system problems)	Miscarriage, premature birth, congenital abnormalities
Toxic metals, lead, mercury, cadmium	Increased susceptibility to poisoning (liver, kidney, blood, and central nervous system problems)	Miscarriage, premature birth, congenital abnormalities

Type of Risk	Potential Effect on Pregnant Worker	Potential Effect on Developing Baby
Physical Hazards		
Biological hazards (e.g., exposure to German measles, measles, mumps, bacteria in a hospital or laboratory setting)		Miscarriage, congenital malformation
Extreme heat and humidity	Increased susceptibility to respiratory, gynecological, and urinary tract infection	Premature birth
Ionizing radiation (e.g., radiology department at a hospital)		Central nervous system abnormalities, mental retardation

- Dress for comfort, not style. You've got the rest of your life to try to squeeze into those high heels and power suits. For now, focus on comfort. Choose loose, comfortable clothing, and dress in layers so that you can remove a layer or two if you begin to feel overheated.

- Eat, drink, and be merry. Make a point of stopping for snacks and meals at regular intervals, no matter how crazy things may be at the office. Keep a bottle of water on your desk so that you can remember to keep yourself well hydrated. And try to keep your stress level to a minimum. (I know, I know: It's easier said than done!)

- Master the art of the power nap. If you're feeling drop-dead exhausted (a not uncommon condition during the first and third trimesters, by the way), then try to squeeze in a nap during your lunch hour or afternoon break. If that's not possible, make flopping out on the couch for half an hour a sacred part of your daily arriving-home-from-work ritual.

- Get your zzzzs. You can't expect to function well on the job if you're sleep-deprived, so be sure to hit the hay early enough to get a good night's sleep. Your sleep needs increase while you're pregnant. Instead of getting away with seven or eight hours a night — what a typical woman of childbearing age requires — you may find that you need nine or ten hours.

🔊 **MOM'S THE WORD**

"You have to be somewhat more assertive about your time and not committing yourself to too many projects when you're pregnant. In this regard, people are usually very understanding. It may be the only time when you can get away with working less than the average person, so take advantage of it!"

—*Janet, 32, mother of one*

Other Things You Need to Know to Keep Your Baby Safe

Up until now we've been focusing on nutrition, fitness, sex, and work during pregnancy. In the remainder of this chapter, we're going to zero in on specific hazards to the developing baby — things that every pregnant woman needs to know in order to keep her baby safe.

- Smoking, drinking, and drugs. Back in Chapter 2, I ran through a whole laundry list of reasons for not smoking, drinking, or using illegal drugs during pregnancy. If you have yet to kick those habits, you owe it to yourself and your baby to run through that list again. One more quick reminder: Dads-to-be also need to be diligent about kicking their smoking habit. After all, you don't want your baby to be exposed to second-hand smoke prior to or after birth.

- Exposure to toxic substances. It's easy to forget just how many toxic substances we come into contact with over the course of a day: paints, solvents, lawn-care products, and other powerful chemicals. Chlorine- and ammonia-based cleaning products can be among the worst offenders: My friend Dianne refers to a popular brand of bathroom tile cleaner as "Spray and Run" because you can't stand to be in the same room with the fumes this product emits! As a rule of thumb, it's best to minimize your exposure to these types of products while you're pregnant.

- Medications that could be harmful to your baby. While you no doubt remembered to ask your doctor if it was safe for you to use your asthma inhaler during pregnancy, you might have forgotten to ask him or her which over-the-counter drug and herbal products that you tend to use routinely are taboo. Before you open up your medicine chest and instinctively pop something in your mouth, you need to check with your doctor, midwife, or pharmacist to find out if that product is safe to use during pregnancy. As Table 6.6 indicates, some of the ingredients in common over-the-counter drug products can be harmful — even toxic — to the developing baby.

- Exposure to radiation. Abdominal X-rays, CAT scans, and diagnostic procedures involving radioactive dyes should be avoided throughout pregnancy. Dental X-rays, on the other hand, are considered relatively safe provided that appropriate radiation shields are used. (Of course, it's always best to avoid any type of X-ray during pregnancy, if at all possible.)

- Exposure to infectious diseases and potentially harmful viruses. You wouldn't dream of hanging out with someone with bubonic plague or some other serious illness, but what you might not realize is that even some normally benign illnesses can pose a threat to the well-being of the developing baby. (See Table 6.7.)

 MOTHER WISDOM

If your job is likely to require some out-of-town travel during your pregnancy, make sure that you bring along a copy of your prenatal record. That way, if you run into unexpected pregnancy complications, the doctor on call at the emergency ward at the nearest hospital will have the information he or she needs to provide you and your baby with the best possible prenatal care. Most airlines have policies prohibiting women from flying during the last two months of pregnancy unless they have a doctor's note — something you'll definitely need to keep in mind when you're scheduling business trips.

FROM HERE TO MATERNITY

You can find a comprehensive chart highlighting the Food and Drug Administration's ratings for hundreds of prescription and over-the-counter drugs in *The Unofficial Guide to Having A Baby* by Ann Douglas and John R. Sussman, M.D. (Hungry Minds, Inc., 1999).

TABLE 6.6

ACTIVE INGREDIENTS IN COMMON OVER-THE-COUNTER MEDICATIONS

Active Ingredient	Possible Problems During Pregnancy
Acetaminophen (found in products such as Actifed Cold and Sinus; Alka-Seltzer Plus; Comtrex; Contac Cold and Flu; Coricidin; Dimetapp Cold and Fever; Drixoral Cold and Flu; Excedrin; Multi-Symptom Formula Midol; Panadol; Robitussin Cold, Cough, and Flu; Sinarest; Sine-Aid; Sine-Off; Sinutab; Sudafed Cold; Sudafed Sinus; TheraFlu; Tylenol; Vicks NyQuil	There is no apparent link to birth defects, but there is a possible association with fetal renal failure.
Aluminum hydroxide (found in antacids such as Gaviscon, Maalox, Mylanta)	There is no apparent link to birth defects, but some studies have indicated that excessive use may be associated with neonatal calcium or magnesium imbalance.
Aspirin (acetylsalicylic acid) (found in aspirin compounds such as Alka-Seltzer, Bayer, Bufferin)	There is no apparent link to birth defects, although there is some conflicting data on that front. Can cause clotting disorders with possible fetal and maternal hemorrhage when taken in large doses close to term. Other possible effects are low birthweight, prolonged gestation and labor, and neonatal cardiac problems. Low-dose aspirin use is recommended,

continued

Active Ingredient	Possible Problems During Pregnancy (Continued)
Aspirin	however, for treatment of certain causes of repeated m scarriage or autoimmune disorders such as lupus.
Attapulgite (found in antidiarrheals such as Donnagel and Kaopectate)	There are no available reports of use during pregnancy.
Bacitracin Zinc (found in antibiotic ointments such as Mycitracin, Neosporin, Polysporin)	There is no apparent link to birth defects.
Benzocaine (found in topical anesthetics such as Americaine, Cepacol, Hurricaine, Chloraseptic)	There are no available reports of use during pregnancy.
Bisacodyl (found in laxatives such as Correctol, Dulcolax)	There are no available reports of use during pregnancy.
Bismuth Subsalicylate (found in products for upset stomach, indigestion, and so on, such as Pepto-Bismol)	Should be used only during the first five months of pregnancy and in amounts that do not exceed the recommended dosages.
Brompheniramine Maleate (found in antihistamines such as Dimetapp, Vicks DayQuil)	There is a possible association with birth defects. What's more, use of antihistamines in last two weeks of pregnancy increases the risk of a neonatal eye problem known as retrolental fibroplasia. Note: If you need an antihistamine, your doctor is most likely to recommend Benadryl.

Active Ingredient	Possible Problems During Pregnancy
Caffeine (found in certain analgesics, including Excedrin)	There is no apparent link to birth defects, although some studies have indicated that high doses may be associated with miscarriage and infertility.
Calcium Carbonate (found in antacids such as Tums)	No adverse effects have been proven with usual dosages.
Camphor (found in anti-itch and local anesthetic products and nasal inhalers such as Afrin, Mentholatum, Vicks VapoRub)	No adverse effects have been proven from topical use.
Chlorpheniramine Maleate (found in antihistamines such as Alka-Seltzer Plus, Chlor-Trimeton Allergy, Comtrex Maximum Strength, Contac, Coricidin, PediaCare, Sinarest, Sine-Off, Sinutab, TheraFlu, Triaminic, Tylenol Allergy)	There is no apparent link to birth defects. See brompheniramine *maleate*.
Clotrimazole (found in antifungal/yeast infection products such as Canesten)	There is no apparent link to birth defects.
Dexbrompheniramine (found in antihistamines such as Drixoral)	There is no apparent link to birth defects. See brompheniramine *maleate*.
Dextromethorphan (found in cough suppressants such as Alka-Seltzer Plus Cold and Cough, Comtrex,	There is a possible link to birth defects. Use as directed by your physician and avoid using preparations containing alcohol wherever

continued

Active Ingredient	Possible Problems During Pregnancy (Continued)
Contac Cold, Dimetapp Cold, Robitussin, Sudafed Cold and Cough, Triaminic, Tylenol Cold, Vicks 44)	possible. (Note: If your doctor recommends that you use a cough syrup that contains alcohol, try not to panic. The amount of alcohol contained in a teaspoonful or two of cough syrup is not sufficiently high to raise serious concerns about fetal alcohol syndrome.)
Dimenhydrinate (found in anti-nausea products such as Gravol)	Generally considered to be safe for use during pregnancy.
Diphenhydramine (found in antihistamines such as Actifed, Benadryl, Contac, Sine-Off Night Time, Tylenol Allergy, Tylenol PM)	This active ingredient may be responsible for cleft palate and other birth defects, but research to date has been inconclusive.
Docusate (found in certain types of laxatives)	Chronic use may cause a fetal magnesium imbalance.
Doxylamine (used as a sleep aid in products such as Alka Seltzer Plus Night-Time Cold, Robitussin Night-Time Cold, Unisom Nighttime, and Vicks NyQuil	This active ingredient may be responsible for skeletal, limb, and cardiac defects; cleft palate; and gastrointestinal malformations. Research to date has been inconclusive.
Ephedrine (used in decongestants such as Primatene Tablets)	This active ingredient may be responsible for heart-rate disturbances, minor birth defects, hernias, and clubfoot, but research to date has been inconclusive.

Active Ingredient	Possible Problems During Pregnancy
Guaifenesin (found in expectorants such as Benylin, Novahistine, Primatene Tablets, Robitussin, Sudafed Cold, Vicks 44E)	There is no apparent link to birth defects.
Hydrocortisone (topical) (used in topical and hemorrhoid sprays and ointments such as Anusol HC-1 Hydrocortisone, Cortaid, Cortizone, Nupercainal Hydrocortisone, Preparation H Hydrocortisone 1%)	There are no available reports of use during pregnancy. Anusol HC-1 and 1% topical hydrocortisone are widely prescribed for use during pregnancy.
Ibuprofen (used in aspirin substitutes such as Advil, Motrin IB, Nuprin)	There is no apparent link to birth defects, but third-trimester use can cause fetal cardiac malfunction.
Magnesium Carbonate/Magnesium Hydroxide/ Magnesium Trisilacate (used in antacids such as Ascriptin, Bufferin, Di-Gel, Gaviscon, Maalox, Mylanta, Phillips Milk of Magnesia, Rolaids, Vanquish)	There are no adverse effects proven with usual dosages, but chronic or excessive use may be associated with neonatal calcium or magnesium imbalance.
Meclizine (used in antinausea products such as Bonamine, Dramamine)	This active ingredient causes birth defects in some animals, but there is no apparent link to birth defects in humans.
Menthol (used in cough and sore throat preparations and in soothing ointments such as Afrin, BenGay, Cepacol, Eucalyptamint, Gold Bond, Hall's Cough Drops, Listerine, Mentholatum, Vicks Chloraseptic, Vicks Cough Drops)	There are no available reports of use during pregnancy.

continued

Active Ingredient	Possible Problems During Pregnancy (Continued)
Miconazole (used in products that treat yeast/fungal infections, such as Lotrimin, Monistat)	There is no apparent link to birth defects.
Oxymetazoline (used in nasal decongestant sprays such as Afrin, Neo-Synephrine, Vicks Sinex)	There is no apparent link to birth defects, but excessive use could impair uterine blood flow.
Phenolphthalein (used in laxatives such as Dialose, Ex-Lax, Phillips Gelcaps)	There is no apparent link to birth defects.
Phenylephrine (used in nasal decongestant sprays and hemorrhoid creams such as Afrin, 4-Way Fast Acting Nasal Spray, Hemorid, Neo-Synephrine, Preparation H, Vicks Sinex)	This active ingredient causes birth defects in animals. May be responsible for minor birth defects: hernia and clubfoot. (These studies do not apply to topical creams.) Excessive use could impair uterine blood flow.
Phenylpropanolamine (used in decongestants and appetite suppressants such as Acutrim, Comtrex, Contac, Dexatrim, Dimetapp, Robitussin-CF, Tavist-D, Triaminic, Vicks DayQuil Allergy)	This active ingredient may cause eye and ear defects and other anomalies, but the research is inconclusive. Excessive use could impair uterine blood flow.
Pseudoephedrine (used in decongestants such as Actifed, Advil Cold and Sinus, Alka-Seltzer Plus, Allerest, Benadryl Allergy/Cold, Comtrex, Contac,	This active ingredient may be responsible for heart rate disturbances, minor birth defects, hernias, and clubfoot, but research is inconclusive.

Active Ingredient	Possible Problems During Pregnancy
Dimetapp, Robitussin Cold, Sine-Off, Sinutab, Sudafed, TheraFlu, Triaminic, Tylenol Allergy, Tylenol Cold, Vicks 44D, Vicks DayQuil, Vicks NyQuil)	
Psyllium (a natural fiber that promotes normal bowel movements), used in laxatives such as Metamucil	There are no available reports of use during pregnancy. Since it's not absorbed into the bloodstream, it's considered safe for use.
Pyrethrins with piperonyl butoxide (used in anti-lice lotions and shampoos such as A-200, EndLice, Pronto, R & C, Rid)	This is the preferred drug for treating lice infestations during pregnancy.
Simethicone (used in anti-flatulents such as Di-Gel, Gax-X, Maalox, Mylanta, 3M Titralac, Tums)	There is a possible association with cardiovascular birth defects, but cause and effect is not likely.
Sodium Bicarbonate (used in antacids such as Alka-Seltzer, Arm & Hammer Pure Baking Soda)	There are no adverse effects proven with usual dosages.
Sodium Chloride (table salt), used in nasal sprays such as Afrin, Ocean Nasal Mist	Considered safe for use during pregnancy.

Adapted from a similar chart in The Unofficial Guide to Having A Baby by Ann Douglas and John R. Sussman, M.D. (Hungry Minds, 1999).

TABLE 6.7

INFECTIOUS DISEASE AND VIRUSES AND THEIR EFFECTS ON PREGNANCY

Type of Infectious Disease or Virus	Possible Effects on the Developing Baby
Chicken pox and shingles	Prematurity, skin lesions, neurological abnormalities, eye anomalies, skeletal abnormalities, gastrointestinal and genito-urinary anomalies, limb deformities, low birth-weight, meningoencephalitis, miscarriage, or stillbirth. Note: 85 to 90% of pregnant women are immune to chicken pox and shingles. If you suspect that you're not immune (e.g., you haven't had chicken pox and you haven't lived in the same house with someone who's had chicken pox or shingles), call your doctor as soon as you're exposed to it. Your doctor can administer a special type of immune globulin (VZIG) to prevent you from getting a severe infection. Chicken pox is most dangerous to the developing baby if you contract it shortly before or after giving birth.
Cytomegalovirus (CMV)	Miscarriage, mental retardation, psychomotor retardation, developmental abnormalities, progressive hearing impairment, respiratory illness, jaundice, intrauterine growth restriction, failure to thrive, or eye infections. Note: CMV is most likely to cause a problem if a woman contracts it for the first time when she's pregnant.
Listeriosis	Miscarriage, stillbirth, or premature labor. Can cause pneumonia, septicemia (a bacterial blood infection), and meningitis in a newborn baby. (See the section earlier in this chapter for a more detailed discussion of listeriosis.) Note: If you've

Type of Infectious Disease or Virus	Possible Effects on the Developing Baby
Listeriosis	previously experienced a miscarriage or other loss because of exposure to listeriosis during pregnancy, this is unlikely to occur in a subsequent pregnancy. Researchers believe that past exposure to listeriosis provides some measure of immunity against the disease.
Measles	Fetal loss and prematurity. Note: Most women have been immunized against this disease, so it's very rare for a pregnant woman to contract it.
Mumps	Increases the baby's risk of developing adult-onset diabetes.
Human parvovirus B19 (Fifth disease)	Miscarriage, stillbirth, or heart failure in the newborn.
Rubella (German measles)	Miscarriage, stillbirth, heart malformations, cataracts, deafness, or infant death.
Sexually transmitted diseases	Can be transmitted to the developing baby during pregnancy or at the time of birth. Chlamydia, syphilis, and herpes are linked to higher-than-average rates of stillbirth, premature labor, and other complications.
Toxoplasmosis	Hydrocephalus, eye problems, psychomotor retardation, convulsions, microphthalmia, and intracerebral calcification (calcium deposits in the brain). Note: Toxoplasmosis can be treated with antibiotics.

- Changing the litter box. Both cat feces and raw meat may contain a parasite called toxoplasmosis, which can be very harmful to the developing baby. (See Table 6.7.) It's best to avoid changing kitty litter at all while you're pregnant, but if you absolutely have to do it because there's no knight in shining armor on hand to do it for you, then wear gloves and wash your hands thoroughly. The same goes for gardening, by the way, because some friendly neighborhood cat may have chosen your perennial garden for a litter box! Wear gloves when you're gardening, and be sure to thoroughly wash the soil off any vegetables that you harvest from your garden, just in case the soil has been contaminated with cat feces.

- Eating foods that may lead to various types of food poisoning. Be on the lookout for improperly canned or preserved food that may lead to botulism; raw or undercooked lamb, pork, or steak that may lead to toxoplasmosis; raw eggs, undercooked eggs, or undercooked chicken that may lead to salmonella; and soft cheeses (e.g., feta, brie, and Camembert), unpasteurized milk, and improperly cooked meat that may be a source of listeriosis (a food-borne illness that can be particularly harmful, even fatal, to the developing baby).

- Douching. Not only does douching increase your chances of experiencing an ectopic pregnancy or of developing pelvic inflammatory disease, but some commercial douching preparations contain substances that can be harmful to the developing baby. Because I've been harping about not douching since the beginning of this book, this time around, for variety's sake, I'm going to hand the microphone over to Natalie Angiers, author of one of my all-time favorite books, *Woman: An Intimate Geography.* Here's what she has to say on the whole subject of douching: "Don't douche, ever, period, end of squirt bottle."

- Allowing your body to become overheated. It doesn't matter what you do to cause your body temperature to shoot sky-high. Whatever it is, it's bad for your baby. That's why it's important to avoid anything that could cause your temperature to climb above 101°F, whether it's vigorous exercise, soaking in a hot tub, or hitting the sauna. It's also important to treat a fever, either by using acetaminophen (provided, of course, that you've got your doctor or midwife's approval) or by using other methods of bringing down your temperature — stripping off layers of clothing, soaking in a lukewarm bathtub, and so on.

- Spousal abuse. You probably don't even want to consider the possibility that you could be beaten up by your partner while you're pregnant, but according to the American College of Obstetricians and Gynecologists and the Centers for Disease Control and Prevention, 4 to 8% of women experience domestic violence during pregnancy. These assaults can result in injury or even death to the pregnant woman and/or her baby. If you find yourself in this situation, you should confide in your doctor, your midwife, or a trusted friend who will support you in whatever decisions you ultimately make. Or pick up the phone and call the National Domestic Violence Hotline (1-800-799-SAFE; TDD for the hearing-impaired: 1-800-787-3224) for information and support.

- Car accidents and falls. While it's best to avoid any sort of abdominal trauma while you're pregnant, you may find it reassuring to know that your baby is well protected from day-to-day tumbles. This is because your body is designed to protect your developing baby. Your uterus is made up of a thick wall of muscle that helps to keep your baby safe. What's more, within the uterus, your baby is cushioned by the amniotic fluid that he or she floats around in. And during the early weeks of pregnancy, your baby has some added protection: The uterus is hidden away behind the thick pelvic bone. Still, you'll want to do whatever you can to avoid slips and falls, and you'll want to get in the habit of wearing both your lap and shoulder belt when you're traveling by car. According to the American College of Obstetricians and Gynecologists, you should buckle the lap belt low on your hipbones (below your belly rather than across your belly) and you should place the shoulder belt between your breasts, making sure that it fits snugly.

FACTS AND FIGURES

Proceed with caution when you get behind the wheel. According to two separate studies in Canada and Norway, pregnant drivers are more likely to be involved in automobile accidents than other drivers. The increased risk is particularly pronounced during the first trimester of pregnancy, perhaps due to increased fatigue.

When you stop to consider all the things that can be harmful to the developing fetus, you may be tempted to hide under the covers for the next nine months. It's easy to become paranoid, but in most cases all you need to do is exercise some common sense. (Of course, that's easy for me to say. I'm not the one who's pregnant and pacing the floor at 2:00 a.m. wondering if the air freshener in the bathroom is emitting any potentially noxious substances!) Take a deep breath and relax. Believe it or not, the odds of ending up with a healthy baby in your arms nine months down the road are decidedly in your favor.

CHAPTER 7

The Worry Zone

"Having a child is so irreversible. Any other decision you make in life can be changed. You can quit a job, grow out a bad haircut, drop out of school, or get a divorce, but nothing stops you from being a parent. I often felt like I was trapped on a speeding train, destination unknown, and I just hoped I'd like where I was when the train finally stopped."
— Tracy, 31-year-old mother of one, quoted in
The Unofficial Guide to Having a Baby, by Ann
Douglas and John R. Sussman, M.D.

Spending a lot of time worrying? You're certainly in good company! After all, worrying is as much a part of pregnancy as stretch marks and popped belly buttons. (Hey, since pregnancy is basically a nine-month apprenticeship in parenthood, it only makes sense that you get the chance to hone your worrying skills before your baby arrives!)

There's so much to worry about during pregnancy, in fact, that I couldn't actually cram a discussion on this topic into a single chapter. That's why you'll find two chapters devoted to the art of worrying in this book — this one and the next. In this chapter, we're going to look at the top ten worries for each of the three trimesters of pregnancy. In the following chapter, we'll zero in on all those pregnancy-related aches and pains that can have you hitting the panic button at 3:00 a.m.: everything from morning sickness to round ligament pain to Braxton Hicks contractions! Then, just in case you're tempted to conclude that getting pregnant is the craziest thing you've ever done, we'll finish off Chapter 8 by considering the joys of pregnancy — and trust me, there are plenty.

Ready to get started? Here we go. Just take your seat, grab your binoculars, and prepare to take a first-class guided tour down Anxiety Avenue.

The Top Ten First-Trimester Worries

Your apprenticeship in worrying starts as soon as the pregnancy test comes back positive. As well as feeling swinging-from-the-chandelier happy about being pregnant, you're likely to find yourself feeling a bit anxious, too. After all, you've just embarked on a nine-month journey that's going to change your life forever!

Don't be surprised if you find yourself experiencing at least one of these classic first-trimester worries.

MOTHER WISDOM

Think pregnant women today have a lot to worry about? A century ago our pregnant ancestors had to concern themselves not only with what they ate or drank, but also any immoral thoughts that happened to pass through their heads. The experts of the day told them in no uncertain terms that their every thought, word, and deed would have lasting effects on the developing fetus: "Low spirits, violent passions, irritability, frivolity, in the pregnant woman, leave indelible marks on the unborn child," warned B.G. Jeffris and J.L. Nichols in their best-selling 1893 family planning manual, *Safe Counsel or Practical Eugenics*.

1. I'm worried that I'll experience a miscarriage.

If there's one concern that's pretty much universal among

newly pregnant women, it's the fear of having a miscarriage. While the majority of pregnant women will go on to have a healthy baby, a significant number of women — somewhere between 15 and 20% of those whose pregnancies are confirmed by a positive pregnancy test — will have their hopes and dreams shattered.

 FACTS AND FIGURES

Your risk of experiencing a miscarriage drops significantly once your doctor or midwife is able to pick up your baby's heartbeat via ultrasound (something that can be performed transvaginally when you're just six weeks pregnant) or Doppler (a hand-held ultrasound device that can usually pick up the baby's heartbeat by the start of the second trimester). One study showed that your risk of experiencing a miscarriage drops to less than 2% if your baby's heartbeat is detected when you're ten weeks pregnant.

Although it is easy to fixate on this figure, it's important to turn it on its head and look at it from the other perspective: You have an 80 to 85% chance of not miscarrying. Yes, I know, it would be a lot more reassuring if those odds were somewhere in the neighborhood of 100%, but they're still pretty good odds nonetheless. I mean, if someone offered you a comparable crack at winning a lottery, you'd be lining up to buy a ticket in a flash.

The fact that some women experience spotting during their first trimester only adds to their worry about miscarriage. While it's only natural to panic if you have bleeding during pregnancy (even spotting that's so light it barely shows up on the toilet paper), as a rule of thumb, light bleeding is generally less worrisome than heavier bleeding accompanied by cramping or the passage of tissue.

Light spotting can be caused by cervical bleeding (e.g., your cervix got bumped during intercourse or started to bleed while your caregiver was performing an internal examination) or by the passage of small amounts of uterine tissue (which occasionally happens in early pregnancy). It can also occur very early on in pregnancy — about seven days after conception — when the fertilized egg first attaches to the uterine wall. (Note: Not all women experience this type of spotting, which is known as "implantation bleeding.")

Because any amount of vaginal bleeding can be a sign of an impending miscarriage, you'll want to report any spotting to your doctor or midwife as soon as possible. He or she may want you to come in for a physical examination, a blood test, and/or an ultrasound to try to figure out if you are, in fact, miscarrying. Until you find out for sure what's going on, however, try not to hit the panic button. Many women who experience first-trimester bleeding end up giving birth to healthy babies eight or nine months down the road.

Here's something else you need to know about another worrying first-trimester symptom: It's not at all unusual to experience period-like cramping around the time your first missed menstrual period was due. This cramping is simply your body's response to the hormonal changes of early pregnancy. As long as it isn't accompanied by any bleeding (one of the warning signs of miscarriage) or sharp pain limited to one side of your abdomen (one of the warning signs of an ectopic pregnancy), there's generally no cause for concern.

MOM'S THE WORD

"Losing the baby had to be my number one concern, right off the bat. I couldn't believe how intense my fear was, or how much I thought about it."

— *Heather, 33, mother of two*

---

2. **I don't feel pregnant any more. Does this mean I've experienced a miscarriage?**

After spending weeks of coping with morning sickness, swollen breasts, and overwhelming fatigue — all the joys of early pregnancy! — you wake up one morning to discover that all your pregnancy symptoms have disappeared. You can't decide whether to celebrate or to start freaking out.

While it's true that a sudden disappearance of pregnancy symptoms can indicate a missed miscarriage (in which the developing baby dies but is not immediately expelled from the mother's body), that's not the only reason your symptoms could have disappeared. They tend to spontaneously disappear around the end of the first trimester anyway.

If you're really concerned, call your doctor or midwife to schedule an extra appointment. Sometimes hearing your baby's heartbeat on the Doppler or seeing it flash on the ultrasound screen is the only thing that will reassure you that the baby is still alive and kicking.

MOM'S THE WORD

"Don't be afraid to bother your doctor about something that's not important or serious. It's important to you."

— *Christina, 25, currently pregnant with her third child*

---

3. **I'm petrified that my baby will be born with birth defects because of the glass of wine I drank the week before I found out I was pregnant.**

Another common worry during early pregnancy is that something you did before you knew you were pregnant will result in permanent injury to the baby. It's a worry that Jennifer, a 32-year-old mother of one, struggled with for much of her pregnancy.

"I conceived in early December, but it was New Year's Day before I even had an inkling I was pregnant. In the meantime, I had celebrated Christmas in the usual way — with lots of rich food, relaxing, and ingesting of my favorite eggnog, which is light on the milk and heavy on the rum and brandy. There was nothing I could do to change what I had done. I read as much as I could on fetal alcohol syndrome and talked to my doctor and found out that there's no sure thing when it comes to drinking during pregnancy: Some alcoholics have normal babies, some casual drinkers have severely damaged babies."

The problem is that the period of greatest vulnerability for the developing baby is when its major organs are being formed — when you're approximately four to ten weeks pregnant (about two to eight weeks after conception). Exposure to a harmful substance during this period can result in birth defects or miscarriage, or it may have no effect at all. If exposure occurs earlier than this (e.g., during the two weeks after conception), either the baby won't be affected at all or you'll have a miscarriage. If exposure occurs later, it's still harmful to the developing baby, but, depending on the substance involved, the effects might not be quite so dramatic.

While it's best to avoid exposing your baby to any potentially harmful substance, you shouldn't immediately conclude that you're going to miscarry or give birth to a severely damaged baby as a result. Not all babies are harmed by prenatal exposure to alcohol or other potentially dangerous chemicals — something that Jennifer learned first-hand. After nine months of worrying about those rum-laced glasses of eggnog, she gave birth to a perfectly healthy baby.

4. I'm worried that my age puts me at risk of giving birth to a baby with a chromosomal abnormality such as Down syndrome.

You've no doubt seen all the scary statistics about how your risk of giving birth to a baby with a chromosomal problem increases as you age (to avoid alarming you unnecessarily, I've tucked this information away in the back of Appendix F). What you might not realize, however, is that the risk of giving birth to a chromosomally abnormal baby increases gradually rather than suddenly as you grow older. A 40-year-old woman has only a 1% greater chance than a 35-year-old woman. What's more, that 40-year-old woman still has a better than 98% chance of conceiving a chromosomally normal child. If you look at the glass as 98% full rather than 2% empty, you'll feel a lot more reassured!

5. I slipped on the ice on my way across the parking lot at work. I'm petrified that I'm going to have a miscarriage because of the fall.

While it's hard not to panic when you slip or fall during pregnancy, it's important to remember that your body is designed to protect your baby from minor accidents like this one. The walls of the uterus are made up of thick, strong muscles. What's more, your baby is floating around in a sea of amniotic fluid, and that fluid tends to provide a cushioning effect. (To get an idea of how much protection the uterus offers your baby, just imagine how hard it would be to break an egg that was floating around inside a water-filled plastic Thermos — short of tossing it out a second-story window, that is.)

FACTS AND FIGURES

The biggest risk to a baby during a high-impact car crash is a placental abruption — the premature separation of the placenta from the uterine wall. If you're involved in a serious car accident you should plan to seek medical attention. Be sure to tell the doctor who's examining you if you're experiencing vaginal bleeding; the leakage of amniotic fluid; severe pain or tenderness to your abdomen, uterus, or pelvis; uterine contractions (abdominal tightening that may or may not be painful); or a reduction in fetal movement (obviously, you won't be able to detect fetal movement changes until you're well into your second or third trimester).

Here are some more reassuring words. During the early part of pregnancy your uterus enjoys some added protection. It's safely tucked behind the pelvic bone — something that helps to minimize the chance of any abdominal injury resulting in harm to the baby. During the second trimester your uterus outgrows its hiding spot, so your baby no longer enjoys quite the same degree of protection. That's why most caregivers want to hear about any falls you experience after the 24th week, particularly ones that result in pain or bleeding, or direct blows to the abdomen. In most cases the baby is fine, but your doctor or midwife may want to monitor the fetal heart rate and/or to do a blood test to check for bleeding from the baby's circulation to yours via the placenta. In most cases, these tests will help to reassure both of you that the baby wasn't injured.

Your best bet, of course, is to prevent these types of accidents from happening in the first place. Here are a few quick tips on minimizing the risk of injury to your baby:

- Keep in mind that your sense of balance will be thrown off as your uterus begins to grow. This can make it easier for you to take a tumble, so be sure to use some extra caution when you're going up and down stairs or when you find yourself in a situation in which there may be a risk of tripping or falling.

- Use extra caution when you're driving. Keep in mind that you're driving "under the influence" of pregnancy hormones that can make you prone to fatigue and make it harder for you to concentrate (the infamous "pregnancy brain"). If you're going to be traveling a great distance, you might want to share the driving duties with someone else to reduce the risk of having an accident and/or make frequent stops so that you can get out of the car and clear the cobwebs from your head. (Don't worry about watching the clock too carefully when it comes to timing these breaks. Your bladder will help to ensure that you make frequent rest stops along the way.)

- Make sure you wear your seatbelt whenever you're traveling by car. While some women fear that the seatbelt will harm their baby in the event of a crash, your baby is actually a whole lot safer if you wear it. Wear the lap portion as low as possible, underneath your belly and across the top of your upper thighs and hipbones, and tuck the shoulder belt between your breasts. (Try tucking a small pillow or pad between the belt and your lap if the lap belt has a tendency to press uncomfortably on the bottom side of your abdomen. And try wrapping the shoulder belt in a soft flannel receiving blanket if it tends to chafe your neck — another common complaint of many pregnant women.)

6. **I'm basically surviving on soda crackers and flat ginger ale, and I'm concerned about depriving my baby of vital nutrients because of all the morning sickness I'm experiencing.**
   This is one anxiety you can scratch off the list fairly easily. For in most cases, morning sickness is far harder on the mother than the baby.
   If your baby had to rely on what you were able to keep down on a meal-to-meal basis, there might be cause for concern. Fortunately, Mother Nature in her infinite wisdom has prepared for just such an emergency by stockpiling nutrients in your body. So even if it's been a couple of weeks since you were able to stomach anything more exciting than soda crackers, your baby is still dining away on nutrients from all the multi-course meals you enjoyed during your pre-morning sickness days.
   Morning sickness poses a threat to the developing baby only if it happens to be particularly severe and unrelenting. In one out of every 300 pregnancies a woman will develop a more serious form of morning sickness known as hyperemesis gravidarum (Latin for "excessive vomiting in pregnancy"). The symptoms of hyperemesis gravidarum include heavy vomiting (e.g., the inability to keep any food or drink down for more than 24 hours); reduced frequency of urination; dehydration; dryness of

the mouth, skin, and eyes; extreme fatigue, weakness, or faint-ness; and confusion. The condition is generally treated with a combination of IV fluids and anti-nausea medications, but it's far better to nip the problem in the bud than to try to treat it after the fact. Be sure to let your doctor or midwife know if you're having a rough time with morning sickness.

Note: You can find out more about both hyperemesis gravi-darum and garden-variety morning sickness in Chapter 8.

FACTS AND FIGURES

Here's a thought to cheer you while you're dashing to the bath-room. Studies have shown that women who are having a lot of trouble with morning sickness are only one-third to one-half as likely to miscarry as women who are experiencing little or no morning sickness.

---

7. I look about ten times as pregnant as my best friend does and we're due the same week. I'm wondering if I could be expecting twins.

It's easy to assume that women who are at the same point in pregnancy should have roughly the same-sized belly, but that's not the way Mother Nature chooses to handle this whole preg-nancy thing. As I've said before and will no doubt say again before this book is finished, pregnancy is not a one-size-fits-all experience!

But if your belly seemed to blossom overnight and everyone's commenting on how pregnant you look, it's only natural to start wondering if you could be carrying more than one baby. Here's what you need to know.

While every woman has the chance of ending up with mul-tiples, some women face higher-than-average odds of hitting the reproductive jackpot. You fall into this category if

- you've previously given birth to twins (if you're a mother of twins, you're five times as likely to experience a multiple birth the next time around as other pregnant women!)

- fraternal twins tend to run in your family

- you've been taking fertility drugs

- your morning sickness is quite severe

- your uterus is growing more quickly than what would normally be expected at this stage of pregnancy

If your caregiver suspects you're carrying multiples, you'll likely be sent for an ultrasound. Since ultrasound is able to detect almost 100% of twin pregnancies, it's the most reliable way of determining whether you're indeed subletting your uterus to more than one tenant. If it turns out you are carrying multiples, you'll be monitored extra carefully for the duration of your pregnancy, since a multiple tends to be riskier than a singleton pregnancy. (See Chapter 11 for details on the joys and challenges of a multiple pregnancy.)

FACTS AND FIGURES

While it's true that women who use fertility drugs or who undergo certain other types of high-tech reproduction methods have a greater-than-average chance of giving birth to two or more babies, don't let the fact that you conceived the old-fashioned way convince you that you couldn't possibly be carrying more than one baby. About one in 90 "natural" conceptions results in the birth of twins!

FACTS AND FIGURES

Up until a generation ago, as many as 40% of twin pregnancies were undiagnosed prior to labor and delivery. It's no wonder so many fathers fainted in the delivery room!

MOM'S THE WORD

"I wanted to know if I was going to have a similar experience this time around. Would my morning sickness last for 22 weeks this time? Would I have to be induced again for delivery? Would my second child be much bigger than my first (he was 10 pounds, 1 ounce!)?"

— *Lara, 33, who is currently pregnant with her second child*

---

8. **I experienced a lot of complications during my first pregnancy and delivery. I'm worried that I'll end up having the same sorts of problems this time around.**

If you experienced a miscarriage, a high-risk pregnancy, or a difficult birth the first time around, you may be particularly concerned about whether history is destined to repeat itself.

If your first pregnancy ended in miscarriage, you may worry that you face a higher-than-average risk of experiencing another miscarriage. But depending on its cause, this may not be the case. While some women experience a series of miscarriages because a hormonal imbalance or other problem prevents them from carrying their babies to term, the majority of women who've miscarried a child in the past go on to have healthy babies the next time around. This is because a significant number of first-trimester miscarriages are caused by random chromosomal abnormalities. In other words, they can happen to any woman in any pregnancy, and these women are no more likely to experience this type of problem again than other pregnant women. You'll find a detailed discussion of the major causes of miscarriage in Chapter 11.

As for pregnancy-related complications, while there are certain types of problems that do tend to recur in subsequent pregnancies (e.g., complications resulting from chronic health conditions, structural problems with the reproductive organs, and so on), other types of problems are less likely to recur. If, for example, you developed pre-eclampsia (high blood pressure and

fluid retention) during the last few weeks of your first pregnancy, you aren't necessarily doomed to repeat this. Studies have
shown that pre-eclampsia tends to be more of a problem in first
pregnancies with the same partner than in subsequent ones.
You'll find a detailed discussion of pregnancy-related complications in Chapter 11.

Now let's talk about birth-related complications. If you
required a forceps delivery or vacuum extraction when your first
baby was born, you may not necessarily need one the second
time around. It's quite possible that your first baby may have
helped to pave the way for his or her younger brothers and
sisters by opening up your pelvis a little. If, like 22% of
American women, you had a cesarean the first time around,
however, you may be at increased risk of requiring one in your
subsequent pregnancies. While 50 to 80% of women attempting a vaginal birth after cesarean (VBAC) manage to avoid a
subsequent cesarean, sometimes the problems that necessitated
it the first time (e.g., a very small pelvis) can recur in a subsequent pregnancy. You'll find a detailed discussion on VBACs in
Chapter 11.

Of course, up until now I've been talking in generalities. The
best way to address your fears about having history repeat itself
is to discuss your concerns with your doctor or midwife.

**9. I thought that having another baby was a good idea. Now
I'm having second thoughts. What if my first child has a
hard time adjusting to the birth of her younger brother
or sister?**

As excited as you may be about your pregnancy, it's only natural to worry about the disruption that may result from adding
another baby to your family. What if your older child resents,
rather than welcomes, the new arrival?

Lori, a 29-year-old mother of four, remembers being
haunted by this worry: "When I became pregnant with my
second child, I began to worry that maybe it was too soon to

have another baby. My son was 13 months old and so I wondered if I'd had enough time with him before bringing another child into the family. I thought it might be unfair to him, that he wouldn't get as much attention and that perhaps he'd feel as if we loved him less when the new baby was born."

After nine months of worrying, Lori found that the problem resolved itself. "By the time the new baby was born, my first child was six weeks away from turning 2, and he had matured a great deal over the course of my pregnancy. He'd gained some independence and actually wanted to do more on his own." What's more, Lori discovered, "The new baby slept a lot and I still had a lot of time to do things with my son — something that helped to make the transition more gradual for him."

If this particular concern has made it onto your worry list, relax. There's plenty you can do both during your pregnancy and after the birth to help make the transition as smooth as possible for baby number one. Here are a few tips:

- Tap into your child's natural curiosity about babies. Even very young children are fascinated by them. Look at picture books together and talk about what's going on inside your body right now and what the baby will be like after birth.

- Find ways to involve your child in your pregnancy. Have him accompany you to prenatal checkups so that he can listen to the baby's heartbeat or help the doctor or midwife measure your growing belly.

- Give your child a sneak preview of what babies are really like by visiting other families who have newborns. Hint: If you don't know anyone who's had a baby recently, drop by the playground, the children's section of your public library, or some other family-oriented spot where there are bound to be tons of moms with new babies. You might also find out whether the hospital in your community offers sibling preparation classes.

- Encourage your child to help you pick out clothes and other items for the baby. Your child will enjoy seeing the new baby wear the sleeper that she "bought."

- Buy your child an inexpensive gift from the new baby. That way, when friends and relatives show up bearing gifts for the new arrival, your child is less likely to feel left out in the cold.

- Don't oversell the new baby. Your child needs to know that it'll be at least a couple of years before the new arrival is able to play ball or go for a ride on a tricycle. Some young children are very disappointed when their new brother or sister who was supposedly going to be a great playmate ends up sleeping all the time.

- Arrange for a friend or relative to give your child some extra time and attention after the baby arrives. A trip to the zoo or the playground with Grandma and Grandpa may be all that's required to let her know that she's still as special as ever.

- Don't try to enforce a totally "hands off" policy. While you obviously don't want to allow your toddler to pick up the new baby, you can teach him to hold the baby's hand gently or to carefully pat the baby's tummy. Babies are just as irresistible to toddlers as they are to adults. Imagine how frustrated you'd feel if no one let you touch this remarkable new addition to the family!

- Don't forget to take photos of your older child when you're snapping shots of the new baby. Otherwise, she may feel very left out when the prints come back from the photo lab and everyone's *oohing* and *aahing* over the infant. Besides, this is the perfect time to capture the ultimate of Kodak Moments: The first time the newborn stares at your older child's face and your child's big grin when she sees the baby's eyes open wide for the very first time.

- Don't panic if sibling love doesn't blossom overnight. It takes time for relationships to develop. Chances are, that special sibling bond will begin to emerge over time.

MOM'S THE WORD

"Sibling rivalry is inevitable. The only way to avoid it is to have one child."

— *Nancy Samalin, author of* Loving Your Child Is Not Enough

---

10. My vaginal secretions have changed. I'm worried that I've developed some sort of infection.

There's no need to be alarmed if you experience an increase in the amount of leukorrhea (the odorless, white, mucusy discharge produced by the vagina) while you're pregnant. The hormonal changes of pregnancy cause your vaginal secretions to become wetter and more abundant.

There is, however, cause for concern if your vaginal discharge becomes greenish-yellow, foul-smelling, or watery. These types of discharges may indicate that you've developed an infection that requires treatment or that your membranes have ruptured prematurely. In either case you'll need to seek medical attention since certain types of vaginal infections can increase your risk of experiencing various pregnancy-related complications. For example, bacterial vaginosis (an infection characterized by a thin, milky discharge with a fishy odor) is associated with an increased risk of premature labor, premature rupture of the membranes (PROM), and/or preterm delivery. Fortunately, bacterial vaginosis and other similar types of infections can usually be treated quickly and easily with oral or vaginal antibiotics. (And, with any luck, the antibiotics won't trigger a yeast infection!)

The Top Ten Second-Trimester Worries

Now that you're into your second trimester, you can scratch at least a few of those first trimester worries off your list. Before you get too complacent, however, let me warn you: There's an army of second-trimester worries just waiting to replace them!

Don't believe me? I guess it's time to take the next leg of our tour through the Worry Zone. This part of the trip will, of course, focus on all those glorious mid-trimester worries.

1. I haven't felt the baby moving yet. Should I be concerned?

Although you can expect to feel your baby's first movements at some point during the second trimester, you shouldn't expect Junior to be doing somersaults by week 14. The point at which these first flutters and kicks can be detected varies considerably from woman to woman and from pregnancy to pregnancy, but are typically felt sometime between the 18th and 22nd weeks of pregnancy.

 FACTS AND FIGURES

Your baby's movements tend to be rather infrequent at first, but then increase steadily until the seventh month of pregnancy, when cramped conditions in the uterus make it more difficult for it to move around. You're most likely to be able to feel its movements in the evening and in the middle of the night. Studies have shown that babies are rocked to sleep by their mothers' movements during the day, and therefore tend to be most active between 8:00 p.m. and 8:00 a.m.

Some women detect fetal movement sooner than others. As a rule, you can expect to feel your baby's kicks sooner rather than later if

• you've been pregnant before and already know what those early flutters are supposed to feel like (believe it or not, it can be hard to differentiate between baby flutters and intestinal gas until your baby's movements become a whole lot more vigorous!)

- you're relatively slim (heavier moms sometimes have a harder time detecting their babies' first flutters)

- you're tuned into what your baby is doing (if you're running around at breakneck speed all day and night, you might not notice those first gentle nudges)

The location of your placenta can also affect how much movement you feel. If your placenta is located at the front of your uterus, it can cushion your baby's movements, making it more difficult for you to sense any intrauterine gymnastic performances. So try not to worry too much if you don't seem to be experiencing a lot of fetal movement. If your doctor or midwife isn't having any trouble picking up your baby's heartbeat and your pregnancy seems to be otherwise proceeding normally, chances are your baby is doing just fine.

One last thing before we lay this particular worry to rest: It's important to keep in mind that some babies are more active than others. The number of kicks a baby makes in the womb at 20 weeks of pregnancy can vary from 50 to 1,000 a day, with most babies coming in around the 250 mark.

MOTHER WISDOM

Don't expect your partner to be able to feel your baby's kicks until toward the end of your second trimester. It's only after about week 24 that those kicks will be strong enough to be felt by anyone but you.

FACTS AND FIGURES

Your baby will be 32 times heavier by the end of the second trimester than it was at the beginning. It will go from weighing in at a mere 1 ounce to tipping the scales at 2 pounds. If a newborn grew at the same rate, she'd weigh about 240 pounds by the time she was three months!

2. I keep having awful nightmares about losing my baby or giving birth to a baby who is severely deformed. Is this "mother's intuition" telling me there's something wrong with my baby?

There's no denying it: Pregnant women tend to experience vivid dreams that can be both intense and disturbing. Sleep researchers pin part of the blame on — you guessed it! — that wacky cocktail of pregnancy hormones responsible for so many other pregnancy-related complaints.

During pregnancy (especially during the last trimester) you spend a greater percentage of your sleep time in REM (the stage of sleep when you're most likely to dream and to wake up easily). And because you tend to wake up more often in the night when you're pregnant — either because you have to make a trip to the bathroom or because your hips are sore from sleeping on your side — you tend to remember more about your dreams, including the parts you'd rather not.

Hormones aren't solely responsible for these often disturbing dreams, however, as studies have shown that fathers-to-be also experience their fair share of pregnancy-related nightmares. Clearly there's so much mental work to be done during the nine months of pregnancy that both parents' brains end up putting in a fair bit of overtime!

Try not to let your dreams worry you. The fact that you've had a baby-related nightmare does not in any way mean that you're destined to experience it in real life. So if you wake up feeling panicked in the middle of the night, go heat up a glass of warm milk in the microwave and focus on how well your pregnancy is going. And don't be afraid to wake up your partner if you need some cuddles and reassurance. (If he grumbles, just remind him that being woken up at 3:00 a.m. is actually good training for all those nights of disrupted sleep that are likely to occur after the baby arrives!)

3. I'm only 14 weeks pregnant and I've already gained ten pounds. At this rate, I'm going to be huge by the time the baby is born!

While a "typical" pregnant woman (whoever she is!) tends to gain somewhere between three and five pounds during the first trimester, it's not unusual to gain a little more or a little less at this stage. Some women gain a lot of weight right away, but then find that their weight gain tapers off a little around the start of the second trimester. Others have a hard time gaining any weight at all during the first trimester because they're feeling so queasy, but then quickly make up for lost time once their appetite returns.

Rather than fixating on how much weight you have or haven't gained by this stage of pregnancy, focus on consuming reasonably sized portions of healthy food and on maintaining an active lifestyle — and let the number on the scale take care of itself. This is no time to be cutting back on your food intake, since the second trimester is a time of tremendously rapid growth for your baby.

4. When I roll over in bed, I feel this awful ripping pain in my lower abdomen. Is this normal?

Ah, the joys of round ligament pain. Most pregnant women learn the hard way that there's no trickier maneuver than rolling over in bed in the middle of the night. If you change positions too suddenly, you're hit with an excruciating, knife-like pain in your lower abdomen.

While this pain can be alarming, there's no real cause for concern. What you're experiencing is simply a sudden stretching of the round ligaments — the two large ligaments that attach your uterus to your pelvis. Round ligament pain tends to be worse between the 14th and 20th weeks of pregnancy, when your uterus is heavy enough to exert pressure on the ligaments and yet not large enough to rest any of its weight on the pelvic bones (something that happens after the 20th week).

You can find plenty of tips on coping with this particular pregnancy complaint by reading the section on round ligament pain in Chapter 8.

5. When I went for a walk last night, I kept feeling this tightness in my abdomen. I was afraid I was going into premature labor.

As I noted back in the previous chapter, exercise can cause your uterus to contract. It can be worrisome and more than a little uncomfortable, but it doesn't necessarily mean that you're experiencing premature labor. Nonetheless, it's a good idea to familiarize yourself with the symptoms of premature labor so that you'll be able to seek medical attention if necessary. You'll find a list of these all-important symptoms in Table 7.1.

TABLE 7.1
THE SYMPTOMS OF PREMATURE LABOR

If you find yourself experiencing one or more of the following symptoms, you could be experiencing premature labor, and you should get in touch with your doctor or midwife immediately.

Uterine contractions (tightening) that may or may not be painful. While it's normal to experience some uterine tightening when you're exercising, you should be concerned if these contractions continue after you stop exercising; if they don't go away when you drink a large glass of water or juice, empty your bladder, and lie down on your side; and if you continue to have more than four contractions over the course of an hour.

Vaginal bleeding or discharge. If you note a change in the quantity or quality of your vaginal discharge; if the discharge is brown- or pinkish-tinged; and if it's more mucusy or watery than normal, it's possible that you're going into labor.

continued

THE SYMPTOMS OF PREMATURE LABOR (Continued)

Vaginal pressure, or pressure in the pelvic area. If you experience a feeling of pressure in the pelvic area or the vagina that radiates toward your thighs, or you feel as though the baby is falling out, you may be experiencing premature labor.

Menstrual-like cramping in the lower abdomen. If you experience menstrual-like cramping in your lower abdomen — either continuous or intermittent — you may be going into labor.

A dull backache. If you experience a dull backache that radiates to the side or the front of your body, and that isn't alleviated by any change in position, you could be going into labor.

Stomach or intestinal cramping and gas pains. If you experience cramping, gas pains, diarrhea, nausea, or feelings of indigestion, you could be going into labor.

A general feeling of unwellness. Don't underestimate your gut feeling. If you feel unwell and your body is telling you that something's wrong, it's possible that you're going into labor.

6. I just failed the one-hour glucose screening test. Does this mean that I have gestational diabetes?

A number of doctors routinely screen their patients for gestational diabetes toward the end of the second trimester or the beginning of the third. The test is designed to indicate whether you're at increased risk of having this condition, not to state definitively whether you actually do. In fact, if you test positive there's an 85% chance that you don't actually have gestational diabetes.

Most caregivers send anyone who tests positive on the one-hour glucose screening test for a three-hour glucose tolerance test, which involves fasting for at least eight hours, consuming a beverage with a very high concentration of glucose (which makes some pregnant women feel quite nauseous), and having your blood sugar levels measured both prior to and at regular intervals after drinking the sugary beverage. Only when your result is positive on this test will you be diagnosed with gestational diabetes.

Other caregivers prefer to do fasting and post-meal blood sugars rather than relying on the glucose tolerance test. If your blood sugar readings are high on this test, you will be instructed to start monitoring your blood glucose levels at home and will be given some tips on modifying your diet. If your blood sugars continue to climb, you may have to start taking insulin.

You can find out more about gestational diabetes by reading the section on high-risk pregnancy in Chapter 11.

FACTS AND FIGURES

According to the American College of Obstetricians and Gynecologists, gestational diabetes affects approximately 100,000 American women each year.

---

7. I am not usually the kind of person who tends to worry, but since I became pregnant I've been worrying about everything. Is this normal?

It's not uncommon for a pregnant woman's brain to go into overdrive, generating an ever-growing list of things to worry about. You may find yourself worrying about your own health, your partner's health, and — of course — the health of your growing baby.

Jennifer, 27, who's expecting her first child, has been surprised by how much time she spends worrying: "I was extra-aware of my driving and the cars around me. I started to worry if my husband wasn't home exactly when I expected him. And, of course, of utmost importance was the health of the baby."

It's only natural to want to do whatever you can to protect your baby-to-be, but sometimes you can drive yourself crazy with anxiety. Talk to your partner or a trusted friend about your concerns. Sometimes the mere act of expressing your fears can help to chase them away.

🔊 **MOM'S THE WORD**

"When my baby started moving inside me — the best feeling in the world, by the way — I'd worry if it was less active or didn't move for a while. One day I was so upset that the baby hadn't moved much that I put on my *Mozart for Mothers-to-Be* CD: one set of headphones for me and another on my tummy. The baby started kicking immediately. I was so relieved."

— *Jennifer, 27, currently pregnant with her first child*

---

8. **I'm worried about how having a baby will affect my relationship with my partner.**

If you and your partner are currently having problems, you may wonder if coping with the needs of a newborn will drive the two of you further apart. And if you're getting along famously, you may wonder if it really makes sense to jinx a terrific relationship by adding a baby to the mix.

The best thing you can do to alleviate this particular fear is to talk it through with your partner. You may find that he's experiencing similar fears. Then, together, the two of you can come up with some strategies for ensuring you remain connected after the birth. (Note: You'll find plenty of practical tips in the final chapter of this book.)

🔊 **MOM'S THE WORD**

"The biggest emotional challenge for me was preparing to become a mother — adapting to the idea that our life wasn't just about Ken and me anymore, preparing for the major life change in our family, and starting to adapt our lifestyle to accept this new little person who was starting to change our life already."

— *Nicole, 29, mother of one*

9. I'm not quite sure what to do about scheduling my maternity leave. I'd like to have as much time as possible to spend with the baby after the birth, but I don't know if I want to work right up until I go into labor.

While most women try to schedule their maternity leave so that they have as much time as possible to spend with their babies after the birth, there's a lot to be said for taking a bit of time off before the baby arrives. The last thing you want, after all, is to head for labor and delivery after putting in a 12-hour day at the office! If you don't want to stop working entirely during the last few weeks of your pregnancy, why not see if your employer would be willing to have you work on a part time basis? That way, you could help to train your replacement and still have time to rest and prepare for your baby's arrival. Just make sure that you can afford to take the financial hit from those smaller-than-normal paychecks and that you won't be penalized in any way for working part time before the birth. You would hate to find out after the fact, for example, that working part time made you ineligible for any paid maternity benefits offered through your employer's employee benefits package.

Here's something else to keep in mind when you're scheduling your maternity leave: No matter how carefully you map out your plans, they're not carved in stone. Pregnancy can be a rather uncertain business. If you develop complications during the final weeks that require you to go on bedrest or to be induced early, you and your employer will have to rethink your maternity leave game plan.

Before you sit down with your employer to work out the details of your maternity leave, make sure you take the time to bring yourself up to speed on your rights as a pregnant worker. That means learning about your rights under both the Pregnancy Discrimination Act and the Family and Medical Leave Act.

The Pregnancy Discrimination Act

While it's unlikely that your employer will attempt to fire you outright when you announce your pregnancy (after all, that would be a sure-fire way to get himself in hot water with the feds!), you could find yourself facing more subtle forms of discrimination in the workplace. That's why it's important to understand what protection you are entitled to under the provisions of the Pregnancy Discrimination Act of 1978 (an amendment to the Civil Rights Act of 1964).

Basically, the Act, which applies to all companies with 15 or more employees, prohibits any form of discrimination on the basis of pregnancy. (Note: If you happen to work for a company that employs fewer than 15 workers, don't worry that you'll automatically become a victim of pregnancy discrimination. In most cases, state legislation kicks in to ensure that employees of smaller operations are provided with protection similar to that offered by the Pregnancy Discrimination Act.) If you are covered by the provisions of the Pregnancy Discrimination Act, it is illegal for an employer to

- refuse to hire you because you are pregnant if it can be proven that you are capable of fulfilling the major requirements of the job

- introduce any policies that discriminate against pregnant employees (e.g. treating a pregnancy-related disability in a different manner than a non-pregnancy-related disability would be treated; or reimbursing pregnancy-related health expenses differently than expenses for other medical conditions)

- limit pregnancy-related benefits to married couples

If you suspect that you have been the victim of pregnancy discrimination, you should keep a detailed log of critical events and gather evidence that might help to substantiate your claim; ask to review the contents of your personnel file and make copies of anything relevant; and discuss your concerns with your employer. If your concerns are not adequately addressed, you may want to file a formal complaint with the U.S. Equal Employment Opportunity Commission (1-800-669-4000; www.eeoc.gov).

 FACTS AND FIGURES

The U.S. Equal Employment Opportunity Commission handled 4,160 complaints of pregnancy discrimination in 2000.

The Family and Medical Leave Act of 1993

The Family and Medical Leave Act of 1993 covers any worker who is employed by a public agency (including state, local, and federal employees, and schools); or a private sector employer engaged in commerce who employs (or who has employed) 50 or more employees for 20 or more workweeks in either the current or prior calendar year. To be eligible for benefits under the Act, you must have worked for an employer covered by the Act for at least 12 months; you must have worked at least 1,250 hours for that employer during the previous 12 months; and you must have been employed at a location that is either inside the United States itself (or any of its territories or possessions) and where at least 50 employees are employed within a 75-mile area. (Whew! Bet no one told you that you'd need a degree in employment law order to take a maternity leave!)

If you meet all of these conditions, you could qualify for up to 12 weeks of unpaid, job-protected leave following the birth of a baby, the adoption of a child, or in certain other circumstances (providing foster care to a child, caring for an immediate family member who has a serious health condition that requires either hospitalization or bedrest at home, or developing a serious health condition yourself such as a pregnancy-related complication that requires that you go on bedrest). In the case of leave following the birth of a baby, you must take this leave within 12 months of your baby's birth. In most situations, your employer must give you back your original position or offer you an equivalent position with equivalent pay, benefits, and employment terms and conditions when you return to work following your leave. (The only exception is if you're deemed a "key employee" — a highly paid employee whose reinstatement at the company following a period of leave would cause "substantial and grievous economic injury to its operations" — in which case your employer might be exempted from this provision of the Act.)

As with anything else government-related, there's a bit of fine print you need to know about. In order to take advantage of family or medical leave, you must (wherever possible) provide your employer with 30 days' notice of your intention to take such leave; supply a medical certificate in support of your application for leave if your employer requests such a certificate; obtain second and third medical opinions if your employer requests them; and have your doctor or midwife periodically report to your employer about your ability and intention to return to work (if your employer requests this type of information).

FROM HERE TO MATERNITY

Some states have family and medical leave programs that are more generous than what's available under the federal Family and Medical Leave Act. For more information on the programs available in your state, as well as general information about your rights as a pregnant employee, contact the Women's Bureau Clearinghouse, U.S. Department of Labor: 1-800-827-5335 or www.dol.gov/dol/wb.

10. I'm not sure we can actually afford to have this baby! Maternity wear is unbelievably expensive, and then there's all that baby gear to buy. I'm starting to panic about all the expenses.

Having a baby can be expensive, but it doesn't have to be a recipe for financial disaster. If you're willing to compare prices, shop secondhand, and beg, borrow, or steal from relatives, you'll find that your dollars will go a whole lot further. Here are some important points to keep in mind when you're shopping for maternity wear and baby gear.

MOM'S THE WORD

"If you plan on having more than one child, invest in some good basics that will be timeless and that you'll be able to wear during subsequent pregnancies — a nice pair of maternity jeans or overalls, a good skirt or dress in basic black — just like what you might do with your regular wardrobe."

— *Carolin, 34, mother of three*

Maternity wear

- Don't hit the stores too soon, or you'll be tempted to overbuy out of boredom. If you're totally sick of your maternity clothes by the time you actually need them, you might be tempted to pick up an extra outfit or two. You can probably get away with wearing most of your regular clothes until at least the start of the second trimester, although you may have to bid a fond farewell to your dress pants and fitted skirts a little sooner than that.

- Don't buy everything all at once. Rather than blowing your entire maternity clothes budget in one go, plan to treat yourself to a new top every now and again to add some variety to your wardrobe.

- Look for bargains and freebies. "Get hand-me-downs from friends and relatives, shop consignment stores, and make a point of hitting the sale racks," suggests Carolin, a 34-year-old mother of three. "Used maternity clothes are usually in really good condition because they're worn for such a short time." As well as checking out the sale racks at the big maternity stores, be sure to check out the maternity wear sections of the major department stores.

- Skip the maternity aisle. You can save yourself a bundle by avoiding anything with the "maternity" label. Try the plus-sized section of your local department store or shop at a plus-sized women's clothing retailer such as Lane Bryant.

📢 **MOM'S THE WORD**

"Be prepared. There seems to be an overriding sentiment among the designers of maternity clothes that all pregnant women lose their fashion sense when they get knocked up. Go figure: snowflakes, flowers, kittens, etc. Just perfect for a board meeting!"

— *Jenny, 31, mother of one*

- Think "mix and match." Look for high-quality pieces that can be mixed and matched at will to create the maximum number of outfits. "I bought only the basics: black pants, two vests, and a skirt and sweater/cardigan set," says Alexandra, a 33-year-old mother of two. "I mixed and matched along with my 'regular' turtlenecks and blouses."

- Look for clothes that will grow with you. Casual pants with drawstring waists are ideal because the waistband can expand with your belly. The more flexible the garment is, the more wear you'll get out of it.

- When in doubt, buy large. If you're torn between two sizes of maternity clothes, buy the larger one. It's difficult to anticipate just how much you'll grow during the months ahead and it can be more than a little disheartening to outgrow your maternity wardrobe when you've got another two months of pregnancy still ahead.

- Don't forget that your breasts will grow too. Choose clothes that have plenty of room across the chest and under the arms. By the time you're ready to give birth, your breasts will each be a full pound heavier. And treat yourself to some decent bras — ones with wide, padded straps that won't dig into your shoulders as the weight of your breasts increases.

- Wear good-quality underwear. Choose loose-fitting cotton underwear that breathes and that won't irritate your increasingly sensitive skin. Since pregnant women are notoriously susceptible to yeast infections, spending nine months in polyester undies is a recipe for disaster. It's up to you, however, whether you go with bikini underwear or traditional maternity briefs. Let comfort be your guide.

MOM'S THE WORD

"Buy proper maternity clothes — especially pantyhose. What a relief it was to slip into a pair of maternity pantyhose after wearing queen size, which were about eight inches too long!"

— *Maria, 35, mother of two*

- Raid your husband's closet. "Large-size men's shirts can be worn over leggings, slacks, tailored skirts, and so on," says Marguerite, a 36-year-old mother of two.

- Seize the moment. Don't get too hung up on trying to find clothes that can be worn again later. While you might think you'll be happy to wear that A-frame sundress long after delivery day, chances are you'll be sick to death of it by the time your baby arrives. Besides, there's always the off-chance that someone will see you wearing it and assume you're pregnant again — reason enough to banish it to the back of your closet!

- Be prepared for some frustration if you're a full-figured gal. The maternity manufacturers have yet to clue into the fact that large women have sex. This is why most maternity lines seem to end at size 14 or, if you're really lucky, size 18. If you can't find "maternity" clothes, you'll have to improvise by shopping in plus-size stores. As a rule, you can get away with wearing casual clothing like leggings and sweaters that are generous in cut and two sizes larger than what you usually wear.

- Beat the heat. Your body's thermostat is cranked up when you're pregnant, so be sure to look for lightweight clothing made of cotton or other natural fibers. Try to choose garments that can be layered so that you can add or remove them to keep your body at a comfortable temperature. "I was pregnant in the winter and was hot the whole time," recalls Jenny, a 31-year-old mother of one. "I bought lots of colored T-shirts and wore maternity vests over them so that I could look reasonable at work, but not be sweltering."

- Think comfort and joy. While we're talking comfort, here's another important point to remember: Anything that binds at the waist or restricts blood flow in your legs (e.g., knee-high pantyhose) isn't going to be particularly comfortable during pregnancy.

- Hit the sewing machine. If you know how to operate a sewing machine, consider whipping up a few simple jumpers and skirts. You'll save a small fortune and you won't find yourself wearing the exact same navy-blue jumper as every other woman in your prenatal class!

- Don't fall into the trap of buying gimmicky products just because you think you might need them. "Combined maternity shirts/nursing shirts seem like a wonderful idea, but in reality they aren't worth the money," insists Maria, a 31-year-old mother of two. "I felt funny wearing a 'nursing shirt' when I was still pregnant, and yet it didn't fit right when I was no longer pregnant but nursing. The shirt hangs lower in the front when you don't have the belly to support it."

- Put your best foot forward. Choose low-heeled, comfortable shoes that won't pinch your feet if they begin to swell. Believe it or not, your feet may grow as much as a full size during pregnancy. If all else fails, think Birkenstocks!

- Look for clothes that will do double duty. "Business casual is a good category to aim for, as it will allow you to dress for work and for your leisure time without turning to two different wardrobes," says Janet, a 32-year-old mother of one.

- Treat thyself. Pregnancy is, after all, a time for indulgence. "Splurge on a few things that make you feel good, like a special sundress or a formal dress to wear to a wedding," suggests 25-year-old Christina, who is currently pregnant with her third child. If you don't want to spend a small fortune on a drop-dead-gorgeous ball gown for New Year's Eve, consider renting it instead. Maternity clothing rental boutiques are springing up in a growing number of large cities.

MOM'S THE WORD

"My partner was more worried, I think, about his ability to 'provide for' the baby. Even though we're equal financial partners in our marriage, he seems to give finances a great deal more thought than I do."

— *Janet, 32, mother of one*

Baby gear

Now that we've talked about how to trim your maternity clothing budget, let's look at ways to reduce the amount of money you end up spending on baby gear. While most new parents get a great deal of pleasure shopping for the new arrival, there's no need to go overboard. The fact that baby superstores stock hundreds of different products doesn't necessarily mean that your baby needs one of each! Here are some tips on getting the maximum value for your dollar. (Note: You'll find some additional advice on stretching your dollars in my book, *Family Finance: The Essential Guide for Parents,* co-written with financial planner Elizabeth Lewin.)

- Don't hit the stores too soon. If you do all your shopping while you're still pregnant, you're going to end up with doubles or triples of some things — great news if you're having multiples, but a bit of an overkill if you're having a single baby. Believe it or not, you're going to be deluged with baby gifts. People who barely gave you the time of day before you were pregnant will show up on your doorstep, baby gift in hand, hoping for a peek at the wee one. And, at the same time, friends and relatives will offer to loan you mountains of baby stuff. A better strategy is to ensure you've got the basics on hand, and then wait to see whatever else comes your way.

- Learn to distinguish between frills and necessities. The juvenile-product manufacturers are always coming up with new things that babies and their parents supposedly need, but some of these items are nothing more than costly extras. A car seat, a stroller, a baby carrier (e.g., a baby sling), and a safe place for your baby to sleep are the only true necessities for a newborn other than clothing and diapers and Mom. Pass on the rest.

- Don't load up on too much furniture. While the baby magazines would have you believe that no baby's room is complete without a bassinet, crib, dresser, and change table, there's no need to put yourself into debt for these things. That bassinet may end up going unused if your baby sleeps with you during the early months. It's a far better idea to earmark those dollars for a good-quality crib instead. The dresser and change table are nice to have, but they're by no means necessary. You can store your baby's clothes in plastic bins or in an extra laundry basket if you have to, and many parents actually find it easier to change a baby on a bed or on the floor than on a change table. Why not wait until after the baby arrives so you can decide what bits and pieces you're most likely to use? Who knows — you may decide to take the change-table money and spend it on a rocking chair instead — an item that's likely to be much more enjoyable for you and your baby!

- Pass on the designer togs when your baby is first born. Rather than loading up on high-priced outfits, stick to basic newborn nighties ($8 a pop) and inexpensive sleepers ($9 or less). Your baby will need at least a dozen outfits and at least as many receiving blankets, unless of course you're planning to do laundry every day. (See Table 7.2.) Your baby will grow at a phenomenal rate during the early weeks and months of life and will likely outgrow his entire newborn wardrobe before he's 6 weeks old! Note: A baby who weighs in at more than nine pounds may have a hard time fitting into the 3-month size of clothing, let alone the newborn size. Be sure to have some 6-month-size clothing on hand, just in case you end up giving birth to a larger-than-average baby.

- Look for clothing that will grow with your baby. Certain brands of sleepers feature adjustable foot cuffs that allow them to be worn longer.

- Stick to unisex clothing as much as possible. That way, if you decide to have another baby, you won't have to go out and buy a whole new wardrobe if he or she happens to be the opposite sex.

- Don't buy clothing more than a season in advance. While you might be tempted to pick up that size-two snowsuit now while it's on sale, you have no way of telling whether it'll fit your baby during the right season. That $30 "bargain" could end up being a $30 waste of money.

- Put safety first. A second-hand crib or car seat is no bargain if it results in injury or death. Don't even think of buying a crib that fails to conform to current crib safety standards (see Table 7.3) and pass on any secondhand car seat unless you know for a fact that it's never been involved in a car accident. (Even minor fender-benders can twist the frame of the car seat, making it unfit for use.)

- Know what you're buying if you're hitting the garage sale circuit. Before you buy any piece of secondhand equipment, make sure you know who manufactured it and when (this information is generally included on a sticker on the product or in an accompanying manual), what the model number is, how many families have used it (e.g., did the person who's selling it buy it new or secondhand), whether it's ever been repaired, whether any of the parts are missing and if so whether replacement parts are still available, and whether the product conforms to current safety standards.

TABLE 7.2

CLOTHING: WHAT YOUR NEWBORN NEEDS

12 newborn nighties (one size fits most!)
3 sleepers
2 hooded towel and washcloth sets
3 sets of fitted crib sheets
3 blankets
12 extra-large receiving blankets
3 pairs of socks
3 sweaters (depending on the season)
2 cotton hats

1 snowsuit or bunting bag (depending on the season)

4 large bibs (only necessary if you're planning to formula-feed or if your baby spits up a lot)

TABLE 7.3
CRIB SAFETY STANDARDS

To be considered safe, a crib must

feature crib slats or spindles that are no more than 2 3/8" apart (none of the slats or spindles should be loose or missing) and corner posts that are no more than 1/16 of an inch above the end panels (unless they are over 16" high for a canopy)

be constructed so that the mattress fits snugly (no more than two fingers' width between the edge of the mattress and the side of the crib)

be free of hazards such as missing, loose, broken, or improperly installed screws, brackets, or other hardware; cutout areas on the headboard or footboard where a baby's head could get trapped; cracked or peeling paint; or splinters or rough edges.

FROM HERE TO MATERNITY

The Juvenile Product Manufacturers Association publishes a 16-page safety brochure, "Safe and Sound for Baby." You can download a copy of the brochure from the association's Web site at www.jpma.org/public/safe-sound.html or request a copy by sending a stamped, self-addressed business-size envelope to Juvenile Product Manufacturers Association Public Information, 17000 Commerce Parkway, Suite C, Mt. Laurel, NJ 08054.

FROM HERE TO MATERNITY

The U.S. Consumer Product Safety Commission (1-800-638-2772; www.cpsc.gov) is an excellent source of product safety information. If you really want to stay in the know where safety is concerned, sign up for the free e-mail alert service, which notifies you of product recalls the same day they occur. See www.cpsc.gov/about/subscribe.html for further information.

The Top Ten Third-Trimester Worries

Now that you're entering the home stretch of pregnancy, you're starting to think ahead to the birth. That gives you a whole bunch of new things to worry about! Time to wrap up our stroll down Anxiety Avenue by looking at the most common third-trimester worries.

MOM'S THE WORD

"I'm afraid of the pain of delivery — but I'm more afraid of an epidural. I figure it will be the most painful but most rewarding thing I'll ever do for the rest of my life. But what I'm really afraid of is the 'other stuff' — that I'll be a weak person and not be able to tolerate the pain; that my labor will be exceptionally arduous; that I'll poop while giving birth; that I'll have an episiotomy, a stillbirth, a cesarean; that I'll be rushed or pressured into decisions I don't need to make; that I'll say nasty things to my husband and not let him feel like he's a part of the birth; and that I'll be a bad Mom. I'm afraid of doing something wrong for the baby and accidentally hurting him or her — holding the baby wrong, not breastfeeding properly. I'm afraid that I'll have an 11-pound baby. I'm afraid of so many things."

—*Jennifer, 27, currently pregnant with her first child*

---

1. **I'm worried that I won't be able to tell when I'm really in labor and that I'll end up waiting too long before I get help.**

   This is one of the most common fears of first-time mothers: That they won't clue into the fact they're in labor until the baby's head is starting to crown!

   Most women who've been through labor will tell you that, while it's hard to be sure at first whether or not it's actually begun, as time goes on you become more and more certain.

   As a rule of thumb, you should assume it's the real thing rather than a convincing imitation if

- your contractions are getting longer, stronger, more painful, and more frequent, and are falling into some sort of regular pattern

- your contractions intensify if you move around and aren't relieved by either a change of position or by consuming two large glasses of water

- the pain is radiating from your lower back and spreading to your lower abdomen and possibly your legs as well

- you feel as though you're experiencing a gastrointestinal upset and are having some diarrhea

- you're passing blood-streaked or pinkish mucus (the goopy stuff that your prenatal instructor likes to call "bloody show")

- your membranes have ruptured

On the other hand, you should assume that you're experiencing a powerful dress rehearsal for the main event if

- your contractions are irregular and are increasing neither in frequency nor severity

- your contractions subside if you rest, change position, or have two large glasses of water

- the pain is centered in your lower abdomen rather than your lower back

- your show is brownish-tinged rather than red-tinged and likely the result of either an internal examination or intercourse within the previous 48 hours

Of course, everyone has at least one friend whose labor broke the rules — who had no idea she was actually in labor until the moment of truth was almost upon her. That's why I must now take a moment to impress upon you the Mother of All Pregnancy Rules: If in doubt, check it out.

MOM'S THE WORD

"During my first pregnancy, I kept wondering how I was going to be able to tell when I was in labor. I had this feeling I wouldn't know what contractions were."

— *Dorothy, 33, mother of two*

2. I'm petrified that I won't make it to the hospital on time to have my baby.

If you live in an urban area and you're giving birth for the first time, there's generally little cause for concern. Since a first labor averages about 12 to 13 hours, you've got plenty of time to clue into the fact that you're in labor, grab your labor bag, and head for the hospital. In fact, even women who are giving birth for the second or subsequent time generally have time on their side: Their labors average about seven hours.

Things can, of course, be a little trickier if you live a little farther off the beaten path and the nearest hospital is a good hour or two away. While you're likely to have enough time to make it to the hospital, you may have to err on the side of caution and make the trip before you're 100% sure that you're really in labor. Don't be surprised if you end up with a couple of false starts. Sometimes the only way to tell whether it's the real thing is to have your caregiver do an internal examination to see if your cervix has begun to dilate. While it can be frustrating and even a little embarrassing to be sent home from the hospital time and time again, it's better to be safe than sorry if you have a considerable distance to travel.

Something else you may have to keep in mind depending on where you live is the possibility of bad weather. If you're due around the end of January — prime snowstorm season for certain parts of the county — you'll want to talk to your doctor or midwife about what arrangements would be made if the roads aren't passable. Would you need to call 911 to request assistance in getting to the hospital? Would the midwife make the trek to your home by snowshoe? Obviously, these are issues best discussed months before you actually go into labor.

3. I'm worried that my water will break when I'm out in public — like when I'm doing my grocery shopping. I can't imagine anything more embarrassing than that, short of giving birth right in the middle of the produce department!

Here's a reassuring statistic, just in case this particular anxiety is keeping you awake at 3:00 a.m.: Only 10% of women experience premature rupturing of the membranes (when they rupture before rather than during labor). So the chances of your water breaking in the middle of the grocery store are decidedly slim.

And even if your membranes do end up rupturing in a public place, you're more likely to experience a constant trickle of amniotic fluid rather than any sudden gushes. That's because your baby's head acts like a cork, blocking the exit to your uterus and slowing the escape of the amniotic fluid. So while you'll know something's happened (you tend to feel this weird popping sensation, followed by the tell-tale trickle of fluid down your leg), chances are no one else in the store is going to clue in. And because amniotic fluid doesn't have a particularly strong odor, you don't have to worry about smelling funny either.

If you're losing a lot of sleep over this one, there's an easy solution. Start wearing a maxi pad when you go out. It'll buy you some time to exit with grace if your membranes do decide to rupture at an inopportune time and you have to abandon your cart in the frozen-food aisle.

4. I'm petrified that I won't be able to cope with the pain of labor.

Given the scary stories pregnant women are subjected to by well-meaning (and not-so-well-meaning) friends and relatives, it's hardly surprising that many of us decide around the eight-month mark that we really don't want to give birth after all! Of course, there's no turning back at this stage of the game. There are only two ways to get that baby out, and neither of them are a picnic!

 MOTHER WISDOM

"I felt powerfully connected to all my ancestresses down through all time. I could literally see the echoes of every woman who ever labored to give forth a new life. I felt triumphant; filled with grace; utterly humbled by my own body and by the miracle that lay wet and sweet and messy on my belly. I was full to the skin with welcome for the new life that so suddenly became real to me."

— *Heather, 32, mother of one, quoted in* The Unofficial Guide to Having a Baby *by Ann Douglas and John R. Sussman, M.D.*

The best way to cope with your labor-related fears is to learn as much as you can about giving birth. Read up on the subject, take some childbirth classes, and talk to your doctor or midwife about pain relief options during labor. It can be reassuring to know about the smorgasbord of natural and medicinal pain relief methods available to laboring women — methods we'll be discussing in greater detail in Chapter 10.

In the meantime, don't underestimate your abilities. Labor is indeed a trial by fire, but you're up to the challenge. Generations of other women have walked this path before and lived to tell. (Heck, some of them even went back and had more babies!) So rather than feeling afraid that you can't do it, focus on the strength you can draw upon to meet this challenge. (I know this sounds all very crunchy-granola, but it's true: There's an inner reservoir of strength just waiting to be called upon when you're in the heat of labor. Trust me on this one, okay?)

5. I'm afraid that I'll lose control during labor.

This is another tremendously common fear — that you'll do or say something unspeakably embarrassing during labor. You may worry that you'll swear or grunt or say something really bitchy to your partner or that you'll end up pooping a bit while you're pushing out your baby.

Most of us spend our entire lives working at maintaining control, so it can be more than a little disconcerting to envision yourself in a situation where it's your body that's calling the shots rather than the "rational" part of your brain.

The first thing you need to realize is that the labor and delivery staff and your doctor or midwife have seen it all, and they certainly won't think any the worse of you if you happen to lose control during labor. In fact, your caregiver may actually encourage you to make grunting noises during contractions if that helps you to cope with the pain. (It never worked for me, but some women swear by it, so there's got to be something to this whole grunting business!)

And as for your partner thinking any the less of you because of something you do or say during labor, you're forgetting one important detail: He's unlikely to notice anything so trivial because he'll be too busy witnessing a miracle.

6. I'm worried that there won't be anyone on hand to take care of my older child when I go into labor.

Since it's impossible to predict exactly when you're going to give birth — unless, of course, you're having a scheduled induction or a cesarean — the question of who will care for your older child during your labor can represent quite a challenge.

You may have to come up with a whole roster of people who are available at various times of day or night. Hopefully, if you recruit enough bodies, you'll be able to catch at least one person at home when the moment of truth arrives!

Once you've made your arrangements, be sure to fill your child in on the details. She needs to know that she could wake up one morning to find Grandma or Uncle Bill sitting at the breakfast table instead of you. And be sure to explain that you'll

be arranging for her to meet the new baby as soon as possible —
that she'll be able to come and visit you while you're in the
hospital, if you'll be sticking around for a day or two, or that
you'll be bringing the baby home as soon as you can after the
birth.

If you're intending to bring your child to the hospital with
you for the birth, be sure to check to find out whether you'll be
expected to bring along an extra adult to care for your child.
Some hospital policies specify that there must be another adult
on hand to care for children under a certain age.

 MOM'S THE WORD

"Toward the end of my pregnancy, my biggest concern was who
was going to take care of my 6-year-old if I went into labor in the middle of
the night. It was a really big worry for me."

— *Kathy, 34, mother of two*

MOTHER WISDOM

Don't make the mistake of assuming that you won't need to
arrange care for your older child if you're planning a home birth or if your
child will be present at your hospital birth. Unless he's of the age where he
can pretty much fend for himself (10 or older) you'll want to make sure
there's someone else on hand to answer his questions about the birth
and/or get him something to eat when mealtime rolls around. You certainly
won't be up to the task yourself when you're in the heat of labor, and your
partner is likely to have his hands full dealing with you.

7. **One of my pregnancy books talks about the importance
   of avoiding horrible labor procedures like enemas and
   perineal shaves. Do hospitals still perform these types of
   procedures?**

This is one of the easiest labor-related worries to deal with.
All you have to do is toss out that book! Thankfully, routine enemas and perineal shaves have pretty much gone the way of the

dodo bird, and books that warn you about these types of procedures are simply causing you needless worry.

While doctors used to believe it was necessary to give a pregnant woman an enema in order to empty her bowels (it was
thought that a large amount of stool might stop labor from progressing), we now know that Mother Nature takes care of this
particular problem in her usual efficient manner. The diarrhea
that most women experience during early labor ensures there's
very little left in the bowels by the time a woman is ready to give
birth.

Perineal shaving has become similarly passé. While doctors
used to believe that it was necessary to shave the perineal area in
order to minimize the risk of infection, we now know that doing
so actually increases the chances that an infection will occur.
Besides, don't women who've just given birth have enough discomforts to contend with without having to cope with soreness
and itching in this particular area?

8. My partner wants to set up the baby's room now, but I'm afraid that doing so might jinx my pregnancy.

Pregnancy is positively steeped in superstition, and no matter
how logical you might be about everything else in your life, it's
easy to get caught up in these sorts of irrational worries. The
best way to cope is to talk about your fears with your partner
and try to come to some sort of compromise. Maybe he could
hang the wallpaper and buy the crib, just as long as it remains
unassembled until after the baby arrives.

The same goes with baby showers, by the way. If you'd feel
more comfortable postponing these until after your baby arrives,
spread the word to family members and friends and ask that
they respect your wishes. You might tactfully point out the
advantages of holding the shower after your baby's birth: Instead
of limiting their purchases to ho-hum, middle-of-the-road, unisex sleepers, they'll be able to buy the cutest imaginable pink
polka-dotted party dresses or blue pinstriped overalls instead.

That pitch is guaranteed to win over all the grandmas in the crowd.

9. I just tested positive for group B strep. I really worry about what this means for my baby.

Group B strep is a strain of bacteria carried by 20 to 40% of pregnant women. Most caregivers screen for the bacteria during late pregnancy because it can cause a serious, possibly even fatal, infection in the newborn if it's transmitted from mother to baby during labor. There is also at least a theoretical possibility that group B strep could be transmitted from you to your baby, even if your membranes are still intact. Approximately 2% of babies born to mothers with group B strep will end up developing group B strep disease (a serious condition with a 6% mortality rate). Fortunately, the vast majority of cases of group B strep can be prevented by administering antibiotics to the laboring woman.

If you happen to go into labor prematurely, you have previously given birth to a baby infected with group B strep, you develop a fever during labor, or your membranes rupture more than 18 hours prior to delivery, your caregiver may decide to prescribe antibiotics during your labor whether or not you've been formally diagnosed with group B strep. An ounce of prevention is, after all, worth a pound of cure — especially where group B strep disease is concerned.

10. I'm worried that I won't be a good parent. I don't know a thing about caring for a newborn!

No ifs, ands, or buts about it: Next to wondering about what horrors await you in labor and delivery, this has got to be one of the biggest fears expectant couples face during the final countdown to birth. Something that seemed like a vaguely good idea nine months ago is now an imminent reality!

MOM'S THE WORD

"I thought being pregnant was supposed to be magical. Everyone kept saying how good I looked and that I had that pregnant glow, but I didn't feel that way at all. I was worried about money, health, how my school/career dreams would be affected, and if I'd be a good parent. My partner is very laid-back and was hardly worried at all. His attitude was that we'll deal with it and it will work out. I think that made me worry even more because I felt that I had to compensate for his lack of worry."

— *Bevin, 27, mother of one*

It's easy to let your imagination run wild — to play out all kinds of crazy scenarios in your head. You might imagine yourself going grocery shopping with your baby only to accidentally leave her in the cart, or failing to detect the signs of some life-threatening illness that could have been prevented if only you'd been a little more on the ball.

These types of fears are very common in late pregnancy. If they don't catch up with you by day, they're likely to make cameo appearances in your nightmares. In many ways, these worries are a dress rehearsal for the awesome yet exciting role you're about to take on. Despite what you might think, they're by no means an indication that you're woefully underqualified for the job of parenting!

Don't fall into the trap, by the way, of assuming that everyone else in your prenatal class is far better equipped to care for a newborn than you are. No matter how many hours of babysitting they clocked as a teenager, how many books they've read and how many courses they've taken on the ins and outs of baby care, nothing can fully prepare anyone for the challenges of parenthood. Despite what that obnoxiously overconfident couple in your class may believe, there's no way to cram for this particular final exam.

Prepare yourself for the fact that you're likely to experience a few moments of panic during the early weeks. You'll probably end up checking on the baby an inordinate number of times, just to be sure that she's breathing; you'll likely end up making at least one unnecessary trip to the emergency ward because you're convinced she's developed some life-threatening disease when she's actually just come down with a case of baby acne. It's all part of the early-parenting turf!

But before you know it, you'll be an old pro. You'll wake up one day and realize that you've mastered the art of detecting a fever by placing your hand on your baby's forehead and that you've learned to distinguish between run-of-the-mill diaper explosions and bona fide diarrhea. All you need is a little time in the trenches — and, as we both know, that opportunity is fast approaching. Boot camp is about to begin!

Now that we've talked about the 30 most common pregnancy-related worries, it's time to talk about another perennial source of worry during pregnancy: the ever-changing parade of aches and pains. It's time to hit The Complaint Department.

CHAPTER 8

The Complaint Department

"I found pregnancy to be a state of constant training. I would just get used to one symptom when another symptom would appear. It was nine months of gradually slowing down, becoming more and more focused on the baby, setting new priorities. It's the most wonderful and amazing and exhilarating and exasperating time."

— Lynn, 41, mother of one

We all know at least one woman who managed to breeze through pregnancy without so much as a single ache or pain. You know the kind of person I'm talking about: one of those Ms. Perfect Pregnancies who asks the prenatal instructor if it's normal to feel so peppy during pregnancy! Unfortunately, most of us mere mortals don't end up getting off quite that easily, finding ourselves battling an ever-changing parade of symptoms — everything from morning sickness to leg cramps to insomnia.

In this chapter, we're going to take a look at the entire smorgasbord of pregnancy-related aches and pains that can crop up at some point during the next nine months. (While I've yet to meet a woman who's experienced every single one of these complaints, it's a rare woman indeed who gets off entirely.) First we'll consider which types of complaints may indicate a possible problem with your pregnancy. Then we'll run through the laundry list of pregnancy-related aches and pains that, while annoying, seldom signal any real cause for concern. Finally, we'll touch on a topic that too many pregnancy books tend to ignore: the joys of being pregnant.

What's Normal and What's Not

Over the course of your pregnancy, you're likely to experience a variety of different complaints — everything from fatigue to round ligament pain to Braxton Hicks contractions. Because these symptoms tend to randomly appear and disappear, it can be difficult to get a handle on whether a particular one falls into the "harmless but annoying" category or whether it could indicate a possible problem with your pregnancy.

As a rule, you should call your caregiver immediately if you experience one or more of the symptoms listed in Table 8.1.

Pregnancy Complaints from A to Z

Now that we've covered all the scary stuff in Chapter 7 (I figured we'd get that over with right away so that it wouldn't be hanging over your head), let's talk about the garden-variety pregnancy complaints that you may experience at some point during your pregnancy.

To make it easier for you to find information about these quickly and easily, I've chosen to organize the list of complaints in alphabetical order rather than arbitrarily assigning each complaint to a particular trimester, as some pregnancy book authors like to do. (What these authors seem to forget is that you can't set your watch by the arrival and departure of these various complaints. For example, even though morning sickness is supposed to be a first-trimester problem, some women have trouble with it throughout their entire pregnancy. Remember: There's no such thing as a one-size-fits-all pregnancy.)

TABLE 8.1

WHEN TO CALL YOUR CAREGIVER

Type of Symptom	What It May Indicate
Heavy vaginal bleeding or clotting, or the passage of tissue from the vagina	You may be experiencing a miscarriage. If this happens later in pregnancy (e.g. during the second or third trimesters), you may be experiencing placenta previa or a placental abruption.
Lighter vaginal bleeding that lasts for more than one day, or is accompanied by pain, fever, or chills	You may be experiencing a miscarriage. If this happens later in pregnancy (e.g. during the second or third trimesters), you may be experiencing placenta previa or a placental abruption. What's more, if there's bleeding behind the placenta, you could be developing chorioamnionitis (an infection of the membranes surrounding the fetus).
Severe abdominal or shoulder pain that may be accompanied by spotting or bleeding or the passage of tissue	Your pregnancy may be ectopic (e.g., the embryo may have implanted somewhere other than in the uterus) and you may be experiencing internal bleeding as a result. This typically occurs at six to eight weeks of pregnancy, but can also occur when your pregnancy is a little further along.
A severe or persistent headache (particularly one accompanied by dizziness, faintness, or blurry vision)	You may be developing high blood pressure or pre-eclampsia (a serious medical condition characterized by high blood pressure). See Chapter 11 for details on pre-eclampsia.

continued

Type of Symptom	What It May Indicate (Continued)
Dehydration (dry mouth, thirst, reduced urine output, low-grade fever)	You may be becoming dehydrated, which puts you at risk of experiencing premature labor.
A fever of more than 101 F	You may have an infection that requires treatment. Even if you don't, your caregiver will want to bring your temperature down because an elevated core body temperature can be harmful to the developing baby and may trigger premature labor.
Painful urination	You may have developed a urinary tract infection, which can trigger premature labor and/or lead to a kidney infection.
A watery discharge from the vagina	Your membranes may have ruptured.
Sudden swelling of the face, hands, or feet	You may be developing pre-eclampsia.
The symptoms of premature labor (uterine contractions, vaginal bleeding or discharge, vaginal pressure or pressure in the pelvic area, menstrual-like cramping, a dull backache, stomach or intestinal cramping and gas pains, a general feeling of unwellness)	You may be experiencing premature labor.
A significant decrease in fetal movement after the 24th week of pregnancy	Your baby may be experiencing problems in the womb.

That said, there are certain complaints that tend to be more of a problem during certain trimesters. That's why I've included a chart that indicates when each problem tends to be the most annoying (see Table 8.2). Just do me a favor and take this table with a grain of salt. Who knows? You could very well be the first woman in the world to experience belly button soreness during the first or third trimester.

TABLE 8.2

THE COMPLAINT DEPARTMENT

Pregnancy-Related Complaint	Month During Pregnancy When It's Most Likely to Be a Problem								
	1	2	3	4	5	6	7	8	9
Abdominal muscle separation				X	X	X	X	X	X
Acne	X	X	X	X	X	X	X	X	X
Backache							X	X	X
Belly button soreness					X				
Bleeding gums (pregnancy gingivitis)	X	X	X	X	X	X	X	X	X
Bleeding or spotting	X	X	X						
Braxton Hicks contractions						X	X	X	X
Breast enlargement	X	X	X	X	X	X	X	X	X
Breast tenderness	X	X	X						
Breathlessness							X	X	
Carpal tunnel syndrome				X	X	X	X	X	X
Constipation	X	X	X	X	X	X	X	X	X
Cramping (abdominal)	X								
Cravings	X	X	X						
Edema (fluid retention) and swelling							X	X	X
Eye changes (dryness and vision changes)	X	X	X	X	X	X	X	X	X
Faintness and dizziness	X	X	X	X	X	X	X	X	X

continued

Pregnancy-related Complaint (Continued)	Month During Pregnancy When It's Most Likely to Be a Problem								
	1	2	3	4	5	6	7	8	9
Fatigue	X	X	X				X	X	X
Food aversions	X	X	X	X	X	X	X	X	X
Gas and bloating	X	X	X	X	X	X	X	X	X
Headaches	X	X	X	X	X	X	X	X	X
Heartburn							X	X	X
Hemorrhoids				X	X	X	X	X	X
Hip soreness				X	X	X	X	X	X
Insomnia	X	X	X	X	X	X	X	X	X
Itchiness		X					X	X	X
Leg cramps							X	X	X
Linea nigra (vertical line down center of abdomen)				X	X	X	X	X	X
Mask of pregnancy (chloasma)				X	X	X	X	X	X
Morning sickness	X	X	X						
Perineal aching									X
Pubic bone pain				X	X	X	X	X	X
Rashes							X	X	X
Rhinitis	X	X	X	X	X	X	X	X	X
Round ligament pain				X	X				
Sciatica							X	X	X
Skin changes	X	X	X	X	X	X	X	X	X
Smell, heightened sense of	X	X	X						
Stretch marks							X	X	X
Sweating, increased				X	X	X	X	X	X
Swelling and edema (fluid retention)							X	X	X
Thirstiness	X	X	X	X	X	X	X	X	X
Urinary incontinence (leaking of urine)							X	X	X
Urination, increased frequency of	X	X	X				X	X	X

Pregnancy-related Complaint	Month During Pregnancy When It's Most Likely to Be a Problem								
	1	2	3	4	5	6	7	8	9
Vaginal discharge, increased	X	X	X	X	X	X	X	X	X
Varicose veins							X	X	X
Weepiness	X	X	X	X	X	X	X	X	X
Yeast infections	X	X	X	X	X	X	X	X	X

Now that I've gotten all the necessary disclaimers out of the way, it's time to hit the Complaint Department.

MOTHER WISDOM

There are considerably more aches and pains to deal with during the first and third trimesters than during the second trimester — the so-called "golden age of pregnancy." So if you're planning a pre-baby romantic getaway for you and your partner, you might want to schedule it for smack-dab in the middle of your pregnancy — after the morning sickness has disappeared, but before third-trimester aches and pains kick in!

Abdominal muscle separation

You don't have to be a rocket scientist to figure out why abdominal muscle separation tends to occur during pregnancy. As your uterus grows, it stretches and pushes apart the two large bands of muscle tissue that run down the middle of your abdomen between your ribs and your pelvic bone. The condition is generally painless, although some women will experience some tenderness in the belly-button region. In fact, the only way you'll know that it's occurred is if you notice a loss of abdominal tone in the middle of your belly or if you make a conscious effort to check for muscle separation by poking around in the middle of your abdomen. (If you try to do a sit-up, there will be a bulge in the middle between the two muscles.) After it's occurred during one pregnancy, it becomes progressively worse in subsequent ones. Fortunately, it corrects itself after each pregnancy.

Acne

Think your problem-skin days are a thing of the past? Unfortunately, the hormonal cocktail of pregnancy can cause skin eruptions that you haven't experienced since your teenage years. Fortunately, pregnancy-related acne doesn't last nearly as long as the adolescent variety. It will disappear shortly after the delivery. In the meantime, you can minimize its severity by using an oatmeal-based facial scrub to help unplug oily pores.

 MOTHER WISDOM

Your skin may be going to pot, but chances are you've got great hair. Pregnancy hormones reduce the rate at which your hair falls out, which can leave you sporting a full, lush head of hair until at least a few months after the delivery.

Backache

During the third trimester, approximately 50% of pregnant women experience some degree of back pain. It's caused by the relaxing of the ligaments in your back, the overstretching of your abdominal muscles, and the changes to both your posture and the curvature of your spine, all of which create additional work for the muscles in your back.

You can minimize the amount of back-related pain you experience during pregnancy by taking steps to protect your back. Here are a few tips:

• Don't jog or participate in any other high-impact sport that may be jarring to your spine.

- Exercise caution when you're bending, lifting, or otherwise changing positions. Let someone else lift the heavy objects.

- If you do have to do some lifting, lift with your legs, not your back.

- Rather than trying to sit up when you're lying on your back, roll over onto your side and then push up with your hands.

- Avoid standing or sitting in one position for long periods of time, as this places an added strain on your back. If you can't change positions as often as you should, put one foot on a stool while you're sitting or standing.

- Pay attention to your posture. The classic swayback position of pregnancy doesn't just make you look about 30 pounds heavier (reason enough to tuck in that gut!), it can also wreak havoc on your back.

- Get in the habit of tucking a pillow between your knees and another under your abdomen when you're sleeping on your side. This will help to take some of the pressure off your lower back.

- Give your back, abdominal, hip, and upper body muscles a workout. According to the American College of Obstetricians and Gynecologists, keeping these muscles strong won't just help to ease back pain: It will help to prepare your body for the Mother of All Marathons — giving birth.

Belly button soreness

I know, I know. It sounds like the most ridiculous complaint in the world. But just wait until it happens to you! Around the 20th week of pregnancy, you may experience some extreme tenderness in the belly button area. This is caused by the pressure of the expanding uterus on your belly button. The tenderness tends to subside as your belly grows, so this is one thing you can strike off the complaint list sooner rather than later.

Bleeding gums

Even if you're not usually a card-carrying member of the International Order of Daily Flossers, you might want to think about taking out a membership for at least the duration of your pregnancy. Pregnant women often develop a condition called pregnancy gingivitis, characterized by inflamed and sensitive gums that bleed more easily than usual. In addition to flossing daily and brushing your teeth after every meal using a gentle-bristled toothbrush, you should plan to take the following steps to minimize pregnancy gingivitis:

- See your dentist at least once during your pregnancy. Having the buildup of plaque that collects at the bottom of your teeth scraped off can help to reduce the severity of your symptoms.

- Rinse your mouth with antiseptic mouthwash several times a day. That will help to keep your mouth sparkling clean.

- Choose foods such as fruit and vegetables that are rich in vitamin C — something that helps to promote healthy gums.

FACTS AND FIGURES

Don't be alarmed if you develop tiny nodules on your gums that tend to bleed easily. These nodules — known as pyogenic granulomas (pregnancy tumors) — are harmless, non-cancerous growths. They usually disappear on their own after you give birth, but if they're causing you a lot of grief in the meantime, your dentist can remove them.

Bleeding and spotting

Any type of vaginal bleeding can be worrisome during pregnancy, but sometimes the light bleeding or spotting you experience is completely harmless and not a symptom of an impending miscarriage. About seven days after conception (when you're three weeks pregnant, counting from the first day of your last menstrual period), you may experience a bit of light bleeding or spotting as the fertilized embryo first implants itself in the uterine wall ("implantation bleeding"). Light bleeding can also occur if the cervix happens to get bumped during intercourse or accidentally grazed during a pelvic exam. While you should always report any vaginal bleeding or spotting to your caregiver, there's generally less cause for concern if the bleeding is very light (unless, of course, you're experiencing cramping at the same time, in which case you could be experiencing a miscarriage). If, however, you experience bleeding later in pregnancy, you'll want to get in touch with your doctor or midwife right away. (See Chapter 7 for a more detailed discussion of bleeding during pregnancy.)

Braxton Hicks contractions

This is the name given to the irregular contractions that occur during the last half of pregnancy. (Just a quick bit of pregnancy trivia: The contractions are named after John Braxton Hicks, M.D., the British doctor who first described them back in 1872.)

While these contractions happen from early pregnancy onward as your uterus begins to train for the main event (labor!), you generally can't feel them until the mid-second or early third trimester. Typically lasting for 45 seconds or less, they feel as if someone has momentarily put a blood pressure cuff around your abdomen and then pumped it up. While these contractions can be quite worrying, the cocktail of hormones of early pregnancy helps to prevent these harmless contractions from progressing into full-blown labor.

Toward the end of pregnancy, they become increasingly uncomfortable and sometimes even painful. In fact, some women have such powerful Braxton Hicks contractions that they have a hard time distinguishing them from "the real thing." They're more likely to be bothersome during subsequent pregnancies, although, like everything else pregnancy-related, that rule isn't necessarily carved in stone.

Breast tenderness and enlargement

The changes that a woman's breasts undergo during pregnancy have to be seen to be believed. One minute you're a woman with an average-sized bosom. The next, you're doing a darned good impression of Pamela Anderson!

Okay, I'm exaggerating a little. The changes generally aren't quite that dramatic. But be forewarned: You're in for a few surprises in the breast department over the next nine months. Let me give you a sneak preview:

- Bigger. You can expect your breasts to grow by one full cup size by the end of your first trimester and by another full cup size by the time you give birth.

- Bolder. You'll also notice some changes to the appearance of your breasts. The areola — the flat area around the nipple — begins to darken; the tiny glands on the areola begin to enlarge and start excreting a lubricating antibacterial oil; and the veins on your breasts begin to look like tiny rivers on a road map. (Your veins are going haywire because of the increased blood flow to your breasts.)

- Super-sensitive. Soon after the pregnancy test becomes positive, your breasts may become sore and swollen. They may feel fuller, tingly, and more sensitive (e.g. taking a simple shower becomes excrutiating!), and you may find yourself experiencing the odd throbbing or shooting pain. The thought of sleeping on your stomach is simply out of the question. (Don't get your heart set on sleeping on your stomach once the extreme tenderness begins to subside, however. By then your growing belly will be well on its way to making tummy-sleeping a virtual impossibility.)

Breathlessness

It's like that song the '50s rocker Jerry Lee Lewis used to sing: "You leave me breathless! Oh baby!" But in this case it actually is a baby that's causing your breathlessness.

As your pregnancy progresses, pressure from your growing uterus makes it increasingly difficult for you to breathe easily. You get a bit of relief when your baby's head begins to descend into your pelvis (during the last month of pregnancy), but you can ease the discomfort in the meantime by using an extra pillow when you're sleeping. (For some reason, breathlessness tends to be particularly annoying at night — yet another tool that Mother Nature uses to prepare you for the sleepless nights of early parenthood!)

To make matters worse, high levels of progesterone leave you feeling short of breath, something that triggers the desire to breathe more deeply. (Is it any wonder that most women heave a sigh of relief when the nine months of pregnancy finally come to an end?!)

FACTS AND FIGURES

Over the course of your pregnancy, your rib cage becomes a few inches wider than usual in order to accommodate the added capacity of your lungs. You're not just eating for two, after all. You're also breathing for two.

Carpal tunnel syndrome

This condition is characterized by numbness or tingling in the hands (either "pins and needles" or an outright burning sensation); pain in the wrist that can shoot all the way up to the shoulder; cramping or stiffness in the hands; weakness in the thumb; and a tendency to drop things. It's relatively common during pregnancy and results from a pinched nerve in the wrist.

In most cases, carpal tunnel syndrome disappears on its own shortly after you give birth. (A few moms do require surgery to correct the problem, however.) While you're waiting for delivery day to roll around you can minimize the discomfort by elevating the affected hand or wearing a plastic wrist splint at night.

Constipation

It's hardly surprising that so many women have trouble with constipation during pregnancy. High levels of progesterone cause the muscles of the intestine to function far less efficiently than normal, resulting in dry, hard stools and infrequent bowel movements.

Fortunately, there's plenty you can do to alleviate this particular complaint. Most pregnant women find the problem takes care of itself if they drink plenty of water, consume large quantities of high-fiber foods, exercise regularly, and use the bathroom as soon as the need arises.

FACTS AND FIGURES

Scientists believe there may be a benefit to having a sluggish intestine during pregnancy. After all, the longer the food remains in your intestine, the more nutrients your body is able to absorb.

Note: If you're taking an iron supplement, it may be adding to your constipation problems. Try taking it on a full stomach and washing it down with plenty of liquids. If that doesn't work, you might want to fall back on the anti-constipation remedy that worked for your grandmother: Two tablespoons of unsulphured blackstrap molasses dissolved in a glass of warm water.

Cramping

It's not unusual to experience period-like cramping (but without any accompanying bleeding) around the time your first menstrual period is due. The cramping is caused by the hormonal changes of early pregnancy and your body's response to the stretching of the uterine muscle, and is considered harmless unless it's accompanied by heavy bleeding (a possible symptom of miscarriage) or a sharp pain on one side of your abdomen (a possible sign of an ectopic pregnancy).

Note: Severe abdominal pain can also be caused by appendicitis, a gallbladder attack, the stretching of adhesions from previous abdominal surgery, or preterm labor, so it's important to get in touch with your caregiver immediately if the pain you're experiencing is severe or long lasting.

Cravings

Some experts pooh-pooh the whole idea of cravings during pregnancy, claiming that they're all in a pregnant woman's head. Others argue that they're actually Mother Nature's way of ensuring you get the nutrients you need. (Of course, this particular argument doesn't do much to explain why some women develop cravings for road salt and other inedible substances during pregnancy — a disorder known as pica.)

One thing the experts do agree on, however, is that cravings can get you into a lot of trouble if you use them as an excuse for overeating during pregnancy — something to bear in mind the next time a truckload of Krispy Kreme doughnuts starts calling your name.

Eye changes

You already know that the changes triggered by pregnancy are rather far-reaching. What you might not realize, however, is that even your eyeballs can be affected.

I know this sounds too crazy to be real, but bear with me while I explain. The fluid retention that occurs during pregnancy changes the shape of your eyeballs, which can cause some pregnant woman to become increasingly nearsighted. And rising levels of estrogen can lead to a condition called dry eye, characterized by dryness and burning, blurred vision, and increased sensitivity to light. (If you find yourself suffering from this latter condition, you'll have to use an artificial-tears product to restore moisture to your eyes and you'll need to wear sunglasses whenever you're out in the sun.) Fortunately, both conditions correct themselves after you give birth, but that can be small solace if eye problems are driving you crazy and you're not even out of your first trimester yet.

Note: Vision problems can also be an indicator of diabetes, so be sure to report any symptoms to your caregiver.

Faintness and dizziness

While the soap opera scriptwriters typically have the heroine fainting long before the pregnancy test comes back positive, real pregnant women don't tend to experience much fainting and dizziness until they're well into their second or third trimesters, when their rapidly expanded blood volume can lead to a decrease in blood pressure. Then, to make matters worse, pressure from the uterus on the major blood vessels in the abdomen during the third trimester can slow the rate of the return of blood to the upper half of the body.

You're less likely to have problems with faintness and dizziness if you

- avoid standing in one position for a prolonged period of time (the blood pools in the lower part of the body, away from your brain)

- don't allow yourself to become overheated

- get up slowly if you've had a hot bath or if you've been sitting or lying down (your cardiovascular system doesn't react as quickly when you're pregnant)

- avoid hypoglycemia and its resulting dizziness by eating at least every two hours and by limiting the number of sugary foods you consume

Fatigue

Fatigue is Mother Nature's way of reminding you that you're pregnant. If you didn't slow down a little, your body would have a hard time directing your energy to where it's needed most — growing a baby. You feel tired because of the increased production of progesterone (which acts as a natural sedative) and the increase in your body's metabolic rate (your body's way of making sure it can provide for the needs of your growing baby).

Some women are shocked by how exhausted they feel during the early weeks of pregnancy. That was certainly the case for Jennifer, a 32-year-old mother of one: "Being so drop-dead tired took me by surprise and reduced me to tears at first. Once I realized and accepted that this was my body's way of dealing with the massive task ahead, I was okay. I lessened my work schedule where I could and gave myself permission to be tired. I also allowed myself to fall asleep whenever I wanted, provided, of course, I wasn't driving or in public!"

The best way to cope with fatigue is to get the rest your body is craving. Hit the hay an hour or two earlier at night and try to squeeze in a nap at some point during the day — either during your lunch hour or afternoon break or after you arrive home from work.

Food aversions

Don't be surprised if the hormones of early pregnancy end up affecting your taste buds. You may experience a mildly metallic taste in your mouth that can make your morning cup of tea or coffee taste downright repulsive. (Maybe it's Mother Nature's way of helping you to kick your caffeine habit.)

Unfortunately, these food aversions are often accompanied by a heightened sense of smell and increased salivation, something that can add to your misery.

Gassiness and bloating

The increased levels of progesterone in your body make your intestines more sluggish during pregnancy, which can cause both gassiness and bloating. The problem tends to be aggravated during the first trimester by the tendency to swallow air as a means of relieving nausea.

Here are tips on minimizing the amount of gassiness and bloating you experience during pregnancy:

- Keep your bowels moving. Drink plenty of liquids, eat a variety of high-fiber foods, and make exercise part of your regular routine. Your body has to push food through your 22-foot-long intestines, so it needs all the help it can get.

- Eat slowly and avoid sipping hot beverages and soup in order to minimize the amount of air you swallow.

- Choose your food wisely. Avoid gas-producing foods such as cabbage, broccoli, cauliflower, Brussels sprouts, beans, green peppers, carbonated beverages, and fried and greasy foods. (High-fat foods are harder to digest, so they stay in your intestines longer, adding to your gas problems.)

Headaches

Headaches are another common pregnancy-related complaint. Some women, like Lori, consider them to be the worst aspect of being pregnant. "They were so severe and I suffered from them every single day from about my third month to about my seventh or eighth month, when they would ease up but not go away completely," the 29-year-old mother of four recalls. "They were just horrible."

While the only true cure for what ails you is giving birth, there are a few things you can do in the meantime to minimize the pain:

- Try to avoid getting headaches in the first place. Little things like changing your position slowly, eating every couple of hours so that you keep your blood sugar stable, and getting plenty of fresh air can help to prevent headaches.

- If you feel a tension headache coming on, apply an ice pack to your forehead right away. This will cause the blood vessels to contract, which will generally help to eliminate your headache within about 20 minutes — roughly the same amount of time it takes a typical painkiller to kick in.

- Put a hot water bottle on your feet. This will cause the blood vessels in your feet to dilate, drawing the blood toward your feet and away from your head.

- Have your partner massage your feet. Since the big toe is the acupuncture point for the head, this can help to relieve your headache.

- If you need to take a pain killer, go for acetaminophen rather than any product containing acetylsalicylic acid (ASA). When taken in large doses close to term, ASA can lead to blood clotting problems that can cause excessive bleeding in the mother and/or the baby. ASA use during pregnancy is also thought to be linked to low birth weight, prolonged gestation and labor, and cardiac problems in the newborn. (Note: There are certain medical conditions that are treated with ASA. If you have such a condition and your doctor recommends that you continue with your ASA regime, it is because the benefits of using ASA outweigh the risks of complications for you and your baby.)

Note: If you experience a severe headache, particularly one that's accompanied by blurry vision, get in touch with your caregiver immediately. You could be developing high blood pressure or pre-eclampsia.

FACTS AND FIGURES

Wondering how pregnancy will affect your migraines? Only time will tell. One-third of migraine sufferers find that their symptoms improve during pregnancy, one-third find that they worsen, and one-third find that they stay the same.

Heartburn

The hormonal changes of pregnancy are to blame for yet another common complaint — heartburn. High levels of progesterone in the body cause the valve at the entrance to the stomach to relax, which can allow stomach acid to pass back up into the esophagus (the tube leading into your stomach) and cause a strong burning sensation in the center of your chest and/or increased burping.

You can minimize your heartburn problems by

- eating smaller, more frequent meals

- avoiding spicy or fried foods

- drinking a glass of milk before you eat (coating your stomach may reduce the amount of acid burn you experience)

- not eating too close to bedtime (you should plan to sit up for at least half an hour after eating in order to give the food in your stomach a chance to digest)

- keeping your head well elevated while you're sleeping

- asking your doctor or midwife to recommend an antacid or medication that's safe for use during pregnancy

Hemorrhoids

Hemorrhoids — itching, soreness, and pain or bleeding in the tissue around your anus when you empty your bowels — are yet another common pregnancy complaint. They occur when pressure from the baby's head causes the veins around the anus to swell. (Just think of them as varicose veins that have shown up in a rather tender part of your anatomy!)

While mild hemorrhoids tend to go away on their own after the baby is born, more severe hemorrhoids may require minor surgery to repair.

Here are some tips on coping with the discomfort of hemorrhoids during pregnancy:

- Avoid straining when you're having a bowel movement, standing for long periods of time, or sitting for long stretches on hard surfaces. Each of these situations can cause your hemorrhoids to worsen.

- Keep the area around your anus clean. Gently wash it after each bowel movement by using either soft, undyed, unscented toilet paper (to avoid irritation), alcohol-free baby wipes, or hygienic witch hazel pads.

- You can relieve the itching of hemorrhoids by applying an ice pack to the affected area or by using an ointment that's been prescribed by your doctor.

FACTS AND FIGURES

Wondering what causes hemorrhoids to become a problem during pregnancy? Blame it on progesterone and your growing uterus. Progestrone causes the vein walls to relax and the growing uterus restricts the return of blood from the lower half of the body to the heart, causing the veins encircling the anal area to enlarge.

Hip soreness

It's also not unusual to experience some soreness in your hips during pregnancy, particularly when you're sleeping on your side at night. The ligaments in your hips stretch and the cartilage softens in preparation for the birth of your baby, which can cause minor hip pain and contribute to that classic pregnancy "waddle."

Insomnia

Sleeping problems are extremely common during pregnancy — the one time in your life when you could really use a good night's sleep! Whether it's anxiety about the upcoming birth, the nighttime trips to the bathroom, your baby's nocturnal gymnastics routine, or the physical challenges of finding a comfortable sleeping position when you've got a watermelon strapped to your belly, you're likely to encounter at least a few sleeping problems at some point during your pregnancy.

You can help to minimize your sleep problems by

- practicing good "sleep hygiene" (going to bed at a regular time, getting up at a regular time, and watching the number of naps you sneak in during the day)

- limiting your caffeine intake or kicking your caffeine habit altogether

- enjoying a mug of warm milk (with cinnamon and honey or sugar, if it tastes too bland on its own) or a cup of herbal tea before you go to bed (milk contains an amino acid that can make you sleepy, and herbal teas like chamomile can help you to unwind)

- exercising regularly (sleep experts have found that 20 to 30 minutes of exercise five days a week can really help to reduce the severity of insomnia)

- not consuming large quantities of liquids within two hours of going to bed (to help minimize the number of middle-of-the-night treks to the bathroom)

- skipping that late-evening snack (eating right before bed boosts your metabolism, which can keep you awake)

- taking time to relax and unwind before you go to bed (listening to soothing music, reading a book, or taking a warm bath)

- keeping your room at a comfortable temperature — neither too hot nor too cold

- surrounding yourself with pillows (tuck one under your belly and one between your legs when you're sleeping on your side to minimize hip and back soreness)

 FACTS AND FIGURES

Think you're the only mom-to-be who's tossing and turning at night? Think again. Researchers at Saint Joseph's University in Pennsylvania found that 97 of pregnant women report having their sleep disrupted at least once per night during the final weeks of pregnancy.

Itching

When you consider how much the skin on your abdomen has to stretch during pregnancy, it's hardly surprising that so many pregnant women have problems with abdominal itching. While the problem tends to correct itself shortly after you give birth and your abdomen returns to its normal size, it can drive you crazy in the meantime. You can reduce the severity of any itching you're experiencing by avoiding strong soaps and rubbing cocoa butter cream and other moisturizers on the affected areas of your belly.

Just one quick word of caution before you reach for the cocoa butter: Don't slather on the creams and lotions right before your prenatal checkup. These substances can interfere with sound transmission when your caregiver is trying to detect your baby's heartbeat — something that can cause your own heart to skip a beat or two!

MOM'S THE WORD

"Toward the end of my pregnancy, sometimes my tummy would itch like crazy. I used to warm some olive oil in the microwave and slowly rub it on my tummy while talking and singing to the baby. It felt absolutely wonderful, and the baby seemed to enjoy the massage. These were powerful bonding moments between mother and child."

— *Alexandra, 33, mother of two*

Leg cramps

Leg cramps are those painful muscle contractions (typically in your calves and your feet) that tend to occur in the middle of the night. They can be totally excruciating, so you'll want to do whatever you can to avoid them: making sure you're consuming adequate amounts of calcium (some experts think the cramps are triggered by a calcium deficiency), and try soaking in a warm tub and stretching out your calf muscles before going to bed (pull your toes up toward your knees while pushing your heel away from you).

If you feel a cramp coming on, point your toes upward toward your knee while pushing your heel downward. Whatever you do, don't make the mistake of pointing your toes or you'll be hit with a massive cramp in the back of your calf. If the cramp does set in, massage the affected area and then walk around on it to improve circulation to the area.

Linea nigra

The term "linea nigra" refers to the brownish line that can show up on your abdomen during pregnancy. (I say "can" because it isn't visible on all women.) The linea nigra — which runs down the middle of your abdomen, from above your belly button to the top of your pubic bone — appears as a result of skin pigment changes during pregnancy (see below). It generally disappears shortly after the birth.

Mask of pregnancy

The term "mask of pregnancy" (chloasma) is used to describe the brownish patch of skin that tends to show up on the face and the neck during pregnancy. Like the linea nigra, it's caused by skin pigmentation changes and tends to disappear shortly after the birth. You can lessen the extent of these changes by avoiding direct sunlight.

While we're talking skin changes, here's something else you need to know: It's not unusual for moles, birthmarks, scars, and freckles to darken during pregnancy.

Morning sickness

What pregnancy book would be complete without a detailed discussion of morning sickness? After all, morning sickness is one of the most annoying pregnancy-related conditions, and definitely one of the most common, affecting between 60 and 80% of pregnant women.

Before we get into a detailed discussion of morning sickness, however, let's talk a bit about the name. While morning sickness does tend to be most severe in the morning, some women experience nausea and vomiting at other times of the day, too — which helps to explain why a growing number of health authorities are ditching the term "morning sickness" and choosing to go with the more medically accurate term "nausea and vomiting of pregnancy" instead.

 MOM'S THE WORD

"At different times, different 'remedies' would calm my stomach. I'd keep cycling through my bag of tricks until something worked: crackers, potato chips, ginger ale, wrist bands, walking in fresh air, getting plenty of rest. We couldn't use garlic until I made it to the second trimester!"

— *Lynn, 41, mother of one*

MOTHER WISDOM

"Morning sickness . . . is the result of an irritation in the womb, caused by some derangement, and it is greatly irritated by the habit of indulging in sexual gratification during pregnancy. If people would imitate the lower animals and reserve the vital forces of the mother for the benefit of her unborn child, it would be a great boon to humanity."

— *B.G. Jeffris and J.L. Nichols, Safe Counsel or Practical Eugenics, an 1893 sex manual*

Bevin, a 27-year-old mother of one, supports the name change: "Morning sickness: Who came up with that term anyway? I was sick morning, noon, and night — sometimes even in the middle of the night when I was sleeping — for the first three months."

Bevin is fortunate that her morning sickness decided to exit on cue. While it tends to be at its worst for most women between the seventh and twelfth weeks of pregnancy, approximately 20% of women experience it beyond that point — and some struggle with it for their entire pregnancy.

Here are some tips on coping with morning sickness:

- Don't allow yourself to get too hungry. Eat smaller, more frequent meals and snack more often. An empty stomach can make nausea worse, which helps to explain why it tends to be more of a problem in the morning than later in the day.

- Don't overeat. Having a stuffed belly will only add to your feelings of nausea.

- Don't have fluids at mealtimes. Some women find that eating and drinking at the same time can trigger nausea. Just make sure you make up for these lost fluids at other times of the day, since dehydration can also cause nausea!

- Eat something before you get out of bed and start moving around in the morning — you're less likely to get sideswiped by a wave of nausea.

- Identify your triggers and avoid them. You may find that you feel perfectly well unless you encounter an offending food (something high-fat and greasy) or odor (perfume, cigarette smoke, coffee, and strong cooking smells are perennial offenders). Some experts advise that you eat your meals next to an open window in order to minimize the number of odors you're exposed to while you're eating.

- Watch when you're taking your prenatal vitamin. If you're taking it on an empty stomach, you're asking for trouble. Try taking it in the middle of a meal instead.

- Choose stomach-friendly foods like yogurt and low-fat, high-carbohydrate foods.

- Avoid hard-to-digest foods like sausages, onion rings, and other fatty fried foods.

- Experiment until you find one or more foods that appeal to you. You may discover that certain categories of foods — salty, bitter, crunchy, sweet, spicy, hot, cold, or thick, for example — also appeal. (See Table 8.3 for suggestions.)

- Don't force yourself to eat foods that make you gag (see Table 8.3) just because they're good for you. It's better to survive on crackers and rice cakes alone than to upchuck all the nutrient-rich veggies you forced yourself to knock back at dinnertime. ("One week, I lived primarily on McDonald's french fries and Kraft Dinner," confesses Jennifer, a 32-year-old mother of one. "That shot my healthy eating plan all to hell, but those were the only two foods that seemed to calm the queasies and leave me feeling satisfied.") You'll have plenty of time to reach for those nutrient-rich foods later in your pregnancy. In the meantime, your baby is drawing upon the stores that you built up before you conceived — the stockpile that Mother Nature saw to in anticipation of just such a "famine."

- Avoid pants with belts and other types of tight-fitting clothing. They'll only add to your discomfort. You may even find that wearing brief-style underwear is too uncomfortable, in which case you may want to switch to bikini style or hip-huggers instead.

- Pick up a set of anti-nausea wrist bands (also known as "sea bands") at your local maternity store. They're designed to apply constant pressure to the acupuncture pressure points on the wrist that control nausea and can therefore help to reduce the severity of your morning sickness.

TABLE 8.3

BITE-SIZED SOLUTIONS: FOODS THAT DECREASE OR INCREASE NAUSEA

Food Group	Stomach-friendly Food Choices	Foods That Tend to Aggravate Morning Sickness
Grain products	Rice cakes, soda crackers, bagels, pasta, cereal, oatmeal	Spicy, high-fat crackers
Fruits and vegetables	Lemons (for sucking on or sniffing), bananas, applesauce, rhubarb, grapes, watermelon, pears, papaya juice, potatoes (baked, boiled, or mashed), avocados, celery sticks, carrot sticks, zucchini, tomatoes	Onions, cabbage, cauliflower
Milk products	Yogurt smoothies, frozen yogurt, puddings	High-fat cheeses
Meat and alternatives	Sunflower seeds	Fried meats, greasy foods, high-fat meats (sausages), fried eggs, spicy foods, foods containing monosodium glutamate (MSG)
Other foods	Ginger (root extract, fresh-ground, capsules, tea, sticks, crystals, pickled, and in other forms), raspberry leaf tea, mints (especially peppermint), lemon drops, licorice, potato chips, chewing gum, pickles, chamomile tea, lemonade, carbonated mineral water with a twist of lemon, sherbet	High-fat foods (e.g., french fries), fried foods (e.g., onion rings), spicy foods (e.g. corn chips), and beverages containing caffeine (e.g., coffee and cola)

- Carry around a slice of lemon inside a small plastic bag. Some women find that sniffing lemon helps to settle their heaving stomach. Other women report similar effects from mint or grated ginger root.

- Know when to seek medical attention. Approximately 1% of pregnant women develop a severe form of morning sickness known as hyperemesis gravidarum, a condition in which vomiting is severe enough to cause weight loss, dehydration, electrolyte imbalances, and other serious and potentially life-threatening complications.

- Don't play the martyr unnecessarily. If you're suffering from a severe case of morning sickness, you may want to talk to your doctor about the advisability of taking an anti-nausea medication that is considered safe for use during pregnancy.

MOM'S THE WORD

"The morning sickness (aka all day and most of the night sickness) was terrible. Nothing alleviated the symptoms entirely. After about three weeks I started taking a medication, which took the edge off the nausea but didn't get rid of it entirely. Eating small amounts on an hourly basis helped a lot. Soda crackers did not help: They made me feel worse!"

— *Janet, 32, mother of one*

It's easy to think that if you're feeling so ill it must mean there's something wrong with your pregnancy, but quite the opposite is true: Studies have shown that women with little or no morning sickness are two to three times as likely to miscarry as those who are feeling totally wretched. What's more, they're more likely to experience a premature birth. (Just a couple of little thoughts to cheer you the next time you find yourself hugging the toilet bowl.)

MOM'S THE WORD

"At about 3 months, I woke up one morning and I wasn't sick any more. I waited and waited, and nothing happened. You'd think I'd have been thrilled about this, but at first I was a little worried. As long as I was sick, I knew the baby was growing and all was well, since hCG [human chorionic gonadotropin] is thought to be what causes the sickness."

— *Jennifer, 27, currently pregnant with her first child*

FACTS AND FIGURES

A recent study in Sweden found that women who experience severe nausea and vomiting during the first trimester are more likely to give birth to a girl. The researchers found that 55.7% of women admitted to the hospital for severe morning sickness were carrying female babies. They believe that high levels of human chorionic gonadotropin (a hormone found in larger concentrations in female babies) may help to explain why these women are more likely to have such severe morning sickness. Of course, before you paint the nursery pink, you'll want to keep in mind that not all scientists subscribe to this theory!

MOM'S THE WORD

"I tried everything before turning to medication to stop the nausea: crackers, flat pop, fruit, small meals, everything that was suggested in any book, and I finally discovered about two months later that, of all things, pepperoni sticks seemed to help."

— *Bevin, 27, mother of one*

Perineal aching

Feel like you're carrying a bowling ball with your perineum? You're not alone. It's not at all unusual to experience aching, pressure, or sharp twinges in the perineal area during late pregnancy. Perineal aching tends to occur during the last month of pregnancy, once the baby's head has descended into the pelvis.

Those Kegel exercises that your prenatal instructor likes to rave about can help to strengthen your perineal muscles, readying them for the challenges of labor.

Pubic-bone pain

While pubic-bone pain is a seldom-mentioned pregnancy-related complaint, it's troublesome to some women nonetheless. The pain is caused by the loosening of the cartilage that joins the two pubic bones together in the middle of your pelvic area. Consider what Chris, a 36-year-old mother of three, has to say about what she experienced during her last pregnancy: "I had excruciating pain at the front of my pubic bone that got worse with each pregnancy. With my second, I could hardly walk after the birth."

While pubic-bone pain disappears on its own after you give birth, sometimes it doesn't disappear quite as quickly as you'd like, so be prepared for some continued tenderness during the first few weeks postpartum.

Rashes

Some women develop rashes during pregnancy. These rashes — which are particularly common in overweight women — are most likely to occur in the sweaty skin folds under the breasts or in the groin area and are caused by a fungal infection known as intertrigo. The best way to cope with intertrigo is by wearing loose-fitting cotton clothing (to reduce sweating), washing and drying the affected areas frequently (using non-perfumed soap to minimize irritation), and applying calamine lotion, baking soda, or zinc oxide powder to the affected areas. This will both relieve the itching and help to decrease some of the moisture in the area. Note: It's important to treat intertrigo early. Left untreated, it can become superinfected with yeast and will require treatment with a specific antifungal cream.

Approximately one in every 150 pregnant women will develop a particularly miserable rash known as pruritic uriticarial papules and plaques of pregnancy (PUPP) — a condition characterized by itchy, reddish, raised patches on the skin. The condition tends to run in families and is more common in first pregnancies. It can be treated with oral medications, anti-itching creams, oatmeal or baking-soda baths, and, in particularly severe cases, cortisone or prednisone, but the most effective cure for this condition is giving birth.

Approximately one in every 500 to 1,000 pregnant women will develop a potentially serious condition called intrapepatic cholestasis of pregnancy. Women with this condition experience severe itchiness caused by a buildup of bile acids in the liver and bloodstream. If you develop this type of rash, your caregiver will want to monitor you closely for the duration of your pregnancy because some studies have shown a link between intrapepatic cholestasis of pregnancy and stillbirth, preterm labor, fetal distress, and postpartum hemorrhage. Researchers at the University of Birmingham in the U.K. believe the disorder is underdiagnosed and that it may be responsible for as many as 4 to 5% of unexplained stillbirths.

MOM'S THE WORD

"During the last two weeks of pregnancy, I broke out in a full body rash. It was extremely itchy, particularly as time went on. I couldn't sleep. Scratching made it worse. I had prescription cream, Aveeno cream, Aveeno oatmeal baths, and baking soda baths. I would get relief for an hour or so and then the itching would start again. Once I gave birth, the rash went away. Hurray!"

— *Teagan, 32, mother of one*

Restless legs syndrome (RLS)

The term "restless legs syndrome" (RLS) describes a variety of unpleasant sensations in the legs: creeping, crawling, tingling, burning, or aching in the calves, thighs, feet, or in the upper portions of the legs. It tends to be most annoying when you're resting, particularly at night, and may even be accompanied by nighttime leg twitching.

The best way to cope with the discomforts of restless legs syndrome is by exercising early in the day, avoiding caffeine, and taking a warm bath and massaging your legs before you go to bed.

Rhinitis

Feel like you've had a runny nose since the moment the pregnancy test came back positive? You're probably suffering from rhinitis — a swelling of the mucus membranes in the nose that's triggered by both your increased blood volume and all the pregnancy-related hormones raging through your body. If your stuffy nose is driving you crazy, you can get temporary relief by using an over-the-counter saline nose spray or steaming your face and nose area with a facial steamer. The best cure, of course, is having your baby: Most women find their rhinitis disappears shortly after they give birth.

Some women also have trouble with nosebleeds during pregnancy. They're typically caused by increased blood flow but can also be a symptom of high blood pressure, so you'll definitely want to let your caregiver know if you're experiencing these.

MOM'S THE WORD

"I had a stuffed-up nose for eight months straight. Then, the day after I delivered, my nose cleared. It was the best feeling in the world, being able to breathe again."

— *Stephanie, 27, mother of one*

Round ligament pain

We talked a bit about round ligament pain back in Chapter 7, but it's worth mentioning again because it tends to be one of the more alarming (although absolutely harmless) pregnancy-related complaints. Round ligament pain is the name given to that awful ripping sensation you experience if you roll over in bed or otherwise change your position too suddenly. Caused by the sudden stretching of the ligaments and muscles that support the uterus, it tends to be at its worst during the first half of the second trimester, when the uterus is large enough to exert pressure on the ligaments, but not yet large enough to rest some of its weight on the nearby pelvic bones.

The best way to cope with round ligament pain is by supporting your belly and moving slowly and carefully when you're changing positions. If you do end up experiencing some pain, you'll find that soaking in a warm tub can help to ease some of the discomfort.

 MOTHER WISDOM

Wish you could tote that heavy uterus around in a sling? A maternity support belt could be the answer to your prayers. Although cumbersome and expensive, these "abdominal bras" help to hold the uterus in place. They're ideal for women with oversized uteruses — women who are carrying more than one baby, or who have fibroids, for example — but they can also provide welcome relief to mothers whose abdominal muscles have long since given up the ghost (e.g., some women who are giving birth for the third or subsequent time).

Sciatica

Sciatica is the name given to the shooting pain, tingling, or numbness that many women experience in their lower backs, buttocks, outer thighs, and legs during pregnancy. (Typically, you'll experience a pain that shoots down your leg to a point below your knee.) It occurs when the baby's head, the enlarging uterus, or the relaxed pelvic joints press down on the major nerves that run from the backbone through the pelvis and toward each leg. After it flares up it can be aggravated by lifting, bending, and even walking.

If you're having trouble with sciatica, you may want to start seeing a chiropractor on a regular basis. Chiropractic treatments can help to relieve some of the pain and discomfort. The only catch is that you have to keep going on a regular basis in order to keep your sciatica under control. Still, if you're hobbling around, unable to put your full weight on your affected leg, trekking off to the chiropractor a few times a week seems like a small price to pay for becoming mobile again.

You can also eliminate a lot of the discomfort of sciatica by changing positions regularly during the day (e.g., getting up and moving around at least once an hour) and by hitting the swimming pool. Floating around in the pool helps to temporarily take the weight of your uterus off your sciatic nerve, a source of much-welcome relief.

MOM'S THE WORD

"During my second pregnancy, starting around the fifth month, I had a lot of problems with my sciatic nerve. It was so bad that there were days when I couldn't walk without crying from the pain, and nights when I had to crawl up the stairs to get to bed. When I was pregnant for the third time, the pain started almost immediately. I went for massage therapy, and the massage got rid of the pain altogether."

— *Lana, 33, mother of three*

Skin changes

We've already talked about a few of the other skin-related problems that you may experience during pregnancy: the so-called "mask of pregnancy"; the linea nigra (that attractive brown line right down the center of your belly!); the darkening of moles, freckles, and scars; and skin rashes galore. Here are a few other types of skin changes you may notice during pregnancy:

- Palmar erythema: The palms of your hands and the soles of your feet may take on a reddish hue. These skin changes are triggered by hormones and disappear spontaneously after the birth.

- Spider veins: Hormonal changes and the increased blood volume can cause spider nevi (spider veins) to pop out on your face, arms, and upper body during pregnancy. Petichiae, small blood spots in the skin or in the whites of your eye that can appear if you push too intensely during delivery. (Labor's hard work, but you don't have to go totally crazy during the pushing stage.) These spider veins usually become less prominent after the delivery, but if they don't, a dermatologist can treat them. Unfortunately, your health plan may not cover the cost of this cosmetic procedure and — to add insult to injury — the spider veins may recur if you become pregnant again, or gain weight, or as you grow older.

- Skin tags: You may develop a series of skin tags (tiny polyps that occur in areas of the body where the skin rubs against your clothing or against itself — in the folds of your neck, along your bra lines, and so on). While these skin tags may disappear a few months after you give birth, they can be annoying in the meantime. If they're causing you a lot of discomfort, you might want to talk to your doctor about the possibility of having them removed. (Once again, you may be on the hook for the cost of this procedure because most health plans don't cover skin-tag removal.)

Smell, heightened sense of

Find yourself being hit by a wave of nausea each time you smell coffee, cigarette smoke, or strong perfume? That's because most women develop a heightened sense of smell during pregnancy. Janis, 31, remembers this as one of the most annoying things she experienced during her pregnancy: "Odors drove me around the bend. I could barely stand to walk down my apartment hall and smell various foods cooking. I was also sensitive to my husband's breath, which seemed so unbearable some nights I felt like sleeping on the couch!"

You'll probably find that your heightened sense of smell is less likely to trigger nausea once the peak period of morning sickness passes (around the end of the first trimester, for most women). In the meantime, you might want to try an old trick: carrying around a handkerchief that's been dipped in lemon juice. Not only does the powerful lemon scent help to block other offending odors, it can also help to relieve nausea.

Stretch marks

Stretch marks occur whenever your skin is forced to stretch more than it's designed to stretch. (Your skin has a certain amount of elasticity, but that elasticity has limits!) These stretch marks appear as red marks on various parts of your body — most commonly your thighs, stomach, and breasts. While they typically fade away to silvery streaks over time, stretch marks seldom disappear entirely.

You can reduce your chances of developing stretch marks by not gaining an excessive amount of weight. As for using special creams and lotions to avoid or get rid of stretch marks, don't waste your money. None of these products have been proven to work.

Sweating

Feeling like you're sweating more than usual? It's not all in your head. High levels of progesterone and increased blood flow boost your body temperature by a full degree Fahrenheit. While your body will do its best to keep you cool by causing you to perspire, there are a few things you can do to help the cause. Wear loose-fitting clothing that breathes (cotton is ideal); dress in layers so that you can peel off an extra layer or two if you start to feel overheated; and drink plenty of extra fluids to replace those you're losing through perspiration.

Don't be surprised if you end up driving your partner a little crazy with this whole temperature thing. He may look at you like you've lost your mind when you insist on turning on the car air conditioner in the middle of November because you're feeling too hot — or when you refuse to sleep in a bed that has anything warmer on it than a lightweight cotton sheet, even though there's a snowstorm outside! Just remind him that a pregnant woman is entitled to have the final say on these matters, end of discussion!

Swelling and fluid retention

Swelling is another common pregnancy-related complaint — and one that tends to become more bothersome as your pregnancy progresses. It occurs because your body retains extra fluid during pregnancy. (Your body needs that extra fluid because your blood volume increases by an astounding 40% when you're pregnant.)

It's not unusual to have slightly swollen ankles, particularly during warm weather or after spending a day on your feet, but you shouldn't experience any pain or discomfort as a result of this swelling. If your symptoms are this severe, you could be developing pre-eclampsia (a potentially life-threatening condition characterized by swelling and high blood pressure).

You can help your body rid itself of extra fluids by lying on your side or sitting with your feet up; soaking in a warm (not hot!) tub; increasing your fluid intake (becoming dehydrated can actually make your fluid retention problems worse); and limiting (but not reducing entirely) your salt intake.

FACTS AND FIGURES

Wondering why your feet are feeling so swollen? Not only does progesterone encourage your body to retain fluid, your uterus puts pressure on the veins that carry blood back from your lower extremities, which can encourage fluids to pool in your feet and ankles.

MOM'S THE WORD

"I had to wear Birkenstock-type sandals because my feet were so swollen — and it was March!"

— *Kathy, 34, mother of two*

Thirstiness

Don't be surprised if you find yourself feeling thirstier than normal while you're pregnant. Your increased fluid intake helps your kidneys get rid of the waste products that are being produced by your baby. What's more, your body needs extra fluids to replenish the supply of amniotic fluid and to maintain your increased blood volume. You should plan to drink at least eight glasses a day of water or other beverages. (Don't count coffee, tea, or other caffeinated beverages because they function as diuretics.)

Urinary incontinence

Urinary incontinence is a common complaint toward the end of pregnancy. You may find that you leak a small amount of urine when you run, cough, sneeze, or laugh. The problem is caused by weak pelvic floor muscles and the weight of your growing baby pressing against your bladder. While there's not much you can do about the weight of the baby, you can do exercises to strengthen your pelvic floor muscles. (You can identify the muscles involved by starting and stopping the flow of your urine the next time you go to the bathroom.) You can also avoid straining those muscles further by avoiding constipation and heavy lifting. (You're not supposed to be doing any heavy lifting anyway, remember?!!)

Since you're likely to be leaking only a small amount of fluid, you can probably get away with using sanitary pads rather than special incontinence products to contain any leaks that occur.

Urination, increased frequency of

While we're talking about the waterworks department, let's deal with the issue of increased frequency of urination. Given that there's a baby camped out on your bladder for much of your pregnancy (a particular problem during the first and third trimesters), an increased need to urinate is hardly surprising. What's more, long before your uterus starts encroaching on your bladder's territory, increased blood flow to the pelvic area can also trigger the need to urinate more frequently.

It's not normal to feel pain during urination. If you experience any sort of pain or burning, get in touch with your caregiver because you may have a urinary tract infection. It's important to seek treatment promptly because these infections can cause premature labor.

Vaginal secretions, increased

Don't assume that you've developed a vaginal infection if your vaginal secretions become wetter or more abundant. It's normal to experience an increase in the amount of leukorrhea (the odorless clear or white mucusy discharge produced by the female body) during pregnancy.

FACTS AND FIGURES

If you're diagnosed with trichomoniasis (a vaginal infection characterized by a yellowish-green discharge with a fishy odor), your infection will be treated with an oral medication or a vaginal gel or suppository. To reduce the risk of re-infection, your partner will be treated with an oral medication at the same time.

There is, however, cause for concern if you're experiencing soreness or pain, or if your discharge becomes greenish-yellow, foul-smelling, or watery. These symptoms could indicate an infection or premature rupturing of your membranes.

You can deal with your more abundant discharge by wearing a light sanitary pad, if necessary. What you shouldn't do, however, is use douching products, vaginal deodorants, or any sort of perfumed soap — all of which could be irritating to your vaginal tissues. (Douching also poses some additional risks, something we talked about back in Chapter 2.)

It's particularly important to report any increased vaginal discharge if you've just had amniocentesis performed, since it's possible that you may have experienced an amniotic fluid leak. Try not to panic, however — these types of leaks frequently repair themselves. Your caregiver will likely recommend that you rest for a day or two to see if the problem resolves itself. (You can find out more about amniocentesis in Chapter 9.)

Varicose veins

Varicose veins are caused by an accumulation of extra blood in and around the valves of the veins. They're more likely to flare up during pregnancy, and are more likely to be a problem if your mother or other female relatives have had them.

Varicose veins tend to occur in the legs (both the calves and thighs) and, less commonly, in the labia region. In both cases, the affected area can become painful and swollen.

If your legs are affected, your caregiver will likely suggest that you elevate your feet whenever you're sitting or lying down. (You can raise the foot of your bed by putting pillows under your mattress.) He or she might also recommend that you do leg exercises if you have to sit for any prolonged period of time and that you get in the habit of wearing support stockings (although, to derive any real benefit from them, you have to put them on first thing in the morning, before you hop out of bed or have your morning shower). Your caregiver will also likely suggest that you avoid wearing any tight-fitting clothing that restricts your circulation, especially knee-high pantyhose and tight calf-height socks.

You should never knead or vigorously massage your varicose veins. Doing so can damage your veins further and may cause a blood clot. And if you happen to notice a red, swollen, tender area that appears to have become infected, elevate your leg and contact your caregiver immediately. You may have developed thromophlebitis, a condition that can lead to a blood clot.

MOM'S THE WORD

"I suffer from varicose veins in my labia when I'm pregnant. When they get very bothersome, I soak a maxi-pad in witch hazel and that seems to help."

—*Jane, 30, currently expecting her second child*

MOM'S THE WORD

"Throughout my pregnancy, I really found myself at odds with society's perspective on being pregnant and having a baby. I just found it very difficult to talk about my fears and my negative feelings with anyone except Scott and my doctor. I think I must have gone through my 'postpartum depression' before I had Norah, but I think a lot of it was because of all the pressure to be happy, to be blissful, and not to question things so much."

— *Myrna, 32, mother of one*

Weepiness

Don't be surprised if you find yourself feeling extra weepy while you're pregnant, even for no particular reason. That wacky, pregnancy-related hormonal cocktail can cause your emotions to fluctuate wildly. "The hormonal ebbs and flows did me in," admits Chris, a 36-year-old mother of three. "I'd be sobbing one minute, laughing the next. Suddenly any bad news, especially if it had to do with babies or children, brought me to tears. There were also very high highs: Feeling the baby move always brought a smile to my face."

While it's normal to have weepy moments — to find yourself with tears streaming down your face because you're just so darned touched by the latest Ivory Snow commercial — it's not normal to experience extreme depression. If you find yourself feeling hopeless and overwhelmed, you could be experiencing prenatal depression — a problem that afflicts more women than most people realize. Be sure to let your caregiver know about the difficulty you're having so that he or she can recommend some possible treatments.

Yeast infections

It isn't hard to figure out why so many pregnant women end up developing yeast infections during pregnancy since the accompanying hormonal changes practically open the door to these. Not only is your vaginal environment less acidic and your immune system less effective, there's an increased amount of sugar stored in the cell walls of the vagina. (And, as we all know, yeast loves sugar!)

You should suspect a yeast infection if you've developed a thick, cheese curd-like, white vaginal discharge accompanied by severe itching; if you develop a very red rash that is surrounded by red spots; or if you experience pain and soreness when you urinate.

You can minimize the discomfort of a yeast infection and reduce the chance of a recurrence by keeping the genital area as dry as possible; wiping from front to back when you use the bathroom; ensuring that your vagina is well lubricated before you have intercourse; wearing cotton or cotton-crotch underwear and avoiding pantyhose, tight jeans, perfumed soaps, and vaginal deodorants; cutting down on the amount of refined sugar in your diet; eating yogurt with acidophilus (active cultures) or taking acidophilus supplements; not spending too much time sitting on vinyl seats in your car, home, or office; and soaking in a warm tub to which one cup of cornstarch and a half cup of baking soda have been added.

The Joys of Being Pregnant

Up until now we've been focusing on all the negative aspects of being pregnant — those worries that have you pacing the floor at 3:00 a.m., and those annoying complaints that can have you counting down the minutes to delivery day!

Despite what you might think, pregnancy is not a nine-month exercise in torture — or at least it's not that kind of experience for most of us. Some women even manage to breeze through the entire nine months without so much as a single complaint. But even if you do end up spending an insane amount of time camped out on your bathroom floor waiting for the morning sickness to pass, you can still feel joyous about being pregnant. (Okay, although it might not be that jump-up-and-down-and-burst-into-song variety, you're probably experiencing a quieter, less stomach-churning kind of joy.)

Here are just a few of the reasons why you may have a cryptic Mona Lisa–type smile on your face even while you're leaning against the toilet bowl:

- You may be thrilled to be pregnant — to have the privilege of witnessing the miracle that's taking place in your very own body. "I've never felt better in my life," says Jennifer, a 27-year-old mother-to-be. "Knowing that I have a baby inside me has given me the best feeling. I'm happier, more energetic, and pretty much always smiling these days."

- You may be feeling better about yourself than you ever have before. That has certainly been the case for 25-year-old Christina, who is currently pregnant with her third child: "Pregnancy is better than I ever could have imagined," she explains. "I feel feminine and beautiful and in touch with my feelings."

- You may feel proud about becoming a mother. Chris, a 36-year-old mother of three, remembers experiencing these types of emotions: "I felt glorious — very much like an Earth Mother — and felt spiritual and connected to nature and cycles of life and stuff like that. Very crunchy-granola!"

 FACTS AND FIGURES

Who's calling who hormonal? It's not just mothers-to-be who experience a hormonal roller coaster ride during the nine months of pregnancy. Researchers at Memorial University in Newfoundland have found that fathers-to-be also experience some noteworthy hormonal changes while their partners are pregnant. An increase in prolactin and a decrease in testosterone ensure that these expectant fathers are programmed to switch into "nurture" mode after their babies arrive.

Pregnancy is a very special time in your life — a time to be savored and cherished. Even if you're not usually the journal-keeping type you might want to make an exception at this point in your life, jotting down your thoughts and feelings about the experience of pregnancy. (If you don't want to get quite that organized, simply make copies of all the letters and e-mails you send to family members and friends, talking about your pregnancy. You'll have some wonderful material for your scrapbook or memory box.)

Maria, a 31-year-old-mother of two, decided to keep a pregnancy calendar during her two pregnancies: "I kept detailed records of signs and symptoms, weight gain, special memories, announcements, prenatal checkups, and many of the firsts — the first kick, the first audible heartbeat, and so on. There's so much to remember about having a baby and how it made you feel that I treasure my pregnancy calendars as much as the baby books that I'm now recording my babies' amazing firsts in."

CHAPTER 9

To Test or Not to Test?

I t's an issue that every pregnant couple will have to grapple with at some point in their pregnancy: whether or not to opt for prenatal genetic testing.

Despite what some of the bossier pregnancy books would have you believe, there's no right or wrong answer when it comes to prenatal genetic testing. There's simply the decision that's best for you and your partner. You may feel strongly about arming yourself with as many facts as possible about the well-being of your future child so that you can consider a variety of options, including pregnancy termination; or you may prefer to avoid the resulting stress and anxiety by skipping the testing and letting nature takes its course.

In this chapter, we're going to talk about what prenatal genetic testing can and can't tell you. Then we'll consider who is and isn't a good candidate for testing. Next, we'll look at the various types of prenatal tests, and their strengths and limitations. We'll conclude by looking at the hard choices you may find yourself faced with if the test results bring bad news.

What Prenatal Testing Can — and Can't — Tell You

While every couple dreams of a storybook happy ending — of bringing home a healthy baby who's perfect from head to toe — not everyone's dream comes true. According to the American College of Obstetricians and Gynecologists, approximately 2 to 3% of newborns are affected by major structural malformations and, contrary to popular belief, the majority of these babies are born to parents with no family history of congenital problems.

While some of these infants will enjoy a reasonable quality of life outside the womb, not all will be so lucky. A number of babies born with serious congenital abnormalities end up experiencing serious health problems or dying during their first year of life. In fact, according to the Centers for Disease Control and Prevention, approximately 22% of deaths occurring during the first 28 days of life (the perinatal period) are caused by congenital problems.

While prenatal genetic testing can help you find out in advance whether your baby is affected by a congenital problem, it's by no means the crystal ball that some expectant couples expect it to be. Even the most sophisticated diagnostic tests have a small margin of error, and what's more, not all problems can be detected through genetic testing. And even if a genetic test does indicate that your child has a particular abnormality, the test can't tell you to what degree your child may be affected, and whether or not you can expect your child to enjoy a reasonable quality of life.

Prenatal genetic tests can, however, be a source of valuable information. If they reveal that your baby is affected by a particular problem, this information can allow you to

- arrange for medical treatment in utero (e.g., a baby with Rh incompatibility problems may be given a blood transfusion)

- make appropriate choices for the delivery (e.g., scheduling a cesarean if you know in advance that you'll be giving birth to a medically fragile infant who might sustain injuries during a vaginal delivery)

- prepare to give birth to an infant with special needs in an appropriate setting (e.g., a hospital with state-of-the-art neonatal facilities)

- accept the fact that you may be carrying a baby who could be stillborn or have life-threatening health problems, or

- make the heart-wrenching decision to terminate the pregnancy

Is Prenatal Genetic Testing the Right Choice for You?

While no one can help you to decide what to do about prenatal genetic testing, it can be useful to find out who is — and isn't — generally considered to be a good candidate for prenatal testing.

Genetic counselors tend to recommend prenatal testing to

- couples who have a family history of genetic disease or who know they are carriers of a particular disease

- pregnant women who have been exposed to a serious infection such as rubella or toxoplasmosis during pregnancy or who have been exposed to a substance known to cause birth defects

- couples who've had three or more miscarriages or who've previously given birth to a baby with a diagnosable birth defect

- couples who are anxious to find out whether or not their baby has any sort of detectable birth defect or other anomaly

On the other hand, prenatal genetic testing is generally not recommended for couples

- who have concerns about the accuracy of certain types of prenatal tests (e.g., the high rate of false positives for the alpha-fetoprotein (AFP) screening test)

- who feel that taking this sort of test will add to rather than alleviate their stress

- who have already decided they wouldn't consider terminating their pregnancy under any circumstances

- who are afraid to undergo certain types of prenatal tests (e.g., amniocentesis) because the procedure may be painful or may cause miscarriage or otherwise harm a normal, healthy baby

Some doctors maintain that all women over age 35 should consider prenatal testing. While your risk of giving birth to a baby with a chromosomal anomaly does increase as you age (see Appendix F), it increases gradually rather than dramatically, and even a 45-year-old woman has excellent odds (25/26 or approximately 96%) of giving birth to a chromosomally normal baby. Besides, what this across-the-board policy fails to take into account, according to John R. Sussman, M.D., co-author of *The Unofficial Guide to Having A Baby,* is the fact that not all women of a particular age will necessarily share the same feelings about giving birth to a baby with a serious — even fatal — birth defect. Bottom line? Don't let your caregiver or other people in your life pressure you into taking prenatal tests that you don't particularly want, just because you've reached the "magic" age of 35 or just because that person thinks you should take these tests.

FACTS AND FIGURES

Despite the fact that older women face an increased risk of giving birth to a baby with a chromosomal abnormality, the vast majority of babies with Down syndrome are born to women age 35 or younger. This is simply because there are many more babies born to women under age 35 than over age 35.

Types of Tests

While a typical set of prenatal classes will go into extraordinary detail about such inane topics as what to pack in your hospital suitcase, more often than not they'll skip over the whole issue of prenatal genetic testing. As a result, most pregnant women don't understand the difference between the two basic types of prenatal tests — screening and diagnostic. Here's what you need to know.

Screening tests are designed to screen a large number of pregnant women in order to identify those who have a greater-than-normal chance of giving birth to a baby with a serious or life-threatening birth defect. They aren't designed to determine whether there is a problem, but rather to alert a pregnant woman and her caregiver that there *could* be a problem. Maternal serum screening is an example of a prenatal screening test. Ultrasound can also be used for screening purposes, although it's frequently used as a diagnostic tool as well. (See Table 9.1.)

FACTS AND FIGURES

According to the American College of Obstetricians and Gynecologists, 70% of pregnant women have at least one ultrasound.

TABLE 9.1
PRENATAL GENETIC TESTS

	Maternal serum screening
	Note: If just alpha-fetoprotein is screened for, this test is known as the alpha-fetoprotein or AFP test. If the AFP test is combined with tests of human chorionic gonadotropin (hCG) and unconjugated estriol, it is known as the triple screen test; and if a fourth substance — inhibin-A — is also tested for, the test is known as the quad-screen test.
When It's Performed	Between the 15th and 18th weeks of pregnancy.
How It's Performed	Levels of alpha-fetoprotein (a substance produced by the fetal liver), human chorionic gonadotropin (hCG), unconjugated estriol (a form of estrogen produced by the placenta), and — in the case of the quad-screen test — inhibin-A (a chemical produced by the ovaries and the placenta) — are measured by analyzing a blood sample taken from a pregnant woman. The results are plugged into a formula that predicts the woman's odds of giving birth to a baby with certain types of birth defects.
What It Can Tell You and How Long It Takes to Get the Results	Can tell you whether you face a higher-than-average risk of giving birth to a baby affected by Down syndrome, a neural tube defect, or certain other types of anomalies (severe kidney or liver disease, esophageal or intestinal blockages, other types of chromosomal anomalies, urinary obstructions, and so on). A high result on the test may also alert your caregiver to the fact that you're at risk for preterm labor, intrauterine growth restriction, and stillbirth. (Women with elevated levels of AFP that are not associated with any identifiable birth defect face a higher-than-average risk of experiencing these types of problems.) You'll generally have your test results within a week. The

Maternal serum screening	
	quad-screen test also gives you information about your risk of giving birth to a baby with another serious chromosome abnormality: trisomy 18.
Accuracy	Capable of detecting more than 80% of open neural tube defects and a significant number of Down syndrome cases. The number of false positives (19 out of 20 positives on this test are false positives) can be reduced significantly if your caregiver does an ultrasound to verify your baby's gestational age.
Risks	No direct risks to the fetus, but a false positive on the test may lead to other, more invasive tests that may carry a risk of miscarriage. It can also massively increase your stress level. False negatives also tend to be falsely reassuring. The test can't tell you for certain that your baby is not affected by the types of birth defects that are tested for. It can only tell you that the odds of the baby being affected are very slim.
Ultrasound	
When It's Performed	Can be used for screening or diagnostic purposes at any point during pregnancy.
How It's Performed	High-frequency sound waves are bounced off the fetus and used to create a corresponding image on a computer screen. The test can be performed by rubbing a transducer across the woman's abdomen or by inserting an ultrasonic probe into her vagina (more common early on in pregnancy when it's more difficult to detect a fetal heartbeat via the abdomen).
What It Can Tell You and How Long It Takes to Get the Results	Early in pregnancy, it can be used to detect a fetal heartbeat or to rule out an ectopic pregnancy (by detecting the presence of an amniotic sac in the uterus). Later on, it can be used to confirm your due date; check for the presence of multiples; monitor the growth and development of your baby;

continued

Ultrasound (Continued)

What It Can Tell You and How Long It Takes to Get the Results	detect certain types of fetal anomalies; locate the fetus, the umbilical cord, and the placenta during amniocentesis and chorionic villus sampling; measure the quantity of amniotic fluid; determine the cause of any abnormal bleeding; assess the condition and position of the placenta; determine the condition of the cervix; check for evidence of miscarriage, an ectopic pregnancy, a molar pregnancy, or fetal demise; determine the baby's sex; assess whether a cesarean might be required; determine the baby's position and size; and so on. If your doctor is performing the ultrasound, you'll have the results immediately. If a technician is performing the test, you may have to wait to see your doctor in order to receive the results.
Accuracy	Accuracy depends on the type of problem being screened for, with detection rates for various disorders ranging from 25 to 71%. In most cases, ultrasound is generally considered to be quite accurate when performed by a skilled technician. Note: The most accurate time to date a pregnancy is during the first trimester. The most accurate time to screen for fetal anomalies is at 18 to 20 weeks of pregnancy.
Risks	While no specific risk factors have been identified, ultrasound is still a relatively new technology and consequently should not be used indiscriminately. The American College of Obstetricians and Gynecologists does not recommend the routine use of ultrasound during pregnancy.

Amniocentesis

When It's Performed	Typically performed at 15 to 16 weeks of pregnancy, although some doctors will perform it at 12 to 14 weeks, in which case it's known as early amniocentesis.

Amniocentesis

How It's Performed	A fine needle is inserted through the abdomen and into the amniotic sac. A small amount of amniotic fluid (less than an ounce) is withdrawn for analysis. Note: The procedure can be done with or without local anesthetic. (Note: Some women find the procedure to be quite painful; others do not find it painful at all.)
What It Can Tell You and How Long It Takes to Get the Results	Can be used to detect chromosomal defects, neural tube defects, certain genetic and skeletal diseases, fetal infections, central nervous system diseases, blood diseases, and chemical problems or deficiencies. It can also be used to determine the sex of the baby (important if a couple is known to be a carrier for a disease such as hemophilia that is only a problem for babies of a particular sex), assess the baby's lung maturity (important if the mother is experiencing premature labor or pregnancy-related complications that may necessitate a premature delivery), and measure the bilirubin count of the amniotic fluid (which can help the doctor determine whether a baby with Rh disease may need a blood transfusion prior to birth). It generally takes 10 to 14 days to obtain the results of your amniocentesis if the purpose of the procedure is to screen for chromosomal abnormalities. Results for amniocentesis that has been performed to assess fetal lung maturity, on the other hand, can usually be obtained within 24 hours.
Accuracy	Generally considered to be highly accurate, although specific accuracy figures vary according to the specific type of test. Note: Sex determination tests are 100% accurate if the result is male and 99% accurate if the result is female because there is a slim chance that maternal cells may have affected the test result.

continued

Amniocentesis (Continued)

Risks	Approximately 1/200 women who undergo amniocentesis will miscarry or go into premature labor as a result of the procedure. The rate of miscarriage is higher for women having early amniocentesis (1/100). There's also a small chance that the fetus, placenta, or umbilical cord may be damaged during the procedure, although it appears that earlier concerns about limb reduction abnormalities were unfounded. Note: If you experience an increased vaginal discharge after amniocentesis, notify your caregiver immediately. You may be experiencing an amniotic fluid leak. Your caregiver will likely recommend that you rest and wait to see if the problem will resolve itself.

Chorionic villus sampling (CVS)

When It's Performed	Between 10 and 12 weeks' gestation (12 to 14 weeks of pregnancy)
How It's Performed	A catheter is passed through the cervix or a needle is inserted through the abdomen to obtain a sample of chorionic villus tissue (the tissue that will eventually become the placenta).
What It Can Tell You and How Long It Takes to Get the Results	Can be used to detect Down syndrome, sickle cell disease, thalassemia, cystic fibrosis, hemophilia, Huntington's disease, or muscular dystrophy. Unlike amniocentesis, however, it cannot be used to measure AFP levels to detect spina bifida. Note: It can take anywhere from a few days to a few weeks to obtain the results.
Accuracy	Less accurate than amniocentesis, due to the risk that the sample may become contaminated with maternal cells.
Risks	The miscarriage rate is approximately 1% — lower than that for early amniocentesis, but higher than conventional amniocentesis. Approximately 30% of women who undergo CVS will experience some sort of bleeding. Note: Some early research that linked CVS to limb reduction abnormalities have since been disproven.

Diagnostic tests, on the other hand, are designed to determine whether a particular baby is affected by a particular problem or problems. Unfortunately, there's no single diagnostic test capable of detecting every possible problem, and there are still a significant number of serious health problems that can't be detected prior to birth. Amniocentesis and chorionic villus sampling are examples of prenatal diagnostic tests.

Many pregnant women mistakenly expect screening tests to perform like diagnostic tests. For example, they may become angry if they receive a false positive on the maternal serum test (i.e., the test says their baby may have a problem when in fact their baby is perfectly healthy). What they're forgetting is that in order to ensure that as many problems are detected as possible, screening tests inevitably end up generating a certain percentage of so-called false positives. The alternative would be to make the testing criteria so rigid that the test would ignore any results that were less than clear-cut, which would dramatically increase the number of false negatives (situations in which the test says your baby is perfectly healthy when in fact there's a problem).

It's also important to keep in mind that a "normal" test result doesn't offer any guarantee that the baby that you're carrying will be perfect. Some conditions cannot be tested for and others occur as the pregnancy progresses and therefore cannot be predicted ahead of time.

MOM'S THE WORD

"My advice to women having amnio? Keep your eyes on anything in the room but the needle!"

— *Susan, 35, mother of one*

What to Do If the Test Brings Bad News

It's something that every couple going for prenatal testing needs to think about up front: what they'll do if the test reveals a serious or even life-threatening birth defect. While some couples will opt to carry the pregnancy to term, others will make the difficult and painful decision to terminate the pregnancy as soon as possible.

If you find yourself faced with heartbreaking news and you're trying to decide whether to carry your pregnancy to term, you'll want to weigh the following factors carefully:

- whether you're prepared to raise a child born with a severe disability or give birth to a baby who may either be stillborn or die shortly after birth

- how much your child would suffer physically and emotionally if he or she were to survive past birth

- whether the baby's disabilities are treatable and, if so, the odds for success

- whether new methods of treating your baby's disabilities are likely to be developed in the near future

- whether the baby would be able to live at home or whether he or she would need to be cared for in the hospital or an institutional setting for an indefinite period of time, perhaps forever

- whether your relationship with your partner is strong enough to survive the emotional and financial stresses of caring for a severely disabled child

- whether you and your partner are opposed to abortion under all circumstances or just under certain circumstances

- whether you'd prefer to cherish the remaining time you have left with your baby by carrying your pregnancy to term or whether you'd find it excruciatingly painful to continue your pregnancy, knowing that your baby would likely die prior to or shortly after birth

- whether you would prefer to have a funeral for your baby rather than a private memorial service or no memorial service at all (more common options for couples who choose termination)

- whether you're concerned that your child may be subjected to painful medical interventions if he or she were to survive beyond birth.

There are no easy answers to these questions, and you'll likely find yourself second-guessing whatever decision you make. So it's important to remind yourself in the weeks and months to come that the decisions you made for your baby, however heart-wrenching and difficult, were made out of love. As Deborah Davis, Ph.D., notes in *Empty Cradle, Broken Heart,* you did the best you could, given the options you had: "You had to make an impossible choice between 'terrible' and 'horrible.'"

Whether your baby dies prior to or after birth or is born with a severe disability, you'll need to take time to grieve the loss of "the perfect baby" you'd hoped for from the moment you first found out you were pregnant. You may want to read the material on grieving that can be found in Chapter 11 and to consult Appendix D for the contact information for associations that may be able to offer support to you and your partner during this difficult time in your lives.

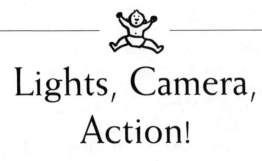

CHAPTER 10

Lights, Camera, Action!

"I think that nine months is the perfect length for pregnancy. By the end, you want to be able to move around easily again and you're so excited and eager to hold your baby."
— *Chris, 36, mother of three*

Starting to feel as though you're going to be pregnant forever? Convinced that you're destined to spend the rest of your days coping with insomnia, back pain, and the other third-trimester aches and pains? Believe it or not, you're in the home stretch now. At some point over the next few weeks, your baby will get tired of using your bladder as a trampoline and will decide it's time to be born.

In this chapter, we're going to talk about the things you're likely to be most concerned about at this stage of the game: whether or not you should attend prenatal classes; why you might want to use the services of a doula (a professional labor support person); what a birth plan can — and can't — do for you; what — if anything — you can do to avoid an episiotomy; the pros and cons of circumcision; the advantages of breastfeeding your baby; the physical changes you can expect to experience as your body prepares for labor; how to tell if you're really in labor; what to bring to the hospital; what types of pain relief (both pharmacological and non-pharmacological) you may wish to use during labor; what to expect from a vaginal delivery and a Cesarean delivery; the facts about vaginal birth after cesarean (VBAC); how to stay sane if you go overdue; what to expect if your labor is induced; and what those first moments after the birth may be like.

Prenatal Classes: Who Needs Them?

There's no denying it: Prenatal classes are a rite of passage for most pregnant couples. If your pregnancy hasn't felt "real" up until now, it will when you find yourself holed up in an auditorium with a room full of pillow-toting pregnant women!

Depending on what's available in your community, you may have the chance to attend one or more types of prenatal classes:

- first- or second-trimester classes that cover such topics as nutrition and exercise during pregnancy

- third-trimester childbirth classes designed to prepare you for the birth (most include a tour of the birthing suite at the hospital where you'll be delivering your baby)

- breastfeeding classes designed to give you a preview of what you can do to get breastfeeding off to the best possible start

---

MOM'S THE WORD

"I can honestly say I didn't learn much from the prenatal classes, but I'm so glad we went because they made it all seem so much more real. I remember the instructors had these round nametags on and they explained to us that these were 10 cm in diameter — the exact size our cervixes would have to dilate to in order to give birth. You should have seen the shocked expressions on everyone's face. It certainly put things into perspective!"

— *Maria, 35, mother of two*

While parents today have a smorgasbord of options — classes that focus on the Lamaze, Bradley, Gamper, Leboyer, Odent, or Kitzinger methods or that are of the Heinz 57 variety: a smattering of this philosophy served up with a side dish of that! — most cover the same basic turf: the physiology of pregnancy, the basic elements of prenatal care, the physical and psychological experience of giving birth, what to expect from a vaginal and a cesarean delivery, laboring positions that can help to reduce pain or encourage your labor to progress more efficiently, the role of pain relief during labor, information on baby care (including breastfeeding), physical changes to expect during the postpartum period, and so on.

Prenatal classes have a lot to offer:

- They can give you a sneak preview of what to expect during both a vaginal and cesarean delivery. (Be sure to pay attention during the cesarean part of the birth movie, by the way, since you may not know ahead of time whether you'll require one!)

- They can provide you with the facts you need about your various birth options (e.g., the pros and cons of using various types of pain relief during labor) so that you can make informed decisions. (Of course, if your prenatal instructor has strong philosophies about particular aspects of the birth, you may end up with a large serving of propaganda rather than anything that could be described as cold, hard facts.)

- They can arm you with breathing, relaxation, and other coping techniques that may help to reduce your perception of pain during labor.

- They can give you the opportunity to ask any questions you may have about pregnancy, labor, birth, breastfeeding, and newborn care.

- They encourage your partner to become involved in your pregnancy.

- They give you the opportunity to meet other couples who are due at roughly the same time you are — contacts that can be pure gold if you find yourself housebound in February with a colicky baby!

Some couples find prenatal classes to be highly beneficial — one of the highlights of being pregnant.

"We had a wonderful experience at our prenatal class," says Nicole, a 29-year-old mother of one. "The group of parents was fun and the instructor was a wealth of information. We came away with a package of information as well as a phone number we could call if we ever had any questions or needed any advice."

Maria and her husband had a similarly positive experience. "I think the classes were very beneficial for my husband," the 35-year-old mother of two explains. "He learned a lot and the classes really helped to demystify the birthing process for him."

Jennifer, a 32-year-old mother of one, enjoyed the opportunity to get to know other pregnant couples — something that made for a fun reunion class a couple of months down the road. "It was amazing to see everyone with flattened bellies and real little people in their laps, and to see everyone casually feeding or changing when a few months earlier most of us didn't have the first clue about how to care for an infant."

Other couples, however, are considerably less enthralled with the whole prenatal class experience.

Jennifer, 27, who's about to give birth to her first child, found the prenatal classes she took left her feeling anxious. "It didn't help that the instructor liked to tell scary stories," she remarks.

Carole, a 33-year-old mother of two, thought the classes she took didn't do an adequate job of preparing her for anything other than a medication-free delivery: "I found the classes a little misleading in that they gave the impression that if you used proper breathing, you wouldn't need medical intervention. That wasn't the case for me. I did require an epidural during my first birth, and because of the class I felt like somewhat of a failure."

If you find you're not particularly thrilled with the prenatal classes offered by the hospital, health unit, and/or childbirth association, there is an alternative. Depending on where you live, you may be able to arrange for a childbirth educator to conduct private classes for you and your partner. You can either ask your doctor or midwife to pass along the names of childbirth instructors in your community who provide this type of service, or you can call the International Childbirth Education Association (ICEA) for referrals to childbirth instructors in your area: 1-952-854-8660.

📢 **MOM'S THE WORD**

"Take a good breastfeeding course before the birth. My son would not latch and it took almost six weeks of pumping and working with a lactation consultant to get nursing fully established. New mothers need to be aware that occasionally babies and mothers don't naturally take to nursing, but that perseverance does pay off."

— *Lara, 33, currently pregnant with her second child*

Decisions, Decisions . . .

Your coffee table is overflowing with pregnancy books and your fridge is plastered with pamphlets about various aspects of prenatal health. Sometimes like you feel as though you've read enough to earn your Ph.D. in motherhood!

Well, believe it or not, you're not finished hitting the books yet. You've still got a few more important issues to read up on before baby arrives, namely, doulas, birth plans, episiotomies, pain relief during labor, circumcision, and breastfeeding.

Doulas are a girl's best friend

Looking for a way to decrease the length of your labor, reduce your need for pain medication, decrease your chances of needing a forceps delivery or a cesarean, and leave you feeling satisfied about your birth experience? What you need is a doula — the birthing world's equivalent of a fairy godmother!

FACTS AND FIGURES

There are two types of doulas: birthing doulas (who offer support during and after the birth) and postpartum doulas (who offer both hands-on assistance and motherly advice during the days and weeks following the birth). Some doulas offer both types of services to their clients.

Think I'm exaggerating? Consider the evidence for yourself! There's a growing body of research proving that doulas can help to improve the birthing outcome for both mother and baby. A study at Case Western Reserve University in Cleveland, for example, found that while 63% of women who did not have the support of a doula required a cesarean after a labor induction, just 20% of those with a doula required a cesarean. And a recent study at the University of Texas Medical School found that women who used the services of a doula were more nurturing toward their babies two months after the delivery.

Here are some other recent findings on the doula front:

• Women who have support from a doula during labor are 40% less likely to require a forceps delivery.

- Women who use the services of a doula are 60% less likely to request an epidural and 40% less likely to require synthetic oxytocin (Pitocin) to keep labor moving along.

- Having the support of a doula may reduce the length of your labor by 25%.

Doulas typically charge $300 to $600 for attending a birth. This fee includes one or more meetings prior to the birth to talk with you and your partner about your plans; helping you to draft a birth plan; making herself available by phone to address any concerns the two of you may have about the birth; providing continuous support during labor; and providing support and breastfeeding help during the first few hours postpartum. Doulas do not, however, perform medical checks (e.g., monitor your blood pressure or do internal examinations), nor are they licensed to deliver babies. Their role is to provide labor support (most doctors are too busy to do this and some birthing unit nurses simply do not have the time) and, if necessary, to advocate on your behalf with the medical staff.

The best way to get a referral to a doula who's practicing in your community is to contact your nearest midwifery practice. If there isn't a midwifery practice in your community, you might want to call Doulas of North America (DONA) at 206-324-5440, or the Childbirth and Postpartum Professional Association at 1-888-548-3672 to ask for the names of certified doulas in your area.

At that point, you'll want to meet with the prospective doula. In addition to ensuring that and your partner "click" with her and asking her to supply you with a list of references, you'll want to find out

- whether she offers labor support services only, postpartum support services only, or both types of services

- what type of training she's had (Is she certified through Doulas of North America?)

- how many births she's attended

- what role she would see herself playing in the birth

- what she charges for her services

- whether you're welcome to call her with questions and concerns before and after the birth and

- whether she will line up a backup doula (in case she is busy at another birth or otherwise unavailable when you go into labor)

Writing a birth plan

Something else you need to think about at this stage is whether you and your partner would like to write a birth plan.

Contrary to popular belief, a birth plan doesn't have to be overly long or complicated. It's not a business plan, for Pete's sake! It could be as simple as a one-paragraph letter addressing a point of particular concern to you, or it could be a more detailed document addressing such issues as

- where you intend to give birth

- your feelings about the use of medication during labor

- whom you'll be inviting to your baby's birth, and what each person's role will be

- what clothing (if any!) you intend to wear while you're in labor

- the atmosphere you hope to create (e.g., dim lights and quiet music)

- where you're intending to do the bulk of your laboring (e.g., in the Jacuzzi or sitting on the toilet)

- what types of birthing equipment you hope to use (e.g., a birthing stool, a birthing bed, a beanbag chair, a squatting bar, or a birthing tub)

- whether you'd like to be present when the doctor or midwife performs the newborn check on your baby

It's important to remember, however, that a birth plan is just that — a plan. It's not a blueprint for labor. The goal of every delivery is to end up with a healthy baby and a healthy mother. Sometimes you have to deviate from your birth plan in order to achieve that goal — something that Stephanie, 27, learned for herself when her daughter was born 2 ½ years ago. She explains: "I had hoped for a non-medicated birth with a midwife, but I found myself in a room with the midwives, an obstetrician, two nurses, and a pediatrician for my child." In the end, what really mattered to Stephanie was the fact that her baby arrived safely.

Despite what some pregnancy books would have you believe, birth plans aren't necessarily for everyone. Marguerite and her husband found that writing one actually contributed to their sense of failure when their first birth didn't go according to plan. Consequently, when it came time to prepare for the birth of baby number two, they decided to pass on the plan. "We discussed the relevant issues with our midwife, but we didn't write a formal plan," the 36-year-old mother of two recalls.

There are, of course, some situations in which a birth plan can be very helpful. If, for example, you have a history of sexual abuse and you're worried you may have flashbacks or begin to disassociate during the birth, you might want to let the birthing unit staff know what will help to reassure you. Similarly, if you've previously experienced the death of a baby either prior to or shortly after birth, you might want to let the birthing unit staff know whether or not you'd prefer to give birth in the same room as the last time around.

If you and your partner want to write a birth plan but aren't sure how to get started, you might want to consult the sample birth plan in Appendix B. You can either photocopy it and use it as is, or modify it so that it's better suited to your individual needs.

MOM'S THE WORD

"I thought the doctor would be in the room from the time I went into labor until the baby was born. Wrong. They come in, check you, and leave again. They only stick around when the actual birth is happening. Once that's over with, they're gone."

— *Rita, 35, mother of two*

MOM'S THE WORD

"For me, the biggest myth about giving birth is that you can read a book and expect everything to happen in a certain way. Every birth is different, and while a lot of what you read may very well happen in some form to you, it may not be exactly the way you thought it would. I guess I'm trying to say that in pregnancy and birth, you have to expect the unexpected and be prepared to roll with the punches — sort of take things as they come and be flexible enough to change your expectations and your strategies for handling things."

— *Joyce, 41, mother of two*

Episiotomy: The unkindest cut of all

You know how squeamish guys get when someone starts talking about vasectomies? The closest thing to that we women will ever experience is reading up on episiotomy — the medical term for the surgical cut that's sometimes made to the perineum (the area between the vagina and rectum) during labor.

And, frankly, there's plenty to be squeamish about. Women who have episiotomies are more likely to experience such complications as blood loss, infection, pain during the postpartum period, pain during intercourse, and the involuntary passage of gas or fecal matter after the delivery. And despite what some pregnancy books will tell you, there's no such thing as a perfect episiotomy. Midline episiotomies (where the incision goes straight up and down) are associated with higher rates of anal incontinence (the involuntary passage of fecal material) and flattus incontinence (the involuntary release of gas from the bowel) following the delivery, while mediolateral episiotomies (where the incision veers slightly to the right or left) are more likely to result in painful intercourse when the couple resumes sexual relations than what is typically experienced by women who have had midline episiotomies.

If you're eager to avoid an episiotomy (and frankly, who wouldn't be, after reading that list of possible complications!), you might want to consider practicing perineal massage. A number of studies have demonstrated quite conclusively that perineal massage can help women giving birth for the first time to avoid episiotomies and severe tearing.

The techniques involved are extremely low-tech. You simply gently massage and stretch the tissues at the opening of the vagina while you're soaking in the bathtub. Or, if you don't mind turning this particular activity into a spectator sport, your partner can help to massage and stretch your tissues when you're lying on a towel on the bed. You might want to use a small amount of olive oil or natural cocoa butter for lubrication if you're going to be doing the perineal massage on dry land. Regardless of where you decide to do your massage, however, you should plan to do it for about 10 minutes a day from the 34th week of your pregnancy onward.

Just one small disclaimer: There are no guarantees. You could massage your little heart out during the weeks leading up to the birth and still end up with an episiotomy or a significant-sized tear. In certain situations an episiotomy may be unavoidable — if your baby is breech, in distress, or in fragile medical condition; your baby's shoulders are too wide to be delivered without an episiotomy (shoulder dystocia); or you're having a forceps delivery. As well, some caregivers will perform an episiotomy if it looks as though you're going to end up with a severe tear or multiple tears. (Others, however, feel it's best to let the tear occur naturally and repair it after the fact.)

If you require an episiotomy, your caregiver will inject anesthetic into the perineum during the height of a contraction (when pressure from the baby's head is helping to numb the area). (Of course, if you've had an epidural or your doctor has injected other anesthetic into the area — e.g., a pudendal block — you won't need to have any additional anesthetic injected at this point.) The incision will also be made during a contraction to take advantage of this natural form of pain relief. Most of the discomfort you experience will occur after the freezing wears off. You can minimize the pain by sitting on one of those doughnut-shaped cushions that work wonders for hemorrhoid sufferers, by squeezing your buttocks together before you sit down, and by pouring water across your perineum while you urinate to prevent the urine from burning. It can take a couple of weeks for your episiotomy to heal — sometimes even longer. Your caregiver will check your episiotomy at your six-week checkup, but don't be afraid to call his or her office sooner if you suspect that it's become infected.

FACTS AND FIGURES

According to the American College of Obstetricians and Gynecologists, an episiotomy is performed during one out of every three deliveries.

Pain relief during labor

Something else you need to consider before the labor contractions kick in is what types of pain relief you'd like to use during labor. You may decide to stick with non-pharmacological methods or you may decide to go right for the hard stuff. Jennifer, a 31-year-old mother of two, opted for Plan B: "I knew I was having an epidural the moment the pregnancy test turned blue."

The following lists present what you need to know about the various types of non-pharmacological and pharmacological methods of pain relief present.

FACTS AND FIGURES

According to the American College of Obstetricians and Gynecologists (ACOG), some health insurance companies are only willing to pick up the tab for pain relief during labor if the attending physician considers that pain relief to be medically necessary. ACOG opposes this practice, arguing that insurance companies should cover the cost of pain relief during labor under *all* circumstances, including the mother's request for pain relief. "The last thing a woman needs to hear during a painful labor is that her insurance company isn't going to cover her epidural," notes Michael Greene, M.D., chair of ACOG's Committee on Obstetric Practice.

Non-medicinal pain relief options:

- Acupuncture. Needles are inserted in your limbs or ears to help to block the corresponding pain signals.

- Hypnosis. Self-hypnosis techniques can be used to promote relaxation during labor, thereby reducing the amount of pain you experience. What's more, some caregivers also have special training in the area of hypnosis.

- Laboring in water. Laboring in water relaxes you and helps to counteract the effects of gravity, something that can make labor less painful.

- Relaxation and positive visualization. Relaxation breathing and/or focusing on an object that you find calming can help to relax you during labor, and so reduce the amount of pain you experience.

- Transcutaneous electronic nerve stimulations (TENS). A TENS machine stimulates the nerves in your lower back, which can help block the transmission of pain impulses to the brain.

- Other techniques. A number of other pain relief techniques can be used during labor: massage (especially the application of counterpressure to the lower back if back labor is being experienced), applying heat and cold, using a birthing ball, changing positions, and so on.

Medicinal pain relief options:

- Sedatives. Sedatives, tranquilizers, and sleeping pills can be used to reduce anxiety and encourage a laboring woman to relax. Unfortunately, these drugs cross the placenta and can affect the baby. Babies whose mothers use sedatives during labor can have breathing and sucking problems after the delivery and may actually remain limp until the effects of the drug wear off.

- Antinausea drugs. Some laboring women take antinausea drugs like Gravol to combat nausea and vomiting triggered by either labor itself or by the use of narcotics such as Demerol. These drugs tend to cause sleepiness and dizziness in the mother.

- Injectible narcotics and narcotic-like medications. Narcotics such as Demerol, morphine, Nubain, and Stadol can provide up to two hours' worth of pain relief. Unfortunately, the doses given to laboring women tend to be relatively low and frequently fail to provide adequate pain relief. What's more, the drugs can cause such undesirable side effects as drowsiness, nausea, vomiting, respiratory depression, and low blood pressure, and can result in breathing difficulties in the newborn if the drugs are used within two hours of the delivery. There's also some evidence that Demerol may make labor longer.

- Epidural. An anesthetic is injected into the space between the covering of the spinal cord and inside the bony vertebrae of your spine, numbing you from the waist down. An epidural provides full relief for 85% of women, partial relief (e.g., pain relief on one side of the body) in 12% of women, and no relief in 3% of women. The side effects of epidurals include longer labors, low blood pressure, a reduced ability to push (which may necessitate a forceps or vacuum extraction delivery), difficulty urinating after the delivery (because bladder catheterization is typically required during the delivery), and — in rare cases — severe postpartum headaches. Epidurals are not considered a good option for women whose labor has not progressed past the three- to four-centimeter mark. Despite what you may have read, the incidence of life-threatening complications resulting from epidurals is extremely rare, occurring in just 1/5000 to 1/10,000 births.

FACTS AND FIGURES

A study reported in *Obstetrics and Gynecology* indicates that women who receive epidurals for pain relief are almost twice as likely to end up with third- or fourth-degree perineal lacerations (tearing of the muscles and connective tissue in the area between the openings to the vagina and the rectum). What's more, a study reported in a recent issue of *Pediatrics* indicated a possible link between use of epidurals and maternal fever during labor — a condition associated with a higher rate of complications in the newborn.

- Spinal. A spinal is similar to an epidural, except that anesthetic is injected into the spinal fluid in the lower back, numbing you from the waist down. Spinals are sometimes used for cesarean deliveries in cases when the anesthetic must be administered in a hurry (e.g., an emergency forceps delivery), if the placenta has been retained, or if you've experienced a severe tear that requires a difficult repair. They're not recommended for women with severe pre-eclampsia or who face a high risk of hemorrhaging (e.g., women with low blood platelet levels, placenta previa, or a major placental abruption). They can cause low blood pressure, severe post-delivery headaches, temporary bladder dysfunction, nausea, and, in rare cases, convulsions or infection.

- Inhalable analgesics (e.g., nitrous oxide). Inhalable analgesics such as nitrous oxide numb the pain center in the brain. The key advantage to this pain relief method is that it's administered by the woman as she needs it and can be used to help a woman to weather a difficult transition stage as she waits for the pushing stage to begin. The key disadvantages are that it can cause drowsiness and nausea, as well as claustrophobic feelings (you have to wear a mask tightly on your face), it does not provide pain relief, it's only suitable for a short period of time (typically an hour or less), its effectiveness varies significantly from woman to woman, and, what's more, some studies have shown that women who use nitrous oxide during labor can aspirate (inhale the contents of their stomachs).

- Local anesthetic. Local anesthetic can be injected into the tissues of the perineum so that an episiotomy can be performed or an episiotomy or tear can be repaired after the delivery. Some studies have demonstrated that injections of local anesthetic may weaken the perineal tissue, which increases the likelihood of tearing in the event that an episiotomy isn't performed after all. Another form of local anesthetic is a pudendal block — local anesthetic that is injected into the middle of the vagina to numb the perineal nerves.

- General anesthetic. A general anesthetic is sometimes used in emergency situations. They're no longer used routinely during delivery, as they were a generation ago, because of the high risk of breathing problems and extreme sleepiness in the newborn and the small chance that the mother might aspirate (breathe) the contents of her stomach while she's under the anesthetic, causing potentially life-threatening complications.

While you should give some thought to the types of pain relief you hope to use during labor, it's important to go into labor with an open mind. If the speedy delivery you envisioned turns out to be a 30-hour endurance test, you may want to rethink your stance on epidurals. Conversely, the epidural you had your heart set on might not be feasible if you're already eight centimeters dilated by the time you arrive at the hospital!

Marguerite found that the natural methods she had planned to use during the birth of her first child weren't particularly helpful: "I couldn't tolerate any of the planned massage or counting techniques," the 36-year-old mother of two recalls. "My poor husband had to remain silent, not touching me and not doing anything else either. I was very irritable and couldn't tolerate any distractions of any kind. All our practiced breathing and massage and relaxation techniques were totally useless to me. I just needed to focus on myself."

Jane ended up changing her game plan when labor dragged on and on. "I expected a textbook labor, and mine wasn't," the 33-year-old mother of two explains. "I stayed at two centimeters after 24 hours of good, strong labor. I don't know how common this is, but I didn't hear much about it from my midwife or from the classes. I became more and more frustrated and less and less able to cope with the pain as the hours went by and I still didn't progress. If I'd been moving forward bit by bit, I think I could have gone on longer without drugs. As it was, I had an epidural after 24 hours. I needed a rest from the pain. I was exhausted and I felt very, very out of control. The contractions had become scary and negative for me because they weren't getting me anywhere."

The circumcision decision

To circumcise or not to circumcise. That is the question.

It's a question that many pregnant couples grapple with during pregnancy — and for good reason. If you sit down and make a list of the pros and cons of circumcision, you'll find the list to be fairly evenly balanced. (See Table 10.1.) On the one hand, circumcision can help to reduce the risk of a variety of health-related complaints and makes hygiene a lot easier; on the other hand, it's painful and stressful to the newborn and can, in rare cases, lead to complications.

TABLE 10.1

THE PROS AND CONS OF CIRCUMCISION

Pros	Cons
Reduced incidence of urinary tract infections, balanoposthitis (inflammation of the skin of the penis caused by either trauma or poor hygiene), sexually transmitted diseases, and penile cancer.	Procedure is both painful and stressful to the newborn and has been shown to affect the baby's behavior for up to 24 hours after.
Prevents paraphimosis (an emergency situation that occurs if the foreskin gets stuck when it's first retracted) (Note: Many cases of balanoposthitis and paraphimosis are believed to be caused by well-meaning caregivers who try to forcibly pull the foreskin back. If the foreskin is generally left alone, the combination of spontaneous erections and masturbation are generally enough to loosen the foreskin.)	Complications occur in approximately 1 in 1,000 circumcisions. In rare cases, severe penile damage can occur. Note: Circumcision is not recommended for infants who are sick, premature, or who have any type of penile abnormality.
Greater ease of hygiene.	In most cases, circumcision is not medically indicated — something which explains why the American Academy of Pediatrics does not recommend routine newborn circumcision.
Newborn circumcision is less risky than circumcision later in life.	

Even the American Academy of Pediatrics acknowledges that the arguments for and against the procedure are about on par (although somes studies have demonstrated some potential medical benefits of circumcision). While it has spoken out against routine circumcision, it acknowledges that parents have to make up their own minds about the issue, factoring in their own personal, religious, or cultural factors.

It's those "personal, religious, and cultural" factors that tend to muddy the waters the most.

FACTS AND FIGURES

According to the National Center for Health Statistics and the American Academy of Pediatrics, approximately 1.2 million babies (64% of male newborns) are circumcised each year.

Lori, a 29-year-old mother of four, found that a lot of people were determined to point out that her uncircumcised sons would look different in the shower than their circumcised father — an argument she felt had little validity. "I decided that even if he was circumcised, he wouldn't look like his father anyway. No small boy could look at his own penis and his father's penis and think they looked the same. So I thought that was a silly argument."

The same issue arose for Jane's partner: "My husband was initially concerned about having to explain a physical difference between him and his son," the 33-year-old mother of two explains. "We decided that we'd deal with that if and when it came up by saying something like, 'Doctors used to believe it was a good idea, but they don't any more.'"

Jane made up her mind about the procedure after watching a video of an actual circumcision. "That was it for me," she recalls. "I decided that no child would go through such a barbaric, unnecessary experience. I figured the foreskin was probably there for some purpose. If, by some remote chance, he had a problem later on that necessitated a circumcision, we decided we'd deal with it then."

There are no easy answers to the whole circumcision issue. If you and your partner want to do more research before you make up your minds, you might want to visit the American Academy of Pediatrics Web site at www.aap.org, where you'll find a copy of the Academy's official position paper on circumcision.

MOM'S THE WORD

"We both wanted our sons circumcised, but I was traumatized by it both times."

—*Jennifer, 31, mother of two*

Breast or bottle?

Another important decision you'll need to make before your baby arrives is whether you intend to breastfeed or bottlefeed.

Unless you've been holed up in a baby-free zone for much of your adult life, you've no doubt heard about all the benefits of breastfeeding for your baby:

FACTS AND FIGURES

Breastfed babies aren't just healthier; they may be smarter too. A recent study revealed that premature babies who were tube-fed breastmilk scored an average of eight points higher on IQ tests administered at age 8.

- Breastmilk is the perfect food for babies, serving up all the nutrients the baby needs in exactly the right proportions. What's even more miraculous, however, is the fact that the "recipe" for breastmilk changes as the baby's needs change. A toddler may be drinking from the same breast he used as an infant, but there's an entirely different beverage on tap!

- Breastmilk is packed with antibodies — something that no artificial baby formula can deliver. Studies have shown that breastfed babies are less likely to develop gastrointestinal infections, urinary tract infections, respiratory infections, middle ear infections, food allergies, tooth decay, pneumonia, and meningitis than bottlefed babies. Breastfeeding even increases the effectiveness of vaccines, which helps to ensure that your baby will get the maximum health benefits from each of his booster shots.

• Breastfed babies are less susceptible to Sudden Infant Death Syndrome (SIDS) than bottlefed babies. They also enjoy added protection against intestinal disease, eczema, thrush, certain types of heart disease, allergies, cancer, and obesity — health benefits that last long beyond weaning.

• Breastfeeding helps to promote normal development of the jaw and facial muscles. Bottlefed babies are more likely to require orthodontic work than their breastfed counterparts.

As if that weren't enough to sell you on the concept, breastfeeding also provides you with significant health benefits:

• It helps your uterus to contract after the birth, which reduces the amount of blood lost after the delivery and allows you to regain your pre-pregnancy shape more quickly.

• It helps you get rid of your extra "baby fat" without dieting, since breastfeeding burns up approximately 500 calories per day.

• It may reduce your risk of developing breast cancer and ovarian cancer later in life.

• It may serve as natural birth control by delaying ovulation. (According to the American College of Obstetricians and Gynecologists, some strict guidelines must be followed if breastfeeding is the sole method of birth control you choose to use.)

Health benefits aside, you need to know that breastfeeding is much more than just a feeding method. It's a whole way of mothering. It fosters a special bond between you and your baby and can increase your confidence in your mothering abilities. Cyndie, a 35-year-old mother of two, notes, "Some of the best moments of caring for my infants were when I was nursing them. I missed it very much when I weaned them."

Yet breastfeeding is not necessarily for everyone, and you shouldn't allow anyone to make you feel as though you're an inferior mother if you're unable to or choose not to breastfeed your baby. Despite what some breastfeeding zealots would have you believe, bottlefeeding is not a form of child abuse. Don't let anyone tell you otherwise.

Eight Months and Counting

While you might feel as though you're in a bit of a holding pattern, waiting for your baby to make his or her grand entrance, there's actually a lot going on inside your body. Here are just a few of the physical changes and sensations you might notice as your body counts down the final days and weeks before your baby's birth:

- Your baby may be doing fewer somersaults than she was a few weeks ago. The reason is obvious: Conditions inside the uterus are getting a little cramped. While a reduction in the number of fetal movements can indicate a possible problem, don't be too concerned if the movements simply become a bit less vigorous and more like rolling than kicking. That's pretty standard at this stage of the game.

- You may be experiencing a lot of pain underneath your ribs. Since she can no longer amuse herself by doing somersaults, your baby's doing some heavy-duty stretching instead. Unfortunately, once she moves into the head-down position (the position that 97% of babies assume before labor), what she likes pushing against most with her feet is the area just under your ribs!

- You may feel some sudden, darting movements. Your baby may be vigorously rooting around, trying to get her thumb back in her mouth (yes, that thumb-sucking habit often starts before birth!); or she may have gulped back enough amniotic fluid to give herself a case of the hiccups.

- You may feel as though your pelvic floor muscles are supporting a cantaloupe. And, frankly, that's not far off the mark! Once your baby descends into your pelvis (which can happen a few weeks ahead of time or right as labor begins), her head begins pressing against your perineum, which can make walking and even sitting rather uncomfortable. You may also notice an odd buzzing sensation — like either a mild electric shock or a tickle. This occurs as your baby raises and lowers her head against your pelvic floor muscles and can be more than a little disconcerting!

- You may feel increased pressure in your pelvis and rectum. This can result in abdominal cramping, groin pain, and persistent lower backache. (Note: You're more likely to experience this particular symptom if this is your second or subsequent baby.)

- You may find that your breathlessness decreases, but that annoying urge to urinate every hour on the hour returns. You may also find yourself experiencing a variety of other pregnancy complaints: sciatica, varicose veins, hemorrhoids, and stretch marks. (See Chapter 8 for the lowdown on these common complaints.)

- Your Braxton Hicks contractions may become increasingly uncomfortable — and perhaps even painful. These practice contractions are busy preparing your body for the hard work that awaits it when "labor day" arrives.

- Your eating habits may change. You may find you need smaller, more frequent meals rather than several large meals each day. Crowded conditions inside your body prevent your stomach from holding a lot of food at one time.

- You may feel more — or less — energetic. Some women get a burst of energy as labor approaches, the so-called nesting instinct. Others are reluctant to do anything more ambitious than lifting their head off the couch. Both reactions are perfectly normal, so don't assume you're never going to go into labor just because you've got absolutely no urge to play Martha Stewart.

- You may lose weight. Even though your baby is still packing on the pounds, your weight may drop by a pound or two during the last month of your pregnancy. This is because the total amount of amniotic fluid in your body is decreasing, a change triggered by the hormonal fluctuations of late pregnancy, and because crowded conditions around your stomach may make it difficult for you to eat as much as you usually do.

You may also notice that your emotional state changes. Even if you've been thoroughly enjoying your pregnancy, you may now be eager to get on with the show. This whole business of being pregnant has long since lost its novelty: Now all you can think about is meeting your baby!

And then there's the business of the impending labor — something that can have you tossing and turning at 3:00 a.m., wondering what on earth you were thinking when you decided to get pregnant eight months ago. After all, the woman in the birth film they showed in prenatal class didn't exactly look like she was having fun.

As your baby's birth day approaches, you may find that you feel increasingly introspective, more tuned into what's going on with your baby and less interested in the world around you. Be sure to treasure this special time before the birth, says Lori, a 29-year-old mother of four. "Enjoy every minute you have your baby to yourself because once the baby enters the world, life becomes a little chaotic and time flies by. When your baby is still being held inside your womb, you can sit back, relax, and appreciate the bond you already have with your child."

How to Tell if It's the Real Thing

You've no doubt heard all the horror stories about women showing up at labor and delivery, convinced they're in full-blown labor, only to be sent home because they hadn't dilated even a single centimeter. Or of women waiting so long to go to the hospital they ended up giving birth at the side of the highway in the middle of rush hour. (Hey, it's one way to end up on the front page of your hometown newspaper!)

MOM'S THE WORD

"At the beginning of my labor there was no pain. I had this uncomfortable feeling and just could not get settled."

— *Rita, 35, mother of two*

Fortunately, these types of scenarios are actually quite rare. Despite what you might think, most women do manage to figure out if the pains they're experiencing are the real thing or just a particularly nasty imitation. Here are a few guidelines to help you decide.

Prelabor symptoms

Despite what the movies would have you believe, labor seldom kicks off with gut-wrenching contractions at two-minute intervals. Most of us gals in the real world experience at least a bit of "prelabor" to warn us that labor day isn't far off. Unfortunately, this prelabor can hurt as much as the early stages of the real thing and — to add insult to injury — it doesn't even guarantee labor any time soon. Does Mother Nature have a twisted sense of humor or what?!!!

That said, you still need to be aware of the classic symptoms of prelabor. They may not guarantee you'll have your baby today, but they sure as heck indicate that the big day is fast approaching. Here's what to look out for:

- Your baby drops. At some point during the last few weeks of pregnancy, you may notice that instead of being pressed against your lungs, your baby is now sitting on your bladder! If you check out your profile in the mirror, you'll see that the change can be quite dramatic. While a first-time mother's baby typically drops sometime during the two weeks leading up to delivery, many women giving birth for the second or subsequent time find their babies don't drop until labor actually starts. (This is because the mother's pelvic muscles have already been stretched during a previous pregnancy, so there's not the same need for a pre-game workout.) Just a quick footnote on terminology before we move on. The terms *dropping, lightening,* and *engagement* are used pretty much interchangeably. So if your doctor or midwife happens to say that your baby's head is engaged, it means your baby has dropped.

- Your Braxton Hicks contractions become stronger. Instead of feeling like a mild tightening sensation, they're starting to resemble menstrual cramps. While they aren't as strong as the contractions you'll feel during labor, they're effective nonetheless. Their job is to thin out (or efface) your cervix, changing it from a thick-walled cone to a thin-walled cup so that it'll be ready to start dilating when you actually go into labor.

- You'll experience some diarrhea and possibly some nausea. As your body prepares for labor your hormones trigger abdominal cramps that cause loose, frequent bowel movements — nature's way of emptying your intestines before labor begins. Unfortunately, these hormones can leave you feeling a bit nauseated. In fact, you might (wrongly) conclude that you're coming down with a touch of the stomach flu!

- Your vaginal discharge thickens. You may notice more egg-white or pink-tinged vaginal discharge as labor day approaches. This is caused by hormonal changes rather than the cervical dilation responsible for the "bloody show."

- You may experience some "bloody show." This is the name given to the blood-streaked mucus that typically passes out of the vagina as the cervix begins to dilate. This mucus plug seals the cervix during pregnancy, protecting your baby from infection. The mucus becomes streaked with blood as some of the tiny blood vessels in your cervix break as your cervix thins. The mucus typically has a pink or brownish tinge. The passage of the mucus plug typically indicates that your labor will start within the next three days, but some women do manage to hang on for another week or two. Note: If there seems to be a lot of blood and not much mucus you could be experiencing potentially serious complications and will need to notify your caregiver immediately.

- Premature rupture of membranes (the rupture of your bag of waters prior to the onset of labor). Approximately 10% of women have their membranes rupture before they're actually in labor. If this happens to you, you can expect your labor to begin within the next few hours or at least within the next day. Due to the risk of infection, your caregiver may want to induce you if your membranes have ruptured and you haven't gone into labor within 24 hours. Note: You should avoid baths and sexual intercourse once your membranes have ruptured.

By the time this period of "prelabor" has ended you'll be approximately one to two centimeters dilated. You'll be ready for "real" labor to begin!

True versus false labor

Don't be surprised if you end up experiencing a few "false starts" before labor actually begins. While there's nothing false about the way these so-called false labor contractions feel, they're categorized this way because they don't actually dilate the cervix.

As a rule of thumb, you're likely experiencing false labor rather than true labor if

- contractions are irregular and are increasing neither in frequency (the length of time between the start of one contraction and the next) nor severity (the amount of pain you experience)

- contractions stop if you change position, empty your bladder, or have two large glasses of water

- the pain from the contractions can be felt in your lower abdomen rather than your lower back

- the show is brownish rather than reddish and so is more likely to be the result of a recent internal examination or sexual intercourse

On the other hand, you should assume this is "the real thing" and double-check that your labor bag's packed (see Table 10.2) if you experience one or more of the following symptoms of true labor:

- contractions that seem to be falling into a regular pattern; that are getting longer, stronger, and more frequent; that intensify with activity; and that don't subside if you change position or drink two large glasses of water

- contractions that start in your lower back and then spread to your abdomen and possibly your legs

- abdominal cramping as if you had a gastrointestinal upset

- diarrhea

- show that's either pinkish or blood-streaked

- the rupture of your membranes

MOM'S THE WORD

"The most unusual thing I brought with me to the hospital was a Tupperware rolling pin. You can fill these with liquid, so I was able to put hot or cold water in it and have my coaches roll it over my back. I had a lot of lower back and hip pain, so it saved my coaches' hands and gave me the exact pressure I wanted over an entire section of my back at a time."

— *Dorothy, 33, mother of two*

TABLE 10.2

WHAT TO TAKE TO THE HOSPITAL

Wondering what you should take to the hospital with you? Here are a few ideas:

Labor Bag	Suitcase
Your health insurance card and proof of any extended health benefits you may have (e.g., semi-private or private room coverage through your health plan at work)	A hairbrush
	Shampoo
	Soap
	Toothbrush
Your hospital pre-registration forms (unless, of course, you've already dropped them off at the hospital)	Toothpaste
	Deodorant
One or more copies of your birth plan	Highly absorbent sanitary pads (unless the hospital provides them)
Sponges (to help keep you cool)	Books and magazines to read (including a good breastfeeding book)
A tennis ball or rolling pin (ideally one that can be filled with hot or cold water) to massage your back	
A frozen freezer pack (small) wrapped in a hand towel	Birth announcements and a pen (fill out as many of these as you can ahead of time, and pre-stamp and pre-address the envelopes)
A picture or other object that you find comforting (you might wish to use it as your focal point during labor)	Earplugs (so you can get some sleep on the noisy maternity ward!)
Massage oil or lotion	A small gift for each of the baby's siblings (unless, of course, this is your first!)
Cornstarch or other non-perfumed powder to reduce friction during massage	Two or more nightgowns (front-opening style if you're planning to breastfeed)
A hot water bottle	A bathrobe
Lip balm or petroleum jelly to relieve dry lips	

continued

Labor Bag

A camera or video camera plus spare batteries and spare film (if you're really paranoid, buy a disposable camera too so that you won't miss out on the ultimate of Kodak moments)

Extra pillows in colored pillow cases (so they won't get mixed up with the hospital pillows)

A portable stereo and some cassette tapes or CDs to listen to during labor or a portable TV/VCR unit with a movie to watch (check with the hospital first to find out which types of electronic devices are and aren't allowed in the hospital, for safety reasons)

Paper and pens

A roll of quarters, a prepaid phone card, or a cell phone

A list of people to phone

Snacks and drinks for your partner

A bathing suit for your partner (so that he can accompany you into the shower or the Jacuzzi to help you to work through contractions)

A change of clothes for your partner (in case your labor ends up being very long)

Books, magazines, a deck of cards, etc.

Suitcase

Two or more nursing bras

Five or more pairs of underwear (disposables or inexpensive ones that can be thrown away if they become badly stained)

Two pairs of warm socks

A pair of slippers

A going-home outfit for you (something that fit when you were five or six months pregnant)

A going-home outfit for the baby (ideally a sleeper or newborn nightie plus a hat)

A receiving blanket

A bunting bag and/or a heavy blanket if it's wintertime

A diaper for your baby to wear home (just in case the hospital uses cloth diapers)

MOM'S THE WORD

"Our child was born in November. My husband was working on a Christmas present for his mom — a cross-stitch birth certificate for the baby. Just as we were about to leave for the hospital, he put it in his bag. I asked him why on earth he'd bring it with him, and he said it was to keep him busy during the slow times. I thought he was nuts, but there was my husband, sitting in the rocker cross-stitching away between contractions. Every time I had a contraction he'd neatly put it all down, come help me through the contraction, and then go back to working on it. He must have done that for a few hours."

— *Stephanie, 27, mother of one*

Of course, there's no such thing as a textbook labor, so you may find that it's not exactly crystal clear whether you're dealing with bona fide labor contractions or not. Sometimes it can be very hard to tell what's really going on.

Maria, a 35-year-old mother of two, had a hard time deciding that her labor contractions were for real, even though her doctor had actually prescribed a cervical gel that was supposed to help ripen her cervix. "Everyone says that when you're really in labor, you'll know. Well, I'm here to tell you that's not always the case. The first time around, I had a prostaglandin gel applied to my cervix to soften it as a preparation for induction. I was told the gel sometimes gets labor rolling, but that it's not that effective in first-time mothers. I went home and started getting these killer menstrual cramps. I mean, they were just horrendous. I remember saying to my husband, 'God, it's so bad and I'm not even in labor yet. What's labor going to be like?' It was awful. I was on my hands and knees trying to get some relief when I threw up all over the floor. And somewhere in the recesses of my brain, a little light went on. 'Oh,' I thought. 'Maybe I'm in labor after all.' Duh!"

Maria was confused because her contractions seemed to defy the "rules" set out by her pregnancy books: "My first labor was nothing like what I expected. I thought labor pains would be sharp and have a beginning and an end. My contractions were dull and grinding and never peaked. I swear, I had one 5 ½- minute contraction."

Like Maria, it took Bevin a while to clue into the fact that she was really in labor: "I was in total denial for the first seven hours of my labor," the 27-year-old mother of one confesses. "It wasn't at all like how they said it would be in prenatal class. All the signs I was having seemed to point to false labor: My pains were centered in my belly, I had no back labor, very little pain, irregular contractions. But seven hours later when the really heavy pains set in, I knew it was really happening."

When to call your caregiver

As soon as your labor is well established, you should let your caregiver know. In general, you should plan to make this call if

- your contractions are strong and regular (generally at five-minute intervals, unless your caregiver has indicated that he or she wants you to call sooner than this)

- your membranes have ruptured or you suspect they've ruptured

- your past experience with labor tells you this is the real thing and you have this nagging gut feeling that it's time to call your caregiver

Rather than letting a family member make the phone call for you, try to make the call yourself so that your caregiver can better assess how far your labor has progressed. She'll know that the contractions are getting pretty intense if you're have a hard time talking during contractions.

Regardless of how well your labor is established, you'll need to notify your caregiver immediately if

- you experience a lot of bleeding (which can indicate premature separation of the placenta or placenta previa — see Chapter 11)

- you notice thickish green fluid coming from your vagina (which can indicate that your baby has passed meconium into the amniotic fluid and may be in distress)

- there's a loop of umbilical cord dangling from your vagina or you think you feel something inside your vagina (a possible indication of a cord prolapse)

FACTS AND FIGURES

If you suspect you've experienced a cord prolapse (an emergency situation in which the cord is presenting in front of your baby's head, leading to a possible lack of oxygen), lie with your head and chest on the floor and your bottom in the air. This will help to prevent your baby's head from compressing the umbilical cord and interrupting the flow of oxygen.

When to go to the hospital

You should plan to head to the hospital when

- your contractions are four minutes apart, lasting one minute, and occurring consistently for one hour or more

- your contractions are so painful that you have to rely on your relaxation breathing or other pain management techniques

- you can no longer talk during a contraction

- your membranes have ruptured (something that should be confirmed just in case antibiotics need to be started)

- you instinctively feel that it's time to go

Of course, if you live a significant distance from the hospital, you're giving birth in the middle of a snowstorm, or you have a history of rapid labors, you'll want to hit the road sooner rather than later. When it comes to labor, it's always better to err on the side of caution.

What Labor Is Really Like

Now we come to the $10,000 question — one of the key reasons why you bought this book. You want to know what labor is really like.

MOM'S THE WORD

"Labor was nothing like I had expected it to be. Nothing I had ever read or been told about it described it accurately. The books tend to make it 'flowery' and it isn't. I thought I would go to the hospital, have a little pain, and that would be it. Nobody prepared me for what it would really be like."

—*Josie, 29, mother of three*

If I could come up with a nice, pat answer, this would become the fastest-selling pregnancy book of all time. Doctors and midwives would be ordering it by the truckload and giving copies to their patients. Maternity stores would be selling maternity T-shirts with my pithy definition of labor printed on the front. The definition would show up on subway ads, the sides of buses, and on the stickers on the apples in the grocery store. PBS would feature public service announcements for kids, offering tips on how to tell if Mom is really in labor. The spinoff possibilities would be endless. . . .

I hate to disappoint you (to say nothing of my publisher), but that's not going to happen. The reason is simple. I'd have to catalogue about 11,000 descriptions of labor per day just to stay on top of things. You see, no two labors are exactly alike, and there are about 11,000 babies born in the U.S. each day, so, in the interests of scientific inquiry, I'd have to interview about 11,000 new moms a day. That would be exhausting, and this book would quickly turn into a multi-volume pregnancy book. (*Encylopedia Pregnanica,* I presume.) See the problem?

Since it's unlikely my publisher would agree to put out a 20-volume pregnancy book set, you're going to have to settle for the next best thing: a privileged, pink-ghetto look at what labor may be like for you. We'll start out by considering the three stages of labor. Then we'll look at what the handy-dandy chart that I've included won't actually tell you: the stuff only your most talkative girlfriends are willing to spill the beans about.

The three stages of labor

The first thing you need to know is that the labor process can be broken down into three distinct stages: the first stage (which lasts from the first contraction until your cervix is fully dilated), the second stage (the so-called "pushing stage"), and the third stage (the delivery of the placenta). (See Table 10.3)

TABLE 10.3

THE THREE STAGES OF LABOR

What Happens During This Stage	How You May Be Feeling Physically	How You May Be Feeling Emotionally	Tips on Coping with This Stage
First Stage (From the Onset of Labor Until the Cervix Is Fully Dilated)			
Early or latent labor (when your cervix dilates from 0 to 3 cm)	Backache, menstrual-like cramping, indigestion, diarrhea, a feeling of warmth in the abdomen, bloody show (the passage of blood-tinged mucus), and a trickling or gushing sensation if your membranes have ruptured	Excitement, relief, anticipation, uncertainty, anxiety, fear	Eat lightly and keep yourself well hydrated, continue with your normal activities as long as possible, ask your partner or labor support person to help you time contractions and to pack any last-minute items before you leave for the hospital or birthing center (unless, of course, you're having a home birth)

First Stage (From the Onset of Labor Until the Cervix Is Fully Dilated)

Active labor (when your cervix dilates from 4 to 7 cm)	Increased discomfort from contractions (suddenly, it's more difficult to talk or walk through a contraction), pain and aching in your legs and back, fatigue, increased quantities of bloody show	Anxiety, discouragement, highly focused on getting through this stage of labor	Remain upright and active as long as possible, experiment with positions until you find one that works best for you when a contraction hits, rest between contractions, empty your bladder regularly (at least once an hour), allow your partner or labor support person to help you with labor breathing and/or relaxation techniques, continue to consume light fluids (as long as you've got your caregiver's go-ahead)

continued

First Stage (From the Onset of Labor Until the Cervix Is Fully Dilated)

What Happens During This Stage	How You May Be Feeling Physically	How You May Be Feeling Emotionally	Tips on Coping with This Stage (Continued)
Transition (when your cervix dilates from 8 to 10 cm)	Increased quantities of show, pressure in your lower back, perineal and rectal pressure, hot and cold flashes, shaky legs, intense aching in your thighs, nausea or vomiting, belching, heavy perspiration	Irritable, disoriented, restless, frustrated	Change positions frequently to see if doing so will provide any measure of pain relief, apply a hot water bottle or cold pack to your back, have your partner or labor support person apply counter-pressure on the part of your back that's hurting, or have him/her apply strong finger pressure below the center of the ball of your foot (an acupuncture point for pain relief).

Second Stage (The Pushing Stage)

Your cervix is fully dilated and your body is ready for the pushing stage.	Expect to experience a series of 60- to 90-second contractions at two- to five- minute intervals. Your baby's head needs to stretch the vaginal and pelvic-floor muscles before the urge to push is triggered, so there can be a delay before you feel that urge. You'll likely experience increased rectal pressure, an increase in bloody show, an urge to grunt as you bear down, a burning or stretching sensation as your baby's head crowns in the vagina, and a slippery feeling as your baby is born.	Excited and energetic or tired, discouraged, and overwhelmed, depending on how your labor is going	Have your partner or labor support person help you move into a squatting or semi-squatting position to make it easier for you to push your baby out, push when you feel the urge, take short breaths rather than holding your breath and pushing through an entire contraction, and be prepared to stop pushing (pant or blow instead) if your caregiver tells you that your perineum needs time to stretch gradually in order to avoid an episiotomy or a tear.

continued

What Happens During This Stage	How You May Be Feeling Physically	How You May Be Feeling Emotionally	Tips on Coping with This Stage (Continued)
Third Stage (The Delivery of the Placenta)			
Your uterus expels the placenta	Mild contractions lasting for one minute or less will gently push the placenta out of your body. Your caregiver will examine the placenta to make sure it's complete, since retained placental fragments can cause hemorrhaging. You'll experience heavy bleeding from the vagina and may pass some large blood clots when you go to the bathroom. (Be sure to tell your caregiver if they're any larger thana lemon.)	Distracted, happy, excited to finally be meeting your baby, exhausted from the delivery, cold, hungry	Your caregiver may give you a shot of oxytocin or methylergonovine to try to prevent any problems with postpartum hemorrhaging. Your baby's nose and mouth will be suctioned and the baby will be assessed using the Apgar test. This test evaluates the baby's appearance, pulse (heartbeat), grimace (response to stimulation), activity (movements), and respiration (breathing). The test is performed twice, at one minute and five minutes after birth. The baby is given up to two points for each attribute. A baby with a score of seven or over is doing well; a baby with a score of five or six may require resuscitation; and a baby with a score of four or less may be in serious trouble.

What other pregnancy books won't tell you

Now let's get to the real nitty-gritty — the things most pregnancy books won't tell you but that you really need to know.

- If you wait to experience each and every labor symptom before you call your doctor or midwife, you'll be giving birth on your kitchen floor. I can practically guarantee it! It could take you two, three, or even a dozen or more pregnancies to experience all these symptoms. Don't get greedy and expect to experience them all the first time around.

- You have an almost endless supply of amniotic fluid. Don't expect it to disappear in one fell swoosh when your membranes rupture. It'll dribble — and dribble — and dribble. In fact, that endless dribbling of the amniotic fluid is one of the most annoying aspects of labor, and one that far too few pregnancy books talk about. It leaves you cold, wet, and frankly quite miserable.

- Your contractions won't feel the way your best friend's contractions felt. There's no such thing as a textbook contraction. Some women have "traditional" contractions with well-defined starts and finishes. Others find that one contraction kind of just blurs into the next. There's no right or wrong way to have a contraction, by the way. Any contraction that ultimately results in the birth of a baby is a good contraction!

MOM'S THE WORD

"I pictured each contraction as a wave crashing on the surf. As each contraction built up in intensity, I imagined a wave building up, building up, and then breaking over me and ebbing away."

— *Carrie, 34, currently pregnant with her second child*

- It's possible to experience uterine contractions primarily as lower back pain. (This is particularly common if, like 10% of babies, your baby is lying in the posterior position, meaning that the back of his head is up against your spine. Most posterior babies make the 180-degree shift into the anterior position at some point during labor, but those that don't can either be delivered naturally or, if necessary, via forceps or vacuum extraction.) Back labor can be long and drawn out and very discouraging. Counterpressure (having your labor support person apply pressure to your lower back), applying a heating pad or a hot water bottle to the affected area, and experimenting with various positions (e.g., tailor sitting, leaning forward while you're standing or sitting, or rocking your pelvis) may help to relieve the pain of back labor.

Sometimes labor can be painstakingly slow or grind to a halt altogether. This can happen if

- your contractions are weak and ineffective

- if there's some sort of fetal obstruction (e.g., your baby is breech or posterior or lying in a transverse or sideways position or oblique or diagonal position, your baby is presenting with its face or forehead first rather than the top of its head, your baby is large in relation to the size of your pelvis, you are delivering twins and they have become entwined, or your baby has a fetal anomaly such as hydrocephalus)

FACTS AND FIGURES

A recent study involving more than 2,000 women in 26 countries concluded that the safest method of delivering a baby in the breech position is via cesarean section. Breech babies delivered vaginally were found to be three to six times more likely to experience serious complications or to die during the first six weeks of life than breech babies who were delivered by cesarean section.

- there's some sort of maternal obstruction (e.g. your pelvis is deformed or unusually small; you have pelvic tumors such as large fibroids or a large ovarian cyst; your uterus, cervix, or vagina is abnormal; or your uterus is contracting in a manner that causes a band of tight muscle tissue to prevent the uterus or cervix from contracting)

- You may feel as though you're on another planet during the most intense part of your labor. Forget about looking lovingly into your partner's eyes while the two of you contemplate the impending birth of your child. You may be just plain zoned out. "Labor was a continual dull ache that consumed my entire being," confesses Bonnie, a 27-year-old mother of two. "I couldn't focus on anything except the next labor pain. I have no idea what was being said or who was in the room. It was almost a delusional state, like when you're very sick. You're in and out of consciousness, it seems."

- Your girlfriends won't be completely honest about their birth experiences until after you're pregnant and likely not until after you've given birth. The reason is obvious. They don't want you to take the vow of celibacy! (Hey, if foot-long stretch marks and 30-hour labors were good enough for them, they're good enough for you, too!) "I think there's a bit of a conspiracy that you don't tell friends who haven't given birth how much it really does hurt because you don't want to scare them," admits Cheryl, 29, who is currently pregnant with her second child (and not saying a word about her first birth to any of her first-time pregnant buddies).

- Pregnancy books are big on euphemisms. Take everything that you read with a grain of salt. "I had a girlfriend who experienced natural childbirth a few months before me," explains Joyce. "Fortunately she tipped me off to this problem.

She told me, 'You know that part in the books that tells you that the mother may experience some burning when the baby's head is crowning? Well, believe me — it's not just a mild burning sensation; it's more like a f — ing blowtorch!'"

- The pushing stage isn't the picnic that so many other pregnancy books make it out to be. Think about it! You're trying to push an 8-pound baby out through an opening that's generally snug enough to hold a tampon in place. You think that's going to be easy? Not according to Cheryl: "I didn't expect it to be so hard to push the baby out. It's a real physical effort and was exhausting." Marinda, a 30-year-old mother of two, agrees: "I was overwhelmed by the pain of the pushing stage. I thought it was hell. For a short time, I didn't even care if I got a baby out of it. I just wanted the pain to end." So the next time a pregnancy book author tells you what a tremendous relief it is to be through transition and into the pushing stage, take a look at the cover and see if a guy wrote the book.

- You'll amaze yourself with your strength and resilience. You'll also dazzle your partner. Joyce was very apprehensive about giving birth, but, in the end, she was pleasantly surprised by her own abilities: "I was so sure I'd be afraid, but what amazed me was how 'natural' the whole thing turned out to be: How we as females and the givers of life have such a reserve of strength we didn't know existed until it's called upon."

 MOTHER WISDOM

"The male sea horse, not the female, gives birth to their babies. The female shoots her eggs into a pouch on his chest, where he fertilizes, then incubates them for two weeks. When it's time to give birth, he will squirt as many as a thousand baby sea horses out of his chest over the course of 24 hours."

— **Kit Carlson,** *Bringing Up Baby: Wild Animal Families.*

MOM'S THE WORD

"I don't think any book can prepare you for labor. It is the most unique experience."

— *Joyce, 41, mother of two*

What to expect during a cesarean delivery

Up until now we've been focusing on vaginal deliveries. Since a significant number of babies are born through cesarean section (22% of babies born in the U.S. in 1999 arrived via cesarean section, in fact) it's now time to talk about what a cesarean delivery involves.

FACTS AND FIGURES

According to a recent Yale University study, male doctors in university hospitals are three times as likely and male doctors in private practice are 1 ½-times as likely to deliver babies via cesarean section as their female counterparts. The study also found that cesarean section rates have quadrupled over the past 20 years: Approximately one in five babies born in the U.S. is now delivered by cesarean section.

At first glance, you might think that a cesarean is the perfect way to have a baby. After all, you get to avoid all those gut-wrenching contractions (unless, of course you get to have the cesarean *after* experiencing a couple of hours of gut-wrenching contractions!), to say nothing of that annoying third-trimester "Am I really in labor or not?" guessing game. Unfortunately, what we moms who have delivered vaginally sometimes forget is that having a cesarean section isn't exactly a picnic. I mean this is major abdominal surgery we're talking about here, complete with a less-than-enjoyable recovery. We're talking killer gas pains, stitches in your abdomen, and — if you require a general anesthesia — feeling somewhat dopey and drowsy when you finally get the chance to meet your baby. And then there are all the possible complications: infection, blood loss, problems related to the anesthesia, blood clots caused by reduced mobility after surgery, and bladder and bowel injuries. It's enough to make you feel damned grateful for that episiotomy, now isn't it?

That's not to say cesareans are a terrible thing. They've helped save the lives of countless mothers and babies, and prevented countless birth-related injuries, after all. And there's something appealing about being able to mark the date of your cesarean on your calendar rather than playing the tortuous game of due-date roulette like most of the moms who are delivering vaginally!

Even if you're 100% convinced that you won't need a cesarean, it's important to read through this section. There's always the chance that an emergency will arise that could see you being wheeled into the operating room. Here's what you need to know about giving birth via cesarean section.

FACTS AND FIGURES

Worried that a baby born through cesarean section is at a disadvantage because he doesn't get the same "squeezing" as babies born vaginally? Most obstetricians agree this is a myth. A fair bit of squeezing occurs as the baby is delivered through the incision in your uterus, something that — like a vaginal delivery — helps to clear amniotic fluid from the baby's lungs and stimulate the baby's circulation.

What will happen before the delivery

- Your doctor will give you some sort of medication to dry the secretions in your mouth and upper airway. He or she will also give you an antacid to reduce the acidity of your stomach contents — important if you end up inhaling some of the contents of your stomach during the delivery.

- Your doctor may give you a single dose of antibiotics to guard against the possibility of infection.

- Your lower abdomen will be washed and possibly shaved as well.

- A catheter will be inserted into your bladder to reduce the risk of injury during the delivery. (A full bladder can be injured more easily.)

- An intravenous needle will be inserted into your hand or arm so that you can be given medications and fluids during the delivery.

- You'll be given an anesthetic (either an epidural, a spinal, or a general).

- Your abdomen will be swabbed with antiseptic solution and covered with a sterile drape.

- A screen will be put in place to keep the surgical field sterile. It also helps to block your view of the delivery. (It's one thing to watch a cesarean being performed on the Discovery Channel. It's quite another to watch it take place live in your own body!)

What will happen during the delivery

- An incision will be made through both the wall of your abdomen and the wall of your uterus as soon as the anesthetic has taken effect. You may still be able to feel some pressure, but you won't feel any pain.

- The amniotic sac will be opened and amniotic fluid will pour out.

- Your baby will be lifted from your body. You may feel a slight
  tugging sensation if you've had an epidural (an obstetrician I
  know says the pressure and sensation you feel during a
  cesarean delivery is similar to what you experience when you
  touch your face or tongue after the dentist has frozen your
  mouth), but you're unlikely to feel any such sensation if
  you've had a spinal. You may also experience some nausea
  and vomiting because tugging on the peritoneum — the
  layer which coats your internal organs — can cause this
  reaction in some women.

What will happen after the delivery

- The umbilical cord will be clamped and the placenta will be
  removed from your uterus.

- Your baby's nose and mouth will be suctioned and the baby
  will be assessed using the Apgar test. The Apgar test evaluates
  the baby's appearance, pulse (heartbeat), grimace (response
  to stimulation), activity (movements), and respiration
  (breathing). The test is performed twice, at one minute and
  five minutes after birth. The baby is given up to two points
  for each attribute. A baby with a score of seven or over is
  doing well; a baby with a score of five or six may require
  resuscitation; and a baby with a score of four or less may be
  in serious trouble.

- Your uterus and abdomen will be stitched up and you'll be
  given the opportunity to hold your baby if both you and the
  baby are feeling up to it.

- You'll be taken to the recovery room so that your vital signs
  can be monitored and you can be checked for excessive
  bleeding and other possible post-delivery complications.

- You may be given antibiotics and/or pain medications at this time.

- You'll be moved to the postpartum floor to continue your recovery.

- About six to eight hours after the delivery, your catheter will be removed and you'll be encouraged to get out of bed.

- You'll be given intravenous fluids for one to two days, until you're able to start eating again. (Basically, you'll be kept on intravenous fluids the entire time you're receiving intravenous drugs and you'll continue to receive these fluids until you're feeling well enough to drink enough fluids to keep your body adequately hydrated.)

- You'll be able to leave the hospital within three to five days after the delivery, unless unexpected complications arise.

Vaginal birth after cesarean (VBAC)

Doctors used to live by the motto, "Once a cesarean, always a cesarean." That's not the case today. More and more often, doctors are encouraging their patients to consider vaginal births after cesarean (VBACs).

While there are clearly some advantages to attempting a VBAC — vaginal deliveries are generally less risky than cesareans, take less time to recover from, and allow you to play a more active role in your baby's birth — there are also some risks involved. There's always the chance, however slight, that the uterine scar tissue from your previous incision may split — a potentially life-threatening complication for both you and your baby. (Your odds of experiencing this sort of complication when you've had a single cesarean delivery are approximately 1 in 1,000.)

Your doctor is unlikely to encourage you to attempt a VBAC if

- you had a vertical rather than a horizontal uterine incision, since there's a higher risk of uterine rupture (Note: The incision on your uterus may not necessarily be in the same direction as the incision on your skin)

- you're carrying more than one baby

- your baby is in either the breech or transverse position

- your baby is likely to have problems fitting through your pelvis

- your baby is showing signs of fetal distress

While you might want to attempt a VBAC in order to have the "ultimate" birth experience, it's important to remember that delivering a baby through cesarean section can be every bit as meaningful as delivering a baby vaginally. What matters most is that you and your baby are both healthy at the end of the day.

Going Overdue

Your due date has come and gone and there's still no baby. Chances are you're feeling pretty cranky! After all, you thought you were signing a 40-week contract when you agreed to this whole pregnancy thing. . . .

MOM'S THE WORD

"We tried having sex close to our due date in an effort to get labor started, and it was just hilarious. In the end, we gave up and decided to let labor start on its own!"

— *A first-time parent*

Here are some tips on maintaining what's left of your sanity until baby makes his grand entrance:

- Remind yourself that it's perfectly normal to be overdue. According to British childbirth expert Sheila Kitzinger, only 5% of babies actually arrive on their due date, and of the 95% who don't, just 3 out of 10 arrive before the due date while 7 out of 10 come after it! And here's another statistic: 9 out of 10 babies manage to make an appearance within 10 days of their due date. So your odds of still being pregnant 10 days after your baby is due are less than 10%.

- Put technology to work for you. If you're sick of fielding all those annoying "Haven't you had that baby yet" phone calls, let your voice mail system pick up the calls. Or better yet, do what one couple I know did and record a message that says, "We're just out. We're not having the baby!"

- Keep yourself busy. Go to a movie. Have lunch with a friend. Do whatever it takes to take your mind off the fact that your baby is L-A-T-E. And don't be afraid to make plans just because you might have to cancel out on your friends. Having a baby is the best excuse ever for standing someone up.

- Pamper yourself. Take advantage of your final baby-free days to get your hair done, soak in the tub, or read incredibly trashy novels. You'll have days like this again, of course — but you'll have to wait another 18 years!

- Enjoy some special time alone with your partner. It may be weeks — even months — before you can both eat dinner at the same time again, so seize the moment!

- Don't expect your doctor or midwife to know how much longer you're going to be pregnant. As much as they'd like to pinpoint the time of your baby's arrival, they don't have a crystal ball.

Is my baby at risk?

You've no doubt heard all the scary stories about the dangers of being overdue — about all the awful things that can happen if your baby ends up spending too much time in the womb. What you might not realize, however, is that there's a world of difference between being overdue (past your due date) and post-date (being more than two weeks overdue). If you're more than two weeks late your doctor or midwife will want to deliver your baby sooner rather than later. Here's why:

- The placenta may start to deteriorate. The placenta — your baby's life support system while he's in the womb — is designed to work for about 40 weeks from the time of conception (i.e., until approximately the 42nd week of pregnancy, counted from the first day of your last menstrual period). Most placentas continue to function for longer than that, but in some cases the placenta will start to deteriorate and will no longer be able to provide the baby with the nutrients he needs to grow. This can cause the baby to lose weight.

- Your baby may become overly large. If your placenta is still working at top capacity, your baby will continue to grow right up until delivery day. If he becomes too large, you face an increased risk of complications during the birth (e.g., you may need to deliver through cesarean section).

- Amniotic fluid levels may drop. After about the 34th to 36th week of gestation, the amount of amniotic fluid that your baby is floating around in begins to decrease. If a pregnancy continues for too long, amniotic fluid levels can drop to the point that your baby is at risk of settling on the umbilical cord and experiencing an umbilical cord compression problem.

- Your baby could inhale meconium. The longer your baby stays in the womb, the greater the odds that he'll pass his first bowel movement — meconium — before birth. If this happens, the baby could end up breathing in some of this black, sticky, tar-like substance, which can result in breathing problems after birth.

FACTS AND FIGURES

There's a growing body of evidence that it may make sense to induce labor at 41 rather than 42 weeks. Research combining 11 different studies on the timing of induction indicates that the perinatal death rate dropped from 2.5 per 1,000 births to 0.3 per 1,000 births when labor was induced at 41 weeks rather than allowed to begin spontaneously. It's something to talk to your caregiver about if you happen to be singing the overdue blues.

While these things don't tend to become a problem until you are two weeks overdue, your doctor or midwife will want to monitor you closely once your due date comes and goes. You may be sent for a non-stress test (which involves monitoring the baby's heart rate via external monitoring equipment for up to 40 minutes), a contraction stress test (monitoring the baby's heart rate during a forced contraction), or a biophysical profile (a detailed ultrasound that assesses the baby's breathing movements, body or limb movements, fetal tone, and the quantity of amniotic fluid). If your caregiver concludes that your baby would be better off being born than remaining in the womb much longer, the decision will be made to induce you.

To induce or not to induce?

Despite what you may have heard about women being induced early so that their doctors don't miss out on important golf games, the decision to induce is rarely taken that lightly.

If your doctor does make the decision to induce, it will likely be for one of the following reasons:

- your baby doesn't appear to be doing particularly well in the uterus and would likely be better off being induced early

- you were diabetic before you became pregnant (there is a high instance of stillbirth in women with pre-existing diabetes and this risk increases once your due date passes)

- a stress test or non-stress test has indicated that the placenta is no longer functioning properly and that it would be better for the baby to be born as soon as possible

- your membranes ruptured more than 24 hours ago, but labor has not yet started

- you've developed pre-eclampsia or some other serious medical condition and an induction is necessary for the sake of the baby's health as well as your own

- you have a history of rapid labor that puts you at high risk of experiencing an unplanned home birth

- you live a considerable distance from the hospital and may not be able to make it there in time to deliver your baby once labor begins

Before inducing you, the doctor will need to determine how ready your body is for an induction. (He or she will likely use the Bishop scoring system, which involves looking for evidence that your cervix has begun to efface and dilate, that your baby has begun to descend into your pelvis, that your cervix has begun to soften, and/or that your cervix is moving into the anterior or forward-pointing position. Basically, you're assigned a score of one, two, or three on each of these five criteria. If you score eight or higher, your body is considered to be ready for induction.) If your body isn't ready, you may need to be induced more than once — something no woman should have to endure! Your doctor also has to ensure that your baby is ready to be born. That means checking your prenatal records to confirm that your due date is accurate and, if there is reason to suspect that your due date may be wrong and your baby may actually be premature, possibly assessing the maturity of your baby's lungs by performing amniocentesis.

MOM'S THE WORD

"My doctor told me we were going to have to induce, and I was just not emotionally ready. I had planned to take the last three weeks before my due date off work, and then I ended up delivering the day after my last day on the job. I felt emotionally and physically unprepared; my baby's room wasn't finished, nor was I emotionally finished with my mental preparations."

—*Jane, 33, mother of two*

What to expect during an induction

Despite what you may have heard, induced labors aren't necessarily more painful than spontaneous labors. Studies have shown that women who are induced are no more likely to require epidurals than women who go into labor on their own.

If your doctor decides to induce you, he or she will likely use one of the following four methods:

- Artificial rupture of membranes (amniotomy). A piece of obstetrical equipment resembling a crochet hook is inserted through your cervix and used to tear a small hole in the amniotic sac. The procedure is virtually painless if you've already started to dilate, but can be quite painful if you're less than one centimeter dilated. What's more, if the induction fails, you'll have to be induced using another method. Once your membranes have been ruptured, there's no turning back.

- Prostaglandin E suppositories or gel. Prostaglandin E suppositories or gel are used to ripen the cervix. In 50% of cases, the woman will go into labor on her own within the next 24 hours.

- Pitocin. Pitocin — the synthetic form of oxytocin (the naturally produced hormone that triggers uterine contractions) — is injected via an intravenous drip and the strength of your contractions is monitored to ensure that you're getting an appropriate dose. If your cervix has not yet started dilating, it can take a couple of attempts to induce labor with Pitocin.

- Cervical dilators. Cervical dilators can be used to manually force the cervix to start to open. Sticks of compressed and dried seaweed or synthetic materials are placed in your cervix. As the sticks begin to absorb moisture and expand, they dilate your cervix.

Meeting Your Baby

The big moment has finally arrived. You get to meet the tiny little person who's been subletting your uterus! If you're expecting your newborn to look like a Gerber baby right away, you're in for a bit of a surprise. Newborn babies are considerably less chubby and pink. In fact, they can look a little odd. Here's what to expect:

- Irregular head shape. Your baby has just made a rather grueling journey through the birth canal. Along the way, his head may have become a little molded or conelike in appearance. What's more, if he ended up pushing against an inadequately dilated cervix, he may have a strange lump known as a caput succedaneum. All these changes are temporary — the molding will be gone within two weeks and the caput succedaneum within a matter of days — but they can be alarming nonetheless.

- Hair. Whether your baby is born with a full head of hair or hardly any at all, he's well within the range of normal. Newborn hair will fall out and be replaced.

- Vernix caseosa coating. Your baby may have remnants of vernix in the folds of his skin. This greasy white substance protected him while he was floating around in the sea of amniotic fluid inside your uterus.

- Lanugo. Your baby may have fine, downy hair on her shoulders, back, forehead, and temples.

- Genital swelling. Your baby's genitals and breasts may be swollen as a result of maternal hormones crossing the placenta. A baby boy will have an enlarged scrotum and a baby girl may pass milky-white or blood-tinged secretions from her vagina.

- Birthmarks. Some babies are born with birthmarks. Reddish blotches are most common in Caucasians, whereas bluish-grey pigmentation on the back, buttocks, arms, or thighs is more common in babies of Asian, south European, or African-American ancestry.

- Newborn urticaria. Your baby may be born with a series of red spots with yellowish-white centers. These spots typically appear during the first day of life but disappear by the time a baby is 1 week old.

- Red marks on the skin or broken blood vessels in the skin or eyes. Your baby may have broken blood vessels or red marks on the skin caused by pressure during the birth. These marks typically disappear within a matter of days.

How you may feel about meeting your baby

After months of anticipation, your baby is finally here. You may feel over the moon with excitement or so tired you can hardly even process the fact that this tiny human being belongs to you. While you may worry that you'll be setting your child up for a lifetime of psychological problems if you don't manage to "bond" right in the delivery room, that's simply not the case.

MOM'S THE WORD

"I did not bond instantly. There were no tears of joy. To be honest, while I loved her dearly, it took a couple of weeks for me to realize that she belonged to me. I wasn't just babysitting! It was the oddest sensation, really."

—*Jane, 30, currently pregnant with her second child*

Lori, a 29-year-old mother of four, remembers what it was like after her first baby arrived: "I wasn't prepared to be as tired as I was. By the time my daughter was born, pain aside, I'd been awake for 32 hours and was completely exhausted. Being in pain and going through labor just intensified that feeling. So by the time my baby was born, all I could think about was sleep."

Stephanie, a 27-year-old mother of one, had a different experience, although it started out the same: "I was so exhausted that I could hardly keep my eyes open," she said. "I remember thinking, 'What's wrong with me? This is my child and I, at this moment, don't even care if I hold her. I just want to sleep.' I took her on my chest and then the midwife came over and helped me to start breastfeeding her. That was the magical moment — to see her instantly take my breast and start sucking. I nursed her for almost half an hour and it was the bonding moment for me."

Alexandra remembers feeling as though she'd just been handed someone else's baby. "I couldn't believe that the little baby on my tummy was mine," the 33-year-old mother of two recalls. "I actually asked the nurses if I could touch her. Although I felt overwhelming love toward my baby, it took a couple of days for me to actually bond with her."

Janet, 32, felt much the same way when her daughter was born. "I was immediately fascinated by her, but I didn't feel like she belonged to us until several days — maybe even a week — after her birth. Initially she seemed like a novelty item of some sort, and it did not sink in that she was with us permanently."

Some women, like Jennifer, do experience that magical, mystical, love-at-first-sight bonding that you hear so much about. "I was amazed at how quickly I bonded with my babies," the 31-year-old mother of two recalls. "There was an instant connection and I felt immediately like their mommy."

Christina, 25, also felt overcome with emotion when she met each of her three children for the very first time. "I felt an instant bond with my children when they were born. It didn't matter that they were wrinkled and funny-looking. They were the most beautiful sight in the world to me. When I held my son in my arms for the first time, I felt something I'd never felt before: unconditional love and an amazingly strong protective instinct."

MOM'S THE WORD

"There isn't necessarily a bright light or a wave of emotion or a band playing when you hold your new child for the very first time. Don't force the situation. Just allow yourself to be happy, tired, relieved, scared — whatever."

— *Jennifer, 32, mother of one*

CHAPTER 11

When Pregnancy Isn't Perfect

*"Not everyone has a textbook pregnancy and delivery and ends up
with a smiling chubby newborn who is breastfeeding with ease.
A problem pregnancy, a preterm delivery, and a failed
breastfeeding attempt do not make you less of a person.
Having a baby is not a contest."*
— *Susan, 35, mother of two children who
were born prematurely*

While some women enjoy the luxury of breezing
through pregnancy with nothing much more
earth-shattering to worry about than whether the
Winnie-the-Pooh wallpaper for the baby's room will arrive on
time, others have considerably more to feel anxious about —
like whether there will, in fact, be a healthy baby to take home
nine months down the road.

This chapter is all about the challenges of coping with a
high-risk pregnancy: why your pregnancy might be classified as
high risk and what you can do to stay sane while you count
down the days to delivery. We'll conclude the chapter by touching on a subject you probably don't even want to think about:
the possibility that your pregnancy could result in a less-than-
happy ending.

What Does the Term "High-Risk Pregnancy" Really Mean?

While it can be pretty scary to have your pregnancy labeled "high risk," it's important to keep in mind that the term tends to be applied quite liberally. Doctors and midwives will consider your pregnancy "high risk" if you face a higher-than-average chance of experiencing complications during pregnancy or birth or of delivering a baby who's in less-than-ideal health. The label is by no means a self-fulfilling prophecy: The vast majority of women to whom it's applied end up giving birth to healthy babies after all.

In general, you can expect your pregnancy to be labeled high risk if

- you have a chronic medical condition that may affect your pregnancy (see Chapter 2 for a detailed discussion of the effects of various medical conditions on pregnancy)
- you have a history of pregnancy-related complications (see Table 11.1) or appear to be developing one of these in your current pregnancy

---

MOM'S THE WORD

"Because of my pre-existing kidney problems, we knew there was a chance we wouldn't be able to continue with the pregnancy. Alport's syndrome is x-linked and is far more serious in males than in females. In affected males, there's a virtual guarantee of kidney failure and the need for a transplant, usually by the late teens or early 20s. In girls, the disease is fairly benign and most affected women can lead a long, full, healthy life. We were going in blind: If we had a son, there was a 50/50 chance that he'd have this disease and a 100% chance that if he did have it, he'd be looking at reduced kidney function, dialysis, and a transplant. Since I'm adopted, there was no likely pool of potential donors. We decided that if the results of the CVS showed we were having a boy, we'd terminate the pregnancy. At 11 weeks we were told we were having a girl, and only then were we able to enjoy being pregnant."

—Jenny, 31, *mother of one*

TABLE 11.1

CONDITIONS THAT CAN ARISE DURING PREGNANCY

Type of Condition	Risks	Treatment
Amniotic Fluid Problems		
Chorioamnionitis (infection of the amniotic fluid and fetal membranes)	Chorioamnionitis increases your risk of premature rupturing of the membranes (PROM) or of premature labor. It can also occur after your membranes have ruptured.	Your doctor will either treat the problem with antibiotics or decide to deliver your baby early.
Oligohydramnios (too little amniotic fluid)	Oligohydramnios can indicate that you're carrying a baby who has missing or malfunctioning kidneys, that you may be leaking amniotic fluid due to premature rupture of the membranes, or that the placenta is not functioning properly.	This condition is generally treated by delivering the baby as soon as possible.
Polyhydramnios (too much amniotic fluid)	Polyhydramnios can indicate that you're carrying a baby with Rh-incompatibility problems, a gastrointestinal anomaly, or diabetes or that you're carrying more than one baby.	If your baby is believed to be at risk as a result of a high amniotic fluid level, excess fluid may be removed through amniocentesis. Your doctor will want to pinpoint the cause of the problem, if possible, in case treatment may improve your baby's outcome. Unfortunately, in almost 50% of cases it's impossible to determine the cause of the problem.

continued

Type of Condition	Risks	Treatment (Continued)
Fetal Health Problems		
Intrauterine growth restriction, also called intrauterine growth retardation (your baby is consistently measuring small for its gestational age)	Intrauterine growth restriction can lead to stillbirth or the growth of a low-birthweight baby with a range of health problems. Note: Intrauterine growth restriction is more likely to occur in women with chronic health problems, who are leading an unhealthy lifestyle, who have high blood pressure, who are carrying multiples, who are on their first or fifth (or subsequent) pregnancy, or who are carrying a fetus with chromosomal abnormalities.	You may be hospitalized or put on bedrest. If your doctor believes the baby would do better outside the womb, labor may be induced or your baby may be delivered by cesarean section.

Type of Condition	Risks	Treatment
Maternal Health Problems		
Gestational diabetes (a form of diabetes that can develop during pregnancy)	Gestational diabetes puts you at increased risk of giving birth to an excessively large baby who may have difficulty adjusting to life outside the womb; of giving birth to a stillborn baby; and of having your diabetes recur later in life. Your baby may also be at increased risk of developing diabetes in adulthood. Note: Women who are overweight, who have high blood pressure, who have recurrent yeast infections, who have a history of polycystic ovarian syndrome (PCOS), who have experienced gestational diabetes in a previous pregnancy, who have a family history of diabetes, who have previously given birth to a baby weighing more than nine pounds, or who have experienced an unexplained stillbirth face an increased risk of developing gestational diabetes.	The condition is controlled through diet, exercise, and — if necessary — insulin injections.

continued

Type of Condition	Risks	Treatment (Continued)
Maternal Health Problems		
Intrahepatic chloestasis (severe itching and mild jaundice)	Intrahepatic chloestasis increases your risk of experiencing either a premature delivery or a stillbirth.	Your pregnancy will be monitored carefully and your baby may be delivered prematurely if it's believed that the baby would do better outside the womb.
Pre-eclampsia (a serious health condition characterized by very high blood pressure)	Pre-eclampsia can develop into eclampsia, a potentially life-threatening condition for both mother and baby. Note: The warning symptoms of pre-eclampsia include swelling of the hands and feet; sudden weight gain; high blood pressure (140/90 or higher or a marked increase over your baseline blood pressure reading); increased protein in the urine; headaches; and nausea, vomiting, and abdominal pain during the second or third trimesters. The condition is more likely to occur in first-time mothers (and in women who are giving birth to their first baby with a new partner), women who are carrying multiples, women who are over 40 or under 18, and women with chronic high blood pressure, diabetes, kidney disease, or a family history of pre-eclampsia. If seizures are present, the condition is known as eclampsia.	Your doctor may recommend bedrest (in cases of mild pre-eclampsia) or an immediate delivery (in situations where both the mother and baby's lives are at risk). Your doctor may also treat you with medication in order to safeguard your own health and to try to buy more your baby some more time in the womb. If you develop serious complications such as seizures or liver or kidney complications, your doctor will have no choice but to deliver your baby as soon as possible.

continued

Maternal Health Problems

Pregnancy-induced hypertension (PIH) (high blood pressure that occurs during pregnancy)	Severe high blood pressure can be dangerous — even fatal — to both mother and baby.	Your doctor will prescribe blood pressure medication to try to bring your blood pressure down. It may also be necessary to deliver your baby prematurely.

Placental Problems

Placental abruption (premature separation of the placenta from the uterine wall)	A placental abruption can result in stillbirth or the birth of a disabled baby and can lead to severe hemorrhaging and even death in the mother. Note: The warning symptoms of a placental abruption include heavy vaginal bleeding, premature labor contractions, uterine tenderness, and lower back pain. Placental abruptions are more common in mothers who've had two or more children, who have pregnancy-induced or chronic high blood pressure, who have experienced a previous placental abruption, who smoke, who use cocaine, or whose membranes rupture prematurely.	Treatment may include careful monitoring and bedrest (if the placental abruption is only partial) or an emergency cesarean (if it appears that a full abruption is inevitable — something that could put both your life and the baby's life at risk). Note: If your baby has already died as a result of the abruption, your doctor will induce labor rather than performing a cesarean section because of the risk of hemorrhage.

Type of Condition	Risks	Treatment (Continued)
Placental Problems		
Placental insufficiency (your baby is not receiving adequate nutrition from the placenta)	Placental insufficiency can be caused by restricted blood flow due to a clot, a partial abruption, a placenta that's too small or underdeveloped, a postdate pregnancy, high blood pressure, cigarette smoking, lupus or lupus antibodies, or maternal diabetes. It can lead to stillbirth or the birth of a small-for-date baby who may have some serious health problems	Treatments include careful monitoring and bedrest or a premature delivery (if it's believed that your baby would be better off being delivered early). You will likely receive two injections of steroids to help mature your baby's lungs if a premature delivery is anticipated. You may also be prescribed baby aspirin to decrease clotting in the placenta.
Placenta previa (the placenta is blocking all or part of the cervix — the exit from the uterus)	Placenta previa may prevent you from giving birth vaginally. In many cases, a low-lying placenta that's diagnosed early in pregnancy will correct itself before you go into labor. The incidence of low-lying placenta in the second trimester is 13%, but only 0.4% at the start of labor. Note: The warning symptoms of placenta previa include bleeding (usually painless) whenever you cough, strain, or have sexual intercourse. The condition is more common in women who've had several children, who have closely spaced pregnancies, who have a history of abortion (multiple D&Cs) and/or cesarean section, or who have endometrial scarring from a previous episode of placenta previa.	Treatment may include bedrest, careful monitoring, hospitalization, and/or delivery via cesarean section. Placenta previa can cause life-threatening hemorrhaging and, in up to 10% of cases of complete placenta previa, a hysterectomy may be required to control the bleeding.

Other Problems

Hyperemesis gravidarum (severe morning sickness)	Hyperemesis gravidarum can lead to dehydration, malnutrition, intrauterine growth restriction, and/or premature labor. Note: Hyperemesis gravidarum is more common in first-time mothers, mothers carrying multiples, and mothers who have experienced this condition in a previous pregnancy.	You may be hospitalized so that intravenous drugs and fluids can be administered. In very severe cases, you may require intravenous feeding (TPN).
Premature labor	Your baby may be born with some medical challenges and possibly some chronic health conditions. If your baby is born too prematurely, he or she may not be able to adjust to life outside the womb and may die shortly after birth. Note: You face a higher-than-average risk of going into premature labor if you smoke, you are younger than 16 or older than 35, your mother took DES when she was pregnant with you, you've been diagnosed with placenta previa or polyhydramnios, you haven't gained an adequate amount of weight during your pregnancy, you've been experiencing some unexplained vaginal bleeding, you've had abdominal surgery or have developed a high fever or kidney infection during your pregnancy, you have high blood pressure, you have an abnormal uterine structure, you have fibroids, or you are experiencing a great deal of physical or emotional stress.	If your baby is very premature, your treatment plan may be designed to hold off labor for as long as possible. Unfortunately, while bedrest, intravenous fluids, and/or drugs can be used to slow down or stop labor, they tend to be ineffective if your cervix has dilated by more than three centimeters or has already begun to thin out (efface). In this situation, your doctor will simply be hoping that these forms of treatment will buy your baby an extra couple of days inside the womb — just long enough for the steroid shots to help mature your baby's lungs prior to delivery.

- you have a history of miscarriage (although most caregivers won't label your pregnancy "high risk" unless you've experienced three consecutive first-trimester miscarriages)

- you have experienced stillbirth

- you've had a baby who died shortly after birth or who was diagnosed with a genetic disorder

- you're a carrier for a genetic disorder

- you're carrying more than one baby (see the section on multiple births later in this chapter)

FACTS AND FIGURES

The rate of complications for women carrying twins is eight times as high as the rate for women carrying a single baby.

- your membranes have ruptured and you're not yet 36 weeks pregnant.

- you have a history of gynecological problems, such as large, symptomatic fibroids (non-cancerous growths in the uterus)

- you have a sexually transmitted disease that could be transmitted to your child during pregnancy or birth (e.g,. herpes, HIV, or hepatitis B or C)

- you have previously delivered a preterm baby

- you conceived using high-tech fertility methods (which may increase your odds of experiencing a multiple birth)

- your mother took an anti-miscarriage drug called diethylstilbestriol (DES) when she was pregnant with you (this increases your odds of a miscarriage or premature birth)

If your pregnancy is diagnosed as high risk, you may find yourself feeling angry and resentful that every other pregnant woman you know seems to be enjoying a blissfully uneventful pregnancy while you have to worry about every little symptom and complaint; or worried and upset about what the pregnancy may mean for you and your baby. You may even experience some guilt feelings if you believe (rightly or wrongly) that you may have done something to put your pregnancy at risk. It's important to talk about how you're feeling with your midwife or doctor or a counselor, or with other women who are currently experiencing or who've been through a high-risk pregnancy in the past. Sidelines National Support Network can match you up with a volunteer who has herself experienced a high-risk pregnancy and who can offer you support and reassurance during the months ahead. (See Appendix D for details on how to contact this non-profit organization.)

Surviving bedrest

If you're carrying three or more babies, you have a medical condition such as pre-eclampsia or a placental abruption, your baby is showing signs of being small for his/her gestational age, or you're threatening to go into preterm labor, your doctor may order bedrest for the remainder of your pregnancy. Bedrest can do all kinds of good things for your pregnancy: reduce the strain on your heart; improve blood flow to your kidneys (something that helps your body get rid of excess fluids); increase circulation to the uterus (which boosts the amount of oxygen and nutrients your baby is receiving); reduce blood levels of catecholamines (the stress hormones responsible for triggering contractions); ease the pressure on your cervix; limit the amount of physical activity you engage in (which helps to reduce the number of contractions you'll experience); and conserve your energy so that you'll have more nutrients available to support your baby's growth.

While you might think that being ordered to watch television, read books, and lie in bed all day might be wonderfully restful, most women find it frustrating and stressful to be confined to bed for an extended period of time. What's more, bedrest can trigger a variety of physical conditions, including increased fatigue, soreness and achiness, and a tightening of the Achilles tendon that can make it painful for you to walk. Because of the risk of blood clots, your doctor may prescribe a blood thinner and recommend a series of leg exercises that can be done while you're in bed.

Here are some tips on staying sane if your doctor recommends bedrest:

• Find out exactly what your doctor means by bedrest. Because the health and well-being of your baby is at stake, it's important to know what you are and aren't allowed to do. (See Table 11.2 for a list of questions to ask your doctor if he or she recommends bedrest.)

TABLE 11.2

QUESTIONS TO ASK YOUR DOCTOR ABOUT BEDREST

If your doctor recommends bedrest, you'll want to find out exactly what you are and aren't allowed to do. Here are some questions you'll want to ask:
How long am I likely to be on bedrest? For a few weeks or months or for the duration of my pregnancy?
How likely is it that I'll be hospitalized at some point during my pregnancy? Under what circumstances might that happen? Could I go to my local hospital or would I have to go to one that has specialized neonatal care facilities?

Am I allowed to rest in a semi-reclined position (e.g., in a chaise lounge in the backyard) or do I have to be lying on my side in bed? (Note: Some doctors will specify that you're to lie on your left side, since that promotes maximum blood flow to the baby.)

What types of fetal monitoring, if any, will be required while I'm on bedrest?

Will I be on full bedrest (e.g., 24 hours a day) or may I be out of bed for a certain number of hours each day?

Am I allowed to get out of bed to walk to the bathroom or do I have to use a bedpan?

Do I need to take precautions to avoid straining due to constipation?

Am I allowed to take a shower or do I have to limit myself to sponge baths?

Am I allowed to walk up and down stairs?

Am I allowed to lift anything? If so, what are the restrictions?

Am I allowed to exercise? If so, what are the restrictions?

Am I allowed to have sexual intercourse? Am I allowed to engage in other activities that could lead to orgasm? Is nipple stimulation permitted?

Will I be allowed to drive a car or be a passenger? If so, what limitations apply?

Source: Adapted from a similar chart in Trying Again: A Guide to Pregnancy After Miscarriage, Stillbirth, and Infant Loss by Ann Douglas and John R. Sussman, M.D. Dallas: Taylor Medical Publishing, 2000.

- Ask your doctor to suggest some exercises you can do in bed or to provide you with a referral to a physical therapist who is trained to work with pregnant women. Depending on the nature of your problems, your doctor may give you the go-ahead to do pelvic tilts; Kegel exercises; gluteal sets; leg, ankle, and heel raises; knee extensions; arm raises; shoulder shrugs; and wrist and neck circles. Don't attempt any type of exercise without checking with your doctor first, however. Many women on bedrest are advised against doing any type of exercise.

- Create a bedrest-friendly environment. Ask friends and family members to help you to gather up all the items that you could possibly need to stay comfortable and sane: a cordless phone; a telephone book; a radio; a cassette tape player or CD player; the remote control for the TV, stereo, or VCR; a variety of movies to watch, music to listen to, and books on tape; the TV guide; a box of tissues; a cooler that's stocked with cold beverages, healthy snacks, and your lunch; a thermos full of decaffeinated tea or coffee or soup; and plenty of reading material.

- Find creative ways to pass the time. This is the perfect opportunity to catch up on your photo albums, start keeping a journal, write letters, or create a pregnancy scrapbook.

- Put out the welcome mat — but do so with caution. While you will want to encourage friends and family to visit to help keep you company, it's a good idea to ask them to call first rather than just dropping by. "Any extra activity such as talking with visitors can bring on more contractions, so you'll want to limit the length of these visits," says Candace Hurley, founder of Sidelines. "If you're uncomfortable asking people you know to keep their visits short, tell them that your physician ordered it." Make sure your visitors are able to let themselves in and out so you won't have to be hopping out of bed to open the door. And if they offer to do something around the house to help you out, take them up on the offer. Let them make meals, fold laundry, and dust and vacuum to their hearts' content.

- Hire a childbirth educator to come to your home to teach childbirth classes to you and your partner. It's a great alternative to attending regular prenatal classes. Or, if your budget won't stretch quite that far, rent some birthing videos and watch them with your partner.

MOTHER WISDOM

Don't be afraid to advertise the fact that you need help. Send out the bedrest SOS to friends, co-workers, and members of any clubs and associations to which you or your partner belong. Ask one person to act as your volunteer co-ordinator and line up people to pitch in with meal preparation, laundry, light housework, and so on.

- Find out if your extended health benefits at work will cover the services of a personal health-care attendant or home-maker for an hour or two each day. Your doctor may need to write a letter on your behalf explaining why you're on bedrest.

- Get online. There are a number of support groups for moms on bedrest. Either check to see whether there's a bulletin board devoted to this topic at your favorite parenting web site or hit the Sidelines National Support Network Web site: www.sidelines.org.

- Keep the lines of communication open between you and your partner. It's easy to nitpick about the condition of the house or lament the fact that there's no clean laundry when you've got all day to come up with a list of grievances. Remind yourself that your partner is going through a very stressful time too: He's worried about you and the baby and he's probably having to pick up a lot of extra slack on the home front.

- Make sure you have a way of contacting your partner or another support person quickly in the event of an emergency. Many beeper companies have cheap, short-term packages for parents, and cell phones are becoming more affordable.

- If you have other children, reassure them that life will return to normal after the baby arrives. They may feel angry and resentful about the upheaval being caused by your bedrest. You can help to smooth things over by making a point of spending as much time as possible with them. Read books, do crafts, have a picnic together in bed, or just have a nice heart-to-heart talk.

- Be prepared for a less-than-enthusiastic response from your employer. You're not likely to get a lot of advance warning if your doctor orders you to go on bedrest, and if you're working outside the home, you may have no choice but to leave work immediately — possibly long before your maternity-leave replacement has been trained or even hired. While most employers generally come around after they get over the initial shock, some make royal nuisances of themselves, badgering their employees about coming back to work.

- If you end up being hospitalized while you're on bedrest, try to arrange for your partner and your children to visit you as often as possible and make an effort to connect with other women on your ward who are feeling just as bored and lonely as you are. If you're feeling really depressed, ask to speak with the hospital social worker or chaplain.

- Remain focused on your goal. The whole reason you're on bedrest is for the well-being of you and your baby. While it's grueling, boring, and frustrating, bedrest is worth it if it results in a happy ending for you and your baby.

The Unique Challenges of a Multiple Pregnancy

There are few things as exciting or overwhelming as discovering that there's more than one baby on the way. You may feel special because you've been blessed with more than one, but you may also feel a bit nervous about the challenges you may face both prior to and after your babies' birth.

You or your caregiver will begin to suspect you're pregnant with multiples if fraternal twins tend to run in your family, you were taking fertility drugs when you became pregnant, you're experiencing excessive vomiting and nausea, your uterus is larger than what would normally be expected for someone at your stage of pregnancy, or you're experiencing a lot of fetal movement. These suspicions will be confirmed if your caregiver is able to pick up more than one fetal heartbeat on the Doppler or ultrasound screen.

If you're carrying multiples, you can expect to face some special challenges during your pregnancy:

- The day-to-day aches and pains of pregnancy tend to be more bothersome if you're carrying more than one baby. You can expect to experience heightened early-pregnancy symptoms such as morning sickness, breast tenderness, and fatigue due to the high level of pregnancy hormones in your body; and, as your pregnancy progresses, you can expect to experience symptoms caused by the pressure of your heavy, stretched uterus on your surrounding organs (e.g., shortness of breath, heartburn, constipation, pelvic discomfort, urinary leakage, back pain, and hemorrhoids).

- You face a higher-than-average risk of experiencing complications during your pregnancy. You're more likely to become anemic, develop pre-eclampsia or gestational diabetes, or experience pregnancy-induced hypertension (high blood pressure) than women who are carrying a single baby.

- You will gain considerably more weight than a woman who's pregnant with a single baby. (See Chapter 6 for details.)

- Multiples face a greater risk of experiencing problems in the womb, including growth discordance (when one baby develops more quickly or slowly than the others) and intrauterine growth restriction. They're also at risk of twin-to-twin transfusion syndrome (a condition that occurs when there's an unequal sharing of nutrients in an identical twin pregnancy with a single placenta, causing one twin to get more than his or her share of nutrients and blood flow).

FACTS AND FIGURES

Approximately 60% of triplet births, 90% of quadruplet births, and 99% of quintuplet births are the result of infertility treatments.

FACTS AND FIGURES

The incidence of multiple births in pregnancies that do not involve fertility treatments is as follows:

- Twins: One in every 90 births
- Triplets: One in every 8,100 births
- Quadruplets: One in every 729,000 births
- Quintuplets: One in every 65,610,000 births

FACTS AND FIGURES

Researchers at the University of Liverpool have discovered that the death of one twin puts the surviving twin at risk of cerebral palsy and other neurological problems. The researchers believe that the death of one baby may affect blood circulation to the other, resulting in damage to the brain. The risk is particularly high in identical twin pregnancies because the circulation of the two placentas is connected.

- You face an increased risk of pregnancy loss. Studies have shown that women carrying twins are twice as likely, and women carrying triplets are four to six times as likely, to experience a stillbirth as women who are carrying singletons. The risks tend to be particularly high if you're carrying monoamniotic twins (twins that share the same amniotic sac): There's a 50% mortality rate with such twins, due to the high risk that the babies will be born conjoined (Siamese twins) or that they'll become tangled up in one another's umbilical cords, cutting off the supply of oxygen.

- You face a higher-than-average risk of going into labor prematurely. A mother carrying twins can expect to deliver her babies about four weeks earlier than a mother carrying a single baby. What's more, moms carrying triplets tend to deliver about seven weeks early, while moms carrying quads tend to deliver about 10 weeks early. It's important to remember, of course, that these figures are averages. Some women deliver sooner or later than this.

- You're more likely to require a cesarean delivery because of presentation problems (problems with the position the babies assume at the time of birth) and because, as the uterus begins to collapse down with the delivery of one of the babies, the risk of a placental abruption increases.

- You face a higher-than-average risk of giving birth to a low-birthweight baby. While a typical singleton weighs about 7 pounds at birth, multiples are considerably lighter, with twins weighing in at 5 pounds, 5 ounces on average, and triplets and quadruplets at 3 pounds, 12 ounces.

- You face a higher-than-average risk of giving birth to a baby with a birth defect. Birth defects are twice as common in multiple pregnancies and, what's more, are far more common in identical twins (twins that develop from the splitting of a single egg) than fraternal twins (twins that develop from two separate eggs).

- You face a higher-than-average risk of having a baby who may die shortly after birth. Twins are three to five times as likely to die during the first 28 days of life as singletons, largely due to health problems associated with prematurity; as well, the risk of Sudden Infant Death Syndrome (SIDS) is twice as high in twins as in singletons.

- You face a higher-than-average risk of experiencing a postpartum hemorrhage. Because the uterus has been severely stretched during pregnancy, it may have more difficulty contracting after the delivery.

- You may be faced with the difficult issue of fetal reduction if you've conceived higher-order multiples (e.g., three or more babies). If you discover you're carrying four or more babies, your doctor may recommend that you consider selectively aborting one or more of the fetuses. (Note: Since the outcomes of twin and triplet pregnancies are relatively similar, fetal reduction is not routinely recommended during triplet pregnancies.) This can be a heartbreaking decision for couples, particularly since there's a 10 to 13% risk that all the fetuses will be miscarried as a result of the procedure. And even if the remaining babies are born healthy, you may feel awful about having been placed in the dreadful position of having to "play God" by choosing which babies should survive.

That's not to say that all women who are pregnant with multiples experience complications, of course. Many end up giving birth to two or more healthy term or near-term babies. If you're concerned about what having multiples may mean to you before, during, or after the birth, you might want to speak to other parents of multiples. There are a number of different groups for parents of multiples that you can turn to for practical advice on coping with the physical, emotional, and financial challenges of raising multiples. See Appendix D for contact information.

FACTS AND FIGURES

As a rule of thumb, you'll need 1.5 times as many clothes for twins as you would for a single baby.

Premature Birth

According to the National Center for Health Statistics, approximately 11.8% of babies decide to make their grand entrance before the 37th completed week of pregnancy. In 40% of these cases there's no apparent reason for the early arrival, while in the remaining 60% the premature birth is triggered by conditions affecting the mother, the baby, or the placenta.

FACTS AND FIGURES

Mothers who've previously given birth to a premature baby have a 15% chance of giving birth to another premature baby in a subsequent pregnancy, while women who have experienced two premature deliveries have a 32% chance of giving birth to another premature baby in any future pregnancies.

Possible health problems

Babies who are born prematurely face a higher-than-average risk of experiencing such complications as respiratory distress syndrome (breathing problems in the newborn), bleeding of the fragile blood vessels in the brain (a stroke-like experience that can lead to developmental delays, cerebral palsy, learning disabilities and/or behavioral problems such as attention deficit disorder), and infection. What's more, according to a recent Canadian study, approximately 25% of children born before 37 completed weeks of pregnancy and approximately 45% of those born before 32 completed weeks of pregnancy will require some sort of special education during their early years at school.

If your baby is born prematurely, she may develop a condition known as respiratory distress syndrome (RDS). This is usually caused by a lack of surfactant (the dish detergent-like liquid that prevents the hollow sacs in the lungs from collapsing and sticking together each time the baby exhales) and can lead to such serious complications as pneumonia (which is particularly common if the baby has contracted an infection prior to or during birth, or if the baby is on a ventilator for an extended period of time), persistent pulmonary hypertension/persistent fetal circulation (a condition that occurs if the pressure in the blood vessels of the lungs fails to drop after birth, thereby reducing the amount of blood that's able to flow through them), bronchopulmonary dysplasia (the abnormal development of the lungs and the bronchial tubes — a condition that's common in babies who've been on ventilators for an extended period of time), and intraventricular hemorrhage (bleeding in the brain).

Because RDS can be harmful or even fatal to a premature baby, babies who are believed to be at risk of RDS are typically treated using one of the following pieces of equipment or methods:

- Oxygen hood (the baby is placed under an oxygen hood so that oxygen can be pumped into her lungs)

- Nasal cannula (the baby is attached to a plastic tube that delivers prescribed amounts of oxygen)

- Continuous Positive Airway Pressure (CPAP) (oxygen and moist air are forced into the lungs)

- Respirator (the baby is hooked up to a respirator so that the respirator can breathe for her until she's able to breathe well on her own)

- Synthetic surfactant (the baby is treated with a synthetic form of the substance that prevents the hollow sacs in the lungs from sticking together)

- Liquid ventilation (fluids are pumped into the baby's lungs to create an "underwater" environment similar to what she experienced prior to birth)

- Nitric oxide (the baby is given a mix of nitric oxide and oxygen in order to prevent blood vessel constriction problems in the lungs)

Risk factors

Studies have shown that certain risk factors are associated with premature birth. You're more likely to give birth to your baby prematurely if

- you're under the age of 20 or over the age of 35

- you've had a cone biopsy performed on your cervix at some point in the past (a cone biopsy involves removing a cone-shaped portion of tissue from the cervix)

- you're pregnant with multiples

- the baby you're carrying has severe congenital anomalies

- you've experienced premature rupture of the membranes (PROM), placenta previa, or a placental abruption

- you've been diagnosed with an incompetent cervix, fibroids, uterine abnormalities, or polyhydramnios (excess amniotic fluid)

- your mother took an anti-miscarriage drug called diethylstilbestrol (DES) when she was pregnant with you

- you have a urinary tract infection or other type of infection (with or without a fever)

- your lifestyle is not as healthy as it should be (e.g., you smoke, use illicit drugs, or are under extreme stress)

- you have pre-existing health problems that put you at risk of experiencing a premature birth (e.g., diabetes, kidney disease, or cardiovascular disease)

- you've previously given birth to a premature baby (According to a study reported in the *Journal of the American Medical Association*, you face a particularly high risk of experiencing a preterm birth if your previous baby was especially premature.)

- your mother gave birth to you prematurely (According to a 1997 study at the University of Utah School of Medicine, women who were premature babies themselves are more likely to give birth to premature babies than other pregnant women. What's more, the more premature they were, the greater the risk they face that any children they bear will be premature.)

Prevention

While researchers have yet to come up with a way to prevent all premature births, there are certain things you can do to reduce your risk of giving birth prematurely:

- seek treatments for conditions that are known to or suspected of triggering premature labor (e.g., bacterial vaginoisis — a vaginal infection characterized by a thin, milky discharge with a fishy odor)

- promptly seek treatment for any urinary tract infections and don't allowing your temperature to climb too high before seeking medical treatment for a fever (a high temperature can cause your uterus to start contracting)

- avoid accidents and injuries that could trigger premature labor

- don't smoke or take illicit drugs, and lead a generally healthy lifestyle during pregnancy

If you've experienced a premature birth in the past, your doctor will monitor any future pregnancies closely. You can expect to be tested for bacterial vaginosis and to have your cervical length measured.

Welcoming a premature baby or a baby with special needs

If your baby is born prematurely or has a lot of health problems, she'll likely spend her first weeks or months in the hospital. This can be very upsetting to you and your partner: After all, your dreams of the perfect birth didn't include watching your baby be whisked away to the neonatal intensive care unit or checking out of the hospital without your baby.

Here are some tips on surviving your premature baby's or special needs baby's hospitalization:

- Spend time getting to know your baby. "It's difficult to bond with your baby when it's in an isolette hooked up to a bunch of machines, but it is possible," says Rita, 35, whose son was born prematurely. "Touch the baby, caress it, talk to it. I didn't think touching the baby did much good until my friend noticed that my son's heartbeat would change when I was with him and he would breathe more relaxed."

- Find out as much as you can about your baby's specific medical condition, either by talking to the medical staff and visiting the hospital library or by asking a friend or family member to do some research on your behalf. (Note: You'll find leads on some excellent health-related Web sites in Appendix E.) "Be realistic about your expectations, however," warns Bonnie, whose second child died at age 9 months. "Denial is your worst enemy."

- Try to master the neonatal intensive care unit (NICU) lingo. Ask a nurse or another parent to explain the terminology so that you won't feel quite so confused and overwhelmed.

MOM'S THE WORD

"We were so surprised when he was born and had the cleft palate because neither of us had a history of it in our families and it was the last thing I was thinking about in terms of his health. Having to live through his surgeries was awful. It's the only time I've seen my husband cry. It was the worst time in our life. I felt guilty that I had somehow caused this, even though I knew I'd taken every possible health precaution when I was pregnant, but I felt like I had ruined his life. I had no one to talk about it with and some of our friends reacted badly. You really learn who your friends are and who are the people you still want to call friends."

—*Jennifer, 31, whose first child was born with a cleft palate*

- Play as active a role as you can in your baby's care, but don't put superhuman demands on yourself. No one expects you to hang out at the hospital 24 hours a day, nor should you expect this of yourself.

- Ask your doctor if you can practice "kangaroo care" (laying your baby against your bare chest). Studies have shown that premature babies respond very positively to this skin-to-skin contact.

- Don't let the fact that your baby is premature discourage you from breastfeeding. While your baby might initially have to drink the breastmilk from a tube, you may be able to gradually switch him over to the breast as he gets stronger and bigger.

- Bring a support person along with you when you're speaking to the medical staff. Not only can this person help you remember all the important details about what the doctor or nurse had to say about your baby's progress, he or she can also help to spread the news to other friends and family members on your behalf. This can really help to alleviate your stress, notes Susan, a 35-year-old mother of two (both born prematurely). "You don't need to be telling the same story over and over again, particularly if the news is not good."

- Start preparing for the day when you'll be able to bring your baby home. The more you participate in your baby's day-to-day care while she's in the hospital, the less intimidated you'll feel when it's time to leave the hospital. And before you check your baby out of the hospital, line up as much support as you can on the home front: Some insurance companies cover the services of a visiting nurse, particularly if you've given birth to multiples.

 MOM'S THE WORD

"Just love your baby. Take things one day at a time or even one hour at a time."

— *Deirdre, 36, whose daughter was born severely disabled as a result of oxygen deprivation during the delivery*

MOTHER WISDOM

If your baby is being cared for at a hospital that's out of town, ask your nurse or the hospital chaplain or social worker to provide you with leads on low-cost accommodations in the area. The hospital may have rooms available within the hospital itself or it may have arranged for a local hotel to provide these sorts of accommodations at a reduced rate.

When a Baby Dies

There are few experiences in life that can compare to the grief of losing a child. Whether that baby is miscarried, stillborn, or dies during or after birth, the loss can be devastating to both you and your partner. As Deborah Davis, Ph.D., notes in her book, *Empty Cradle, Broken Heart:* "While the death of a parent or friend represents a loss of your past, when your baby dies you lose a part of your future. You grieve not only for your baby, but for your parenthood. Times you had looked forward to — maternity leave, family gatherings, and holidays — can seem worthless or trivial without your baby."

Pandora, 45, whose second child died of SIDS, feels that expectant parents are ill prepared for anything other than a storybook happy ending to their pregnancies: "Western society fill us with 'great expectations' and we have no preparations for the empty crib, the unused baby clothes and diaper coupons, and the calls from baby photographers for months afterwards."

MOM'S THE WORD

"I loved being pregnant . . . watching my tummy get bigger and feeling tiny movements inside of me late at night. I loved wearing maternity clothes and looking at tiny cotton dresses and miniature denim overalls at Baby Gap. I loved reading *Little House in the Big Woods* aloud at night, hoping the baby would hear. I loved the excitement in my mother's voice when I called her, and the big smile on my father-in-law's face every time he saw me. I started noticing pregnant women everywhere. I felt like I had finally joined this sort of sacred sisterhood, this exclusive club I had longed to be a part of for so long. And then, as another bereaved mother ruefully put it to me, 'I got kicked out of the club.' "

— *Lori, 39, whose daughter was stillborn at 26 weeks*

What can go wrong

While you might feel as if you're the only person to experience the death of a baby, miscarriage, stillbirth, and infant death are far more common than most people realize:

- Between 20 and 25% of pregnancies end in miscarriage, ectopic pregnancy (a pregnancy that occurs outside the uterus), molar pregnancy (a pregnancy that results in the growth of abnormal cells rather than the development of a healthy placenta and embryo), or stillbirth. This means that approximately 3,600 American women a day experience the heartache of losing a baby.

- Miscarriages (the death of a baby before the 20th week of pregnancy) are the most common type of loss, occurring in 15 to 20% of confirmed pregnancies.

- Ectopic pregnancies occur in 1 to 2% of pregnancies.

- Stillbirth occurs in approximately 1% of pregnancies. Some of these babies die during labor, in which case their deaths are classified as intrapartum deaths.

- Molar pregnancies occur in one out of every 1,500 to 2,000 pregnancies.

The following sections present what you need to know about each of these types of losses.

Miscarriage

Miscarriage is the term used to describe the spontaneous death of an embryo or fetus prior to the 20th week of pregnancy. (Medically, miscarriages are referred to as "spontaneous abortions" — a term that many couples who've lost a baby find upsetting and insensitive.) Some hospitals also use the term *miscarriage* to describe the deaths of babies who are less than 500 grams at birth — something that can apply to babies whose mothers are as much as 23 or 24 weeks into their pregnancies.

While most women who are having a miscarriage experience heavy bleeding and other symptoms (see Table 11.3), other women who've had a "missed abortion" (see Table 11.4) have no idea that they've had a miscarriage until many weeks after the fact, when their caregiver is unable to detect a fetal heartbeat using a Doppler or ultrasound. (Note: An ultrasound can detect the fetal heartbeat as early as six weeks after the first day of your last menstrual period while a Doppler can detect the fetal heartbeat about 12 to 14 weeks into your pregnancy, although it may take a little longer than that if you are overweight.)

MOM'S THE WORD

"I had a miscarriage in my third pregnancy. I was only eight weeks along when I lost the baby, but it was devastating to me. You feel a bond with this child right away and you've already got them growing up in your mind. You need to grieve. You've experienced a great loss. It will forever change the way you look at babies and pregnancy."

— *Christina, 25, who has experienced both miscarriage and the birth of two healthy babies*

TABLE 11.3

THE SYMPTOMS OF MISCARRIAGE

You should seek medical attention if you're experiencing one or more of the symptoms of miscarriage:

spotting or light bleeding with or without menstrual-like cramping
heavy or persistent bleeding (with or without clots) accompanied by abdominal pain, cramping, or pain in the lower back
a gush of fluid from the vagina (an indication that your membranes may have ruptured)
the sudden disappearance of all pregnancy symptoms (e.g., morning sickness or breast tenderness)
Note: It's normal for morning sickness and other first-trimester complaints to disappear around the beginning of the second trimester of pregnancy, so try not to hit the panic button if your symptoms disappear at this point in your pregnancy.

TABLE 11.4

HOW MISCARRIAGES ARE CLASSIFIED

Your caregiver may use one or more of the following terms when describing your miscarriage. (Note: "Abortion" is the medical term for "miscarriage.")

Term	What It Means
Threatened abortion	You appear to be miscarrying (you're likely experiencing some vaginal bleeding and possibly some pain as well), but the miscarriage is not yet inevitable. Up to 50% of these pregnancies are carried on successfully.
Inevitable abortion	Your cervix has begun to dilate and a miscarriage is in progress.

Term	What It Means
Incomplete abortion	You have experienced a partial miscarriage. Some of the so-called "products of conception" (the gestational sac, the fetus, the umbilical cord, and the placenta) remain in the uterus. Generally, a dilation and curettage (D & C) or suction curettage are perfomed to remove the remaining material.
Complete abortion	You have miscarried and all the products of conception have been expelled from your uterus.
Missed abortion	Your baby has died, but neither the baby nor the placenta have been expelled from the uterus. You may not realize there's a problem with your pregnancy until your caregiver is unable to detect the fetal heartbeat. Note: The term "blighted ovum" is used to describe missed abortions in which a fetus did not develop.
Early miscarriage	The term "early miscarriage" is used to describe a miscarriage that occurs prior to the 12th week of gestation.
Late miscarriage	The term "late miscarriage" describes a miscarriagethat occurs between 12 and 20 weeks gestation. (Sometimes miscarriages that occur at this stage of pregnancy are referred to as second-trimester miscarriages or fetal deaths.)

The causes of miscarriage

While there's still much that medical science doesn't know about the causes and treatment of miscarriage, scientists have identified some of the major causes of these early pregnancy losses:

- Chromosomal abnormalities. Chromosomal abnormalities are thought to be responsible for approximately 60% of miscarriages. These randomly occurring genetic errors happen either prior to conception (if there's a defective egg or sperm cell) or during the earliest stages of cell division. Researchers estimate that the incidence of congenital anomalies in newborns would jump from 2-3% to 12% if miscarriages did not occur.

- Maternal disease. Certain types of health problems in the mother increase her risk of experiencing a miscarriage. These conditions include immune system disorders such as lupus, congenital heart disease, severe kidney disease, uncontrolled diabetes, thyroid disease, and intrauterine infection. (See Chapter 2 and the section on stillbirth below for additional information.)

- Hormonal imbalances. Hormonal imbalances can also cause a woman to miscarry. If, for example, she has a luteal phase defect (her body doesn't secrete enough progesterone to sustain the pregnancy), she may end up miscarrying.

- Rhesus (Rh) disease. Rh incompatibility occurs when the mother's blood is Rh-negative and the father's is Rh-positive. If the baby has Rh-positive blood too, this can pose problems during the pregnancy. The mother may become Rh-sensitized if some of the baby's blood cells get into her bloodstream, which can cause her to develop antibodies that may attack the baby's red blood cells, leading to anemia and possibly even the death of the baby. Rh-negative women with Rh-positive partners can generally avoid Rh-sensitivity problems by receiving a shot of Rh immune globulin (Rhogam) whenever there's any sign of bleeding or suspected bleeding during pregnancy (e.g., following amniocentesis or in cases of placenta previa); during the 28th week of each pregnancy; and following each birth or miscarriage. Note: Fetal deaths caused by Rh disease are most likely to occur during the second trimester of pregnancy.

- Immune system disorders. Immune system disorders are believed to be the cause of 5 to 10% of recurrent miscarriages. They occur when a pregnant woman's immune system mistakenly concludes that her baby is an "intruder" and starts attacking the baby. Some forms of treatment are available.

- Allogeneic factors. It's also possible to develop antibodies to your partner's leukocytes (white blood cells), which can lead you to miscarry the baby that the two of you have conceived together. Sometimes this condition can be treated by immunizing you with either your partner's or a third party's leukocytes — a technique believed to trick your body into producing the blocking antibodies that prevent your body from rejecting the developing baby.

- Anatomical problems of the uterus and cervix. Congenital abnormalities of the uterus and the cervix, uterine adhesions and fibroids, complications arising from an elective abortion (e.g., infection or cervical trauma), and an incompetent cervix (a grossly insensitive term that simply means your cervix opens prematurely) are just a few of the problems that can lead to miscarriage or stillbirth. Some of these problems can be treated with surgery.

- Viral and bacterial infections. Viral and bacterial infections have been proven to play a role in miscarriage. Some of them are unlikely to recur during a subsequent pregnancy (e.g., chicken pox) while others are more likely to be a problem again (group B strep). (Note: Group B strep is more likely to be a problem during late pregnancy or during labor itself.)

- Recreational drug and alcohol use. Women who use recreational drugs or consume large quantities of alcohol during pregnancy face a higher-than-average risk of miscarriage.

- Exposure to harmful substances. Exposure to high-dose radiation, certain types of chemicals, chemotherapeutic drugs, cigarette smoke, and moderate to heavy doses of caffeine (more than five cups a day, according to a recent article in the *New England Journal of Medicine*) may increase the risk of miscarriage.

- Maternal age. A woman's chances of experiencing a miscarriage increase as she ages. While women in their 20s have just a 10% risk of miscarrying during any given pregnancy, the risk for women in their 40s is believed to be approximately 50%.

MOM'S THE WORD

"It's amazing how many people kind of dismissed our grief — saying things like, 'Oh well, thank goodness you weren't that far along' and 'Oh, you can try again.' Yes, these things are true, but, at the same time, we had suffered a great loss and it should have been acknowledged as such."

— *Joyce, 41, whose first pregnancy ended in miscarriage*

Recurrent miscarriage

While doctors used to wait until you had experienced three or more consecutive miscarriages before launching an investigation into their cause, many caregivers are now willing to start looking into the problem after your second consecutive loss, particularly if you're over age 35. Your doctor may recommend blood tests (to detect any hormonal or immune system problems that could be causing you to miscarry), genetic tests (to determine if you or your partner are carriers of any genetic disorder that could be causing you to miscarry), a genital tract culture (to look for the presence of any sort of infection that could be causing you to miscarry), an endometrial biopsy (to assess whether your uterine lining is sufficiently thick to allow for implantation), a hysterosalpingography (an X-ray of the uterus and fallopian tubes) or a hysteroscopy (an examination of the inside of the uterus using a telescope-like instrument inserted through the vagina and the cervix) to look for blockages and other problems, or an ultrasound or sonohysterograpy (to look for any structural problems and/or fibroids or adhesions that could be causing you to miscarry).

Depending on what your doctor is able to uncover during this investigation, he or she may recommend one or more of the following treatments:

- surgery to remove large (e.g., grapefruit-sized) or problematic fibroids or to correct any uterine abnormalities that may be causing you to miscarry

- the insertion of a stitch in your cervix (cerclage) at the beginning of the second trimester to help stop the cervix from opening prematurely during your next pregnancy

- a course of antibiotics to cure any infections that may be causing you to miscarry repeatedly

- the improved management of chronic diseases such as diabetes or lupus that may be causing you to miscarry

- hormone therapy to correct any hormonal imbalances that may be causing you to miscarry

- treatment for immune system problems

- treatment for allogeneic problems

FACTS AND FIGURES

Less important than how many miscarriages you've had is whether or not you've been able to give birth to at least one living baby. Women who've had two or more miscarriages and who've never given birth to a living baby have a 40 to 45% chance of miscarrying the next time around, whereas women who've given birth to a living baby but who've experienced as many as four miscarriages in the past have just a 25 to 30% of miscarrying the next time around.

Ectopic pregnancy

An ectopic pregnancy occurs when the fertilized egg implants somewhere other than in the uterus. In 95% of ectopic pregnancies the fertilized egg implants in one of the fallopian tubes, and in the remaining 5% of cases it implants in the abdominal cavity, the ovaries, or the cervix.

An ectopic pregnancy can pose a significant threat to a woman's health. It can put her very life at risk if the fallopian tube ruptures and results in massive internal bleeding. That's why it's so important to be aware of the warning signs of an ectopic pregnancy (see Table 11.5) and to seek treatment before a rupture occurs. An ectopic pregnancy is classified as unruptured or subacute if it's detected before a tubal rupture occurs, and ruptured or acute if it isn't detected until after the tube has burst, causing pain, internal bleeding, and shock.

TABLE 11.5

THE WARNING SIGNS OF AN ECTOPIC PREGNANCY

You should seek medical treatment immediately if you experience one or more of the signs of an ectopic pregnancy:

vaginal bleeding (especially bleeding that's either lighter or heavier than what you'd experience during a normal menstrual period)
abdominal pain (either sudden and acute or sharp and aching), especially pain that's felt more on one side of the body than the other
shoulder pain (caused by the pooling of blood in the abdomen)
weakness, dizziness, fainting, and/or a weak but rapid pulse (caused by substantial blood loss).

Familiarize yourself with the risk factors for an ectopic pregnancy so that you'll know whether you face a higher-than-average risk of experiencing this type of problem:

- a history of tubal infections caused by pelvic inflammatory disease, sexually transmitted diseases, postpartum endometritis, or post-abortion infections (all of which can damage the mucus surface of the fallopian tubes and make it more difficult for the fertilized egg to pass through the tube and into the uterus)

- a history of tubal or pelvic surgery such as surgery to deal with endometriosis or a ruptured appendix (which can lead to tubal adhesions)

- a structural abnormality of the fallopian tubes

- abnormal hormone levels (e.g., insufficient progesterone — the hormone that causes the fallopian tube to contract and propel the egg toward the uterus)

- conceiving while you're using Depo-Provera or another progesterone contraceptive (your fallopian tube's ability to contract and propel the fertilized egg toward the uterus is affected)

- conceiving through in vitro fertilization (there's a possibility that you could have both a uterine and ectopic pregnancy simultaneously)

- smoking (nicotine is thought to interfere with the fallopian tube's ability to contract and propel the fertilized egg)

- douching

- becoming pregnant with an IUD in place or after a tubal ligation (sterilization)

- a past history of ectopic pregnancy (you're 12 times as likely to experience an ectopic pregnancy if you've already experienced one in the past).

Molar pregnancy

The terms molar pregnancy, hydatidiform mole, and gestational trophoblastic disease are used to describe a pregnancy that results in the growth of abnormal tissue rather than a healthy placenta and embryo. Researchers believe that molar pregnancies result from a genetic error at the very beginning of pregnancy.

There are two types of molar pregnancies: complete molar pregnancies and partial molar pregnancies. In a complete molar pregnancy, thousands of fluid-filled cysts develop instead of a fetus. In a partial molar pregnancy, there's an abnormal fetus as well as thousands of these fluid-filled cysts. In very rare situations — approximately one in every 22,000 to 100,000 births — a normal twin is also present and will be born very prematurely.

In most cases, a molar pregnancy is miscarried spontaneously. In some cases, however, it's diagnosed only when a woman begins to experience its symptoms: vaginal bleeding during the first trimester, a uterus that grows too quickly, enlarged ovaries, extremely high levels of hCG, and severe nausea, vomiting, and high blood pressure (possibly even preeclampsia) caused by unusually high hormone levels. Once a diagnosis has been made, the pregnancy is terminated and the uterus is carefully emptied to ensure that no abnormal tissue is left behind.

In rare cases, a molar pregnancy will become cancerous. While the prognosis is good if the cancer is treated right away, it can spread to other parts of the body, including the lungs and brain, if it's not treated quickly enough. The key way of detecting a cancerous molar pregnancy (choriocarcinoma) is by measuring the level of human chorionic gonadotropin (hCG) in your blood during the months following your delivery. You won't be able to become pregnant during this time because it would be impossible for your doctor to determine whether your hCG levels were rising because of the choriocarcinoma or because of your new pregnancy. If your hCG levels are normal for six months to one year after your molar pregnancy, your doctor will likely give you the go-ahead to try again.

Certain women are more likely to experience a molar pregnancy than others:

- women of Southeast Asian descent

- women with a family history of molar pregnancy

- women who have previously experienced a molar pregnancy (there's a 1.3 to 2.9% chance of recurrence)

Stillbirth

Stillbirth is the name given to losses that occur after the 20th week of gestation. It occurs in approximately 1% of pregnancies and is more common in women under the age of 15 and over the age of 35; in pregnancies that last for longer than 42 weeks; in multiple pregnancies; and in pregnancies involving a male fetus.

While approximately 60% of stillbirths are unexplained, researchers have been able to come up with a few clues about the causes of the other 40%. Here's what's known about the most common causes:

MOTHER WISDOM

"I have talked, once or twice, to other parents who have lost babies at birth. Once unleashed, their grief is like a flood. I recognize the sandbags that they keep stacked between it and the rest of life. It does not recede, this flood. It is on the other side, always and forever. It is a peculiar grief, a pregnancy that never ends."

— Beth Powning, *Shadow Child: An Apprenticeship in Love and Loss*

- Chromosomal abnormalities. Babies with chromosomal abnormalities are more likely to be miscarried than chromosomally normal babies. While just 2 to 3% of liveborn infants have chromosomal problems, 6 to 13% of stillborn babies have chromosomal problems.

- Maternal health problems. As we noted back in Chapter 2, certain types of maternal health conditions increase the risk of stillbirth. These conditions include diabetes, epilepsy, high blood pressure, heart disease, kidney disease, liver disease, lung disease, parathyroid disease, sickle-cell disease, systemic lupus erythematosus, and pre-eclampsia. (Note: You'll find detailed information on the specific risk factors associated with each of these conditions in my book, *Trying Again: A Guide to Pregnancy After Miscarriage, Stillbirth, and Infant Loss.* See Appendix G for bibliographic information.)

- Infection during pregnancy. Some types of infections are able to cross the placenta and harm the developing baby. In severe cases, they may result in stillbirth or cause labor to begin before the baby is capable of surviving outside the womb. These infections include group B streptococcus (the leading cause of fatal infection in newborns), cytomegalovirus (CMV), human parvovirus B19 (fifth disease), listeriosis, rubella (German measles), chicken pox, toxoplasmosis, and certain types of sexually transmitted diseases.

- Problems with the placenta. The placenta is the baby's life-support system prior to birth. If serious problems arise, the baby may not be able to survive. There are three major types of problems that can arise with the placenta: placental insufficiency and placental failure (when the placenta is unable to meet the baby's need for nutrients and oxygen), placental abruption (when the placenta begins to separate prematurely from the uterine wall), and placenta previa (when the placenta blocks all or part of the exit to the womb).

- Problems with the uterus. You're at increased risk of experiencing a stillbirth if you've been diagnosed with an incompetent cervix (a cervix that opens prematurely), fibroids (non-cancerous growths of tissue that occur in the wall of the uterus), or uterine abnormalities (e.g., a bicornate uterus or septate uterus).

- Umbilical cord problems. The umbilical cord is the baby's
  lifeline prior to birth, carrying oxygen and nutrients to the
  baby and carrying away waste products. A problem with the
  umbilical cord can result in the death of the baby. The most
  common types of umbilical cord problems include two-
  vessel cords (a normal umbilical cord has three vessels),
  straight umbilical cords (which are more likely to tangle than
  telephone-cord-like umbilical cords), umbilical cords that are
  abnormally inserted into the placenta, prolapsed cords
  (umbilical cords that slip into the vagina ahead of the baby
  during labor), umbilical cord knots, umbilical cord around
  the neck (generally a problem only if the cord has been
  wrapped around the neck a number of times), torsion of the
  umbilical cord (twisting that cuts off the supply of oxygen),
  cord strictures (a cord with insufficient amounts of
  Wharton's jelly — the thick substance that prevents the cord
  from becoming constricted), and amniotic band syndrome (a
  condition that can prevent oxygen from reaching the baby if
  the amniotic bands happen to be located on the umbilical
  cord).

- Complications resulting from a multiple pregnancy. As we
  noted earlier in this chapter, women who are carrying multiples face an increased risk of losing one or more of their
  babies.

MOM'S THE WORD

"I did not know that babies could die during labor or birth in this
day and age."

— *Monique, 27, whose first child was stillborn*

Intrapartum death

Most stillborn babies die before labor begins, but a few die during labor itself. This is more likely to occur in a labor that's prolonged; in which there are excessively frequent contractions; when there are problems with the placenta or the umbilical cord; or if the baby is in medically fragile condition (perhaps due to a congenital anomaly).

Infant death

Despite all the amazing advances in neonatal medicine we've witnessed over the past few decades, there are still a number of problems that medical science is unable to treat or prevent. As a result, approximately one in every 139 liveborn infants dies during the first year of life.

Approximately two-thirds of infant deaths occur during the first month of life — during the so-called neonatal period. The two leading causes of neonatal death are conditions originating in the perinatal period (e.g., respiratory distress syndrome; problems associated with prematurity and/or low birthweight; maternal complications of pregnancy, such as gestational diabetes or pre-eclampsia; problems with the placenta, umbilical cord, and amniotic sac; complications of labor and delivery; slow fetal growth and fetal malnutrition; birth trauma; intrauterine hypoxia and birth hypoxia — when the baby is deprived of oxygen prior to or during birth; hemorrhage; and perinatal jaundice) and congenital anomalies (e.g., neural tube defects such as anencephaly, spina bifida, and hydrocephalus; heart and other circulatory system defects; problems with the respiratory, digestive, genitourinary, and musculoskeletal systems; and chromosomal anomalies such as Down syndrome). The two leading causes of post-neonatal death (deaths occurring between 1 month and 1 year of age) are Sudden Infant Death Syndrome (SIDS) and congenital anomalies. (See Appendix F for more detailed information on the causes of infant death in 1999.)

MOM'S THE WORD

"I lost my first child. He was born at 27 weeks and was just too premature to survive. He lived for 72 hours. The hardest thing was having to go home from the hospital with no baby and facing all the baby stuff. I think first-time parents should wait until they're at least 32 weeks along before getting any baby stuff, and then don't set up anything. Dad can do that while Mom's recovering in the hospital."

—*Josie, 29, mother of three living children*

Some parents know ahead of time that their babies are going to be born with medical conditions that are incompatible with life. If you find out in advance that your baby has a serious health problem that will not allow her to survive for very long after birth, you'll want to decide in advance how you'd like to spend your baby's few short days or hours of life. Here are some questions you'll need to consider:

- Would you like to spend that time alone with your baby and your partner?

- Would you like to have your baby's grandparents or any other children you may have there as well?

- Would you like your baby to receive pain relief if she seems to be experiencing a lot of discomfort or pain?

- Would you like to hold your baby as she passes away?

- Would you like to spend some time alone with your baby after her death?

- Do you intend to donate her organs?

MOTHER WISDOM

"The fullness of motherhood was compressed into that day. A mother's deep love for her son, her tender concern, her exquisite pain of separation, her comforting touch for a lifetime of scraped knees, her worry for a lifetime's danger, her peace in their inseparable bond, all came together in that rich moment as she gazed upon her precious little boy."

— *Pediatrician Alan Greene of DrGreene.com, recalling the experience of a patient who lost a baby to trisomy-13 shortly after birth*

Sudden Infant Death Syndrome

The term Sudden Infant Death Syndrome (SIDS) is used to describe the death of an infant that remains unexplained after a thorough investigation has been completed. It's responsible for the deaths of approximately 1 in every 1,500 liveborn infants in the U.S.

FROM HERE TO MATERNITY

The National Sudden Infant Death Syndrome Resource Center is an excellent source of information and support. See Appendix D for contact information or visit its Web site, www.sidscenter.org.

While there's still much we don't know about SIDS, researchers have identified some risk factors involved and have recommended some strategies for minimizing the number of SIDS-related deaths. Here's what we know so far.

Some babies face a greater risk of dying as a result of SIDS than others. The key risk factors for SIDS include prematurity (especially babies with birthweights of less than 4.4 pounds); being a multiple as opposed to a singleton; abnormal or irregular breathing in the newborn (particularly if the baby periodically stops breathing); a minor respiratory infection in the newborn (one-third of infants who die of SIDS had a runny nose or slight cough in the two to three days prior to their deaths); maternal smoking or illicit drug use during pregnancy; sex (male babies are more likely to die from SIDS than female babies), ethnicity (African-American and aboriginal babies face a greater SIDS risk); age (the peak risk period for SIDS deaths is between two and four months); the time of year (SIDS deaths are more common during the winter months than at other times of the year); and placental problems during pregnancy.

While there's nothing you can do to guarantee that your baby won't die from SIDS, there's plenty you can do to reduce the risk:

- Place your baby to sleep on his back unless your baby has a specific medical condition that requires that he sleep on his stomach. The risk of SIDS is higher when your baby sleeps on his front or side than on his back. Note: You'll want to ensure that everyone who cares for your baby is aware of the importance of putting your baby to sleep on his back. Researchers at the Children's National Medical Center in Washington, D.C., found that infants who are unaccustomed to sleeping on their stomachs face an even higher risk of SIDS if they are placed to sleep in this position.

- Create a safe sleeping environment for your baby. Make sure the mattress is firm but not soft and that the crib, bassinet, or bed where your baby will be sleeping is free of pillows and other soft bedding that could increase the risk of suffocation or cause large quantities of carbon dioxide to pool around your baby's head. (A lack of oxygen or an excess of carbon dioxide is thought to be responsible for some SIDS deaths.) Do not allow your baby to sleep on a waterbed.

- Proceed with caution when it comes to co-sleeping. You might want to rethink your decision to have your baby sleep in your bed if you and/or your partner smoke, have been drinking, or have been using drugs (either legal or illicit) that might result in increased drowsiness. There's also some evidence that severely obese parents should avoid co-sleeping due to an increased risk of accidentally rolling on top of the baby.

- Don't smoke when you're pregnant and don't expose your baby to secondhand smoke after the birth. Secondhand smoke doubles a baby's chances of dying from SIDS, while babies whose mothers smoked during pregnancy are three times as likely to succumb to SIDS.

- Create a drug-free environment both prior to and after birth. That means avoiding alcohol, marijuana, crack, cocaine and heroin while you're pregnant or breastfeeding; and ensuring that your baby isn't exposed to any secondhand smoke from marijuana and other drugs.

- Watch your caffeine intake while you're pregnant. Researchers have found that babies whose mothers drank large amounts of caffeine (400 milligrams per day, the equivalent of four cups of coffee) during pregnancy are twice as likely to die from SIDS as other babies.

- Don't allow your baby to become overheated. Some studies have shown that infants who are overdressed or bundled in too many blankets may face a greater risk of SIDS. What isn't clear, however, is whether it's the overheating or the fact that an infant's head may have been inadvertently covered by the blankets or clothing that's to blame. The easiest way to monitor your baby's temperature is by placing your hand on the back of your baby's neck. If she's sweating, she's too warm. As a rule of thumb, babies need at most one more layer than their parents.

- Breastfeed your baby. Some research has found that breast-feeding may help to reduce the risk of losing a baby to SIDS.

If the unthinkable happens and you do lose a baby to SIDS, don't fall into the trap of blaming yourself for what has happened. Since the cause or causes of SIDS remain unknown, you should not conclude that you were somehow responsible for your baby's death.

Coping with SIDS-related fears

While most worries are relatively easy to chase away once you've pulled out your baby books or made a quick call to your doctor's office, some of them are a lot more resilient, keeping you awake at 3:00 a.m. when you know you should be sleeping. At the top of the list for most parents is the fear that their baby will become a victim of SIDS.

According to Deborah Davis, co-author of *The Emotional Journey of Parenting Your Premature Baby: A Book of Hope and Healing,* the key to learning to live with SIDS-related fears is to accept the fact that there are some aspects of parenting that are beyond your control: "With regard to feelings of vulnerability to tragedy, their intensity does fade as you are able to accept that life and death just happen. And when you realize that the death of your child has no bearing on your worth as a parent or as a person, then you can accept that you truly do have little control over many circumstances. Not everything is your fault or deserved. You can just try to control the things you can, and let go of what you can't. Peace comes from experiencing that feeling of 'letting go.'"

Grieving the Loss of Your Baby

It's a topic that prenatal classes tend to skip over and pregnancy books tend to ignore: the possibility that pregnancy could result in anything other than a happy ending. Regardless of when you lose your baby — prior to or after the birth — you'll need to take time to grieve the death of your baby.

You may find that you experience many of the psychological and physical symptoms of grief: Preoccupation with thoughts of the baby you lost, irritability, restlessness, anxiety, fear, yearning, hopelessness, confusion, shortness of breath, tightness in the throat, fatigue, crying spells, an empty feeling in your abdomen, sleeplessness, a change in appetite, heart palpitations, and other physical symptoms of anxiety. Some bereaved parents experience some additional symptoms: Empty, aching arms and having illusions about seeing, hearing, or feeling the presence of the baby.

You may feel shocked and overwhelmed that this has happened. You may feel as though you're making the motions of everyday living even though your mind is preoccupied with the task of making sense of something that makes no sense at all. You may also find yourself denying that your baby has died or wishing desperately that he hadn't; blaming yourself or others for his death; and coping with feelings of depression and despair.

Some parents who have lost a baby are afraid to work through their grief, believing that doing so will cause them to forget about the baby they lost. Here are some reassuring words from Deborah Davis, Ph.D., author of *Empty Cradle, Broken Heart*: "You will never forget your baby. Many people mistakenly believe that resolution means you stop grieving, forget about the baby, and meekly abandon your baby to death. To the contrary, grief does not end. You will always feel some sadness and wish that things could have turned out better. But, with time, the denial, failure, guilt and anger fade; the sadness becomes manageable. . . .The peaceful feelings that come with resolution are a blessed change from the ravages of grief."

MOM'S THE WORD

"I had known women who had suffered miscarriages, but I never knew how painful it was until I went through it. It took months to 'get over' it. I cried so much and was so desperately sad. It was horrible. I asked my midwife to collect all the medical records from the E.R. and O.R. and I made an appointment at the hospital records department to read through my chart to see what the doctors and nurses had found. To see what might have caused the miscarriage or to see exactly what was wrong. I spoke with the obstetrician who did the D & C and with my midwife and no one could tell me anything. It was just 'one of those things.' I think the worst part was not knowing how it happened or why."

— *Lori, 29, mother of four*

Here are some suggestions on surviving the first few weeks and months after the death of your baby:

- Make sure that you have been given a clear explanation of the circumstances that led to your baby's death (assuming, of course, that it's possible for your doctor to provide you with a medical explanation). You may have a difficult time grasping this information when you're dealing with the shock of your baby's death, so you might wish to have a support person accompany you to meetings with the doctor or the coroner so that your support person can try to absorb some of the information for you. And don't be afraid to set up a follow-up appointment with the health-care practitioners involved if you find that you still have unanswered questions weeks or months later.

- Plan to spend some time with your baby's body after her death. In addition to holding and dressing your baby, you might want to take some photographs of her in your arms, in your partner's arms, with other special people in your life (e.g., her grandparents), and, in the case of a twin pregnancy, with her surviving twin. These photos may become some of your most treasured mementos of the time you spent with your baby. Note: If you decide to take photos, you might want to use black and white rather than color film. The redness of the skin of a baby who was miscarried or stillborn quite prematurely and the skin changes that happen after a baby dies are less apparent if you take black and white photos.

- Think about what other mementos you might want to have of your baby: perhaps a lock of hair or a set of handprints or footprints. A growing number of hospitals are starting to make handprints or footprints available to bereaved parents, so don't be concerned that the hospital staff will think it's odd if you make this type of request.

- If you decide to dress your baby in a special outfit or you choose to have your baby buried along with a toy or other memento, you might want to take photos of these items with your baby and/or to purchase duplicates so that you'll have these special keepsakes.

MOM'S THE WORD

"Keep one thing that belonged to your baby or that you bought for your baby. If you can, take a picture of your baby so that when you're grieving and no one else will talk about it with you, you'll have something tangible to hold on to and cry with."

— *Liz, 36, mother of four, who has experienced two miscarriages*

- Find ways to collect other memories of your pregnancy or your baby's short life. You might want to start a scrapbook and include cards you received when you found out you were pregnant, pictures of yourself when you were pregnant, and so on. Or you may decide to write a letter to your baby, reflecting on the joys of your pregnancy and letting your baby know how much she is missed.

- Recognize that there's no one "right" way to grieve. You may spend a lot of time crying or you may find that you feel numb and frozen. Your grief may come in waves or it may be with you 24 hours a day. There's no such thing as "normal" when it comes to grief.

- Accept the fact that your partner may grieve differently from you. Don't automatically assume that he's less affected by the loss just because he's less willing to express his emotions. Many bereaved fathers feel tremendous pressure to "hold it together" when their partners are falling apart.

- Be prepared to make some difficult decisions. If you know ahead of time that you will miscarry, you will have to decide whether you prefer to miscarry naturally at home or go to the hospital for a D & C. If your baby is stillborn or dies shortly after birth, you'll have to decide whether to have an autopsy performed and what to do about a baptism, a burial, a memorial service, and so on.

MOM'S THE WORD

"It seems that women get more closely attached to a pregnancy earlier on than men do. Everything changes for a woman the moment you find out you're carrying a new life. Generally, I thought about that baby during every waking moment and thought about what I could do to give it the best chance possible."

— *Tammy, 31, mother of one living child and two very premature babies who died shortly after birth*

- Find ways of involving your living children in the grieving process. They may wish to help pick out flowers for the funeral bouquet or to draw a picture for the baby who died. Remind yourself that they are grieving, too, even though they may express their emotions in unexpected ways. One mother who thought that her 7-year-old son was unaffected by the baby's death was very touched to inadvertently discover that he'd drawn a "sad face" in crayon on the ceiling above his bunk bed. Whatever you do, don't make the mistake of telling your children that the baby has "gone to sleep" or been "lost": These types of statements may cause them to become unnecessarily fearful.

- Reach out for support from other women who have experienced the loss of a baby. Lori, a 29-year-old mother of four who's also been through a miscarriage, feels that support groups have a lot to offer: "There are so many shoulders to cry on — so many people to listen to. And it helps tremendously when you can help another person," she explains.

(Note: You can find the contact information for a number of perinatal loss and grief-oriented support groups in Appendix D, and leads on sources of online support and information in Appendix E.)

- Resist the temptation to bury your grief by turning to alcohol or prescription drugs or by throwing yourself into your work and refusing to face your feelings. You can't avoid working through your grief — you can only postpone it.

- Accept any and all offers of help. Family members can prepare meals for you, help you to make funeral arrangements, make phone calls for you, and so on. Note: Most parents find that they prefer to handle at least some of the funeral preparations themselves since this is one of the last things they'll ever have the opportunity to do for their baby.

- Take care of your physical needs as well as your emotional needs. Get the sleep you need, exercise regularly, and make a point of eating nutritious, well-balanced meals. Don't forget that you'll also need time to recover from the delivery if your baby was miscarried or stillborn, or died shortly after birth. If you had a miscarriage, you'll need about six weeks to physically recover from the experience. If your baby was stillborn or died shortly after birth, you can expect to experience all the usual postpartum discomforts associated with a vaginal or cesarean delivery on top of trying to cope with your grief. (See Chapter 12 for information about the postpartum recovery period.)

 MOTHER WISDOM

If your baby is stillborn or dies shortly after birth or after breastfeeding has already been established, you'll also have to cope with breast engorgement (overly full and uncomfortable breasts). Having milk leaking from your breasts after your baby has died can be both physically and emotionally stressful. You may feel as though your entire body is mourning the loss of your baby — which, in fact, it is. The period of engorgement tends to last for about 48 hours. You can relieve your breast tenderness in the meantime by expressing a small amount of milk. (Don't express too much or your body will start producing more milk.) Binding your breasts tightly, applying ice packs to your breasts, and wearing a snug bra at all times can also help to reduce your discomfort. Note: If you notice red, warm, hard, or tender areas in your breasts; develop a fever of more than 100°F, notice that the lymph nodes under your arms are becoming uncomfortable, or feel generally ill, it could be because you're developing a breast infection. Contact your doctor or midwife to talk about treatment options.

- Find ways to honor your baby's memory. You might wish to make a donation to a charity in your baby's name or to buy a piece of equipment for your hospital's neonatal ward in your baby's memory.

 MOTHER WISDOM

If you're worried about the costs of burying your baby, talk to your doctor or midwife about burial options for families with modest incomes. You may find that a local funeral home offers a significant discount or waives its fees entirely for families who have experienced the death of a baby.

- Be prepared for insensitive comments from people who fail to understand the extent of your grief. "Don't let anyone tell you you'll 'get over it,'" insists Lori, 39, whose daughter was stillborn at 26 weeks due to intrauterine growth restriction. "You never get over it. You just learn — gradually — to live with your loss. In time, it does get easier to cope with day-to-day life, but you never, ever forget."

- Accept the fact that you may always have questions about your baby's death. The one question that parents want answered most is the one that is generally the most difficult to find an answer to: Why did this happen to *my* baby?

- Remind yourself that you have the strength to get through this — that as painful as it is to have to say goodbye to a baby you desperately wanted, you can survive this heartbreak. As hard as it may be for you to believe it right now, you will find joy in your life again.

MOM'S THE WORD

"I wrote in a journal to get my feelings out. Since we didn't want to tell anyone about the pregnancy right away, I couldn't talk to my friends about my anxiety. I tried not to be negative but, at the same time, if something made me nervous (e.g., dyeing my hair), I didn't do it. In between my miscarriage and my new pregnancy, I stayed in prenatal mode: I kept taking my vitamins, I didn't drink coffee, I watched what I ate."

— *Christina, a 25-year-old mother of two whose third pregnancy ended in miscarriage, and who is now pregnant again*

Preparing for Another Pregnancy

It takes courage to start trying again when your previous pregnancy has ended in heartbreak. As you know only too well, there are no guarantees when it comes to conception, pregnancy, and birth.

Physical healing

Your doctor or midwife will likely suggest that you give yourself time to heal before you embark on another pregnancy. If you had a miscarriage or an uncomplicated vaginal delivery, you'll likely be advised to wait until you've had two to three normal menstrual cycles before you start trying to conceive. This will help to reduce your chances of experiencing a miscarriage since, if you conceive right away, your uterine lining may not have had the chance to build back up to healthy levels again. If you had a cesarean section, on the other hand, you'll be advised to wait for six months before you start trying to conceive again. It takes a couple of months for your uterine scar to heal, and becoming pregnant too quickly could increase your odds of experiencing a uterine rupture or other complications during your subsequent pregnancy.

Emotional readiness

You can't base your decision about whether or not to start trying again on physical factors alone, however. You also need to assess your emotional readiness for another pregnancy. That means considering whether you've had the opportunity to work through some of your grief, whether you'd be able to cope if you were to have trouble conceiving or experience another loss, whether you're ready to cope with the stress of a subsequent pregnancy (a major consideration if your next pregnancy is likely to be classified as high risk), whether you actually want another baby — or whether what you really want is the baby who died, and how your partner feels about trying again.

You may be eager to start trying again right away, or you may decide that it's important for you to let certain key milestones pass before you become pregnant again — the due date of the baby you lost, the anniversary of your baby's death, and so on. You'll find a detailed discussion of these issues in my book *Trying Again: A Guide to Pregnancy After Miscarriage, Stillbirth, and Infant Loss.*

Getting pregnant again won't make all your worries go away. In fact, it'll make a whole bunch of new worries appear on the horizon! Here are some tips on weathering the emotional highs and lows of pregnancy after a loss:

MOM'S THE WORD

"It took us almost an entire year to conceive after our loss. I think the most bothersome aspect of the whole experience was that, once your baby dies, the medical establishment doesn't want to understand what you both are going through. If only one of the doctors or specialists had said to either of us, 'I know how demoralizing this is for you. I know how much despair you must be feeling. If you need to talk about it and discuss your options about trying to conceive again, I'm here.' But no one ever did."

— *Pandora, 45, mother of two living children and a baby who died of SIDS*

- Be prepared to experience a range of emotions — everything from joy at being pregnant again, to fear that something could go wrong this time too, to guilt at "betraying" the baby you lost by moving on with your life.

- Surround yourself with people who are prepared to support you during your subsequent pregnancy. You might wish to join a pregnancy-after-loss support group (if there's one available in your community) or an online support group. (I highly recommend the Subsequent Pregnancy After a Loss support e-mail list. I joined it after my daughter was stillborn and it kept me sane during my subsequent pregnancy with my now two-year-old son. You'll find the contact information for this group in Appendix E.) At the very least, you should arrange for a friend or family member to accompany you to your prenatal appointments and/or ultrasound appointments in case you need some additional support.

- Make sure you've got a supportive caregiver. You need a doctor or midwife who will understand that you'll likely need extra reassurance — and perhaps even extra prenatal visits — this time around. If you're not getting that kind of care and support from your current caregiver, it's time to consider making a change.

- Find out as much as you can about the cause of your previous loss and what, if anything, can be done to prevent the problem from recurring this time around. The more knowledge you have about the medical aspects of your pregnancy, the more in control you'll feel.

- Take things day by day — hour by hour, if you have to. Rather than dwelling on the fact that there are 40 weeks of pregnancy ahead of you, focus on achieving the next milestone — making it to the end of the first trimester, passing the point at which you lost your previous baby, and so on. Cyndie, a 35-year-old mother of two, found that taking this approach was the only thing that kept her sane when she became pregnant again after experiencing three consecutive losses: "It was like holding your breath for nine months, afraid to breathe, afraid to let your guard down," she recalls. "Every waking moment was lived literally from moment to moment. Every internal twinge or sensation signalled a rush of adrenaline as a surge of panic raced through my bloodstream. How I lived through nine months' worth of seconds like this I still have no idea. I guess because I never allowed myself to live in the future. Every day, every hour, even every minute, was only that and nothing more."

- Expect certain milestones to be particularly tough: The anniversary of your previous baby's due date or death, the week of pregnancy when you lost your previous baby, and so on. You might want to schedule your prenatal visit around this time so that you'll have the reassurance you crave when you need it most.

- Rather than focusing on all the scary things that could go wrong, try to remain positive. The majority of couples who have experienced miscarriage, stillbirth, or infant death go on to give birth to healthy babies the next time around.

MOM'S THE WORD

"When Renée was born — 5 $^1/_2$ years after the birth of my first child, and following three losses — she brought me completion. She gave me pure satisfaction and joy. I smile inside every day. She alone numbs the pain of my losses and makes 3 $^1/_2$ years of hell worth every step. I'd do it all again if I knew she'd be the reward. Now I take nothing for granted and I enjoy every moment with my children. They are my priority, my happiness, my life."

— Cyndie, 35, mother of two

CHAPTER 12

Life After Baby

*"The time immediately following birth is precious. . . . A child is
born, and for a moment the wheeling planets stop in their tracks,
as past, present, and future meet."*
— *Sheila Kitzinger, in her book,* Homebirth

*"I remember driving home with our new son and marveling how
much everything looked the same. It felt so different, but it was
the same. We got home and the house was quiet, almost eerie. I
felt there should have been something special, like in the
movies — huge crowds of cheering people, balloons, jugglers —
something."*
— *Jennifer, 32, mother of one*

No matter how many hours of baby-sitting time you
logged as a teenager and how many pregnancy and
baby-care books you've read over the last nine months,
nothing can ever fully prepare you for those first few weeks after
your baby's birth. Most women describe the postpartum period
as the best of times and the worst of times, all wrapped in one:
a time to celebrate the joys of becoming a mother and to mourn
the loss of your pre-baby freedom. Add to that the fact that your
hormones are crashing, you haven't had a good night's sleep

since your second trimester (if then!), and you're aching from head to toe, and you can see why the first few weeks postpartum are likely to be one of the most challenging periods of your life.

We'll begin this final chapter by talking about the physical aspects of postpartum: the types of aches and pains you may be experiencing and what you can do to get your body back in shape. Then we'll consider the emotional aspects of life after baby: how you may feel about becoming a mother and how your relationship with your partner may change after you give birth. We'll conclude the book by getting down to the nitty-gritty of what you can do to weather the storms of this weird yet wonderful time in your life.

MOTHER WISDOM

"After the birth of the baby, the mother should be kept perfectly quiet for the first 24 hours and not [be] allowed to talk to anyone except her nearest relations, however well she may seem. She should not get out of bed for 10 days or two weeks, nor sit up in bed for nine days.... She should not work a sewing machine with a treadle for at least six weeks and avoid any unusual strain or over-exertion."

— Advice given to new mothers a century ago by authors B.G. Jeffris and J.L. Nichols in their bestselling book Safe, Counsel or Practical Eugenics, published in 1893.

Your Postpartum Body: What to Expect

Don't be surprised if you do a double-take the first time you catch a glance of your naked body in the mirror. It takes time for your body to reverse the dramatic changes that occurred over the previous nine months. Here's the scoop on what you can expect from your body during the first days and weeks after the birth:

MOM'S THE WORD

"I was shocked by how I looked, and I felt disgusting, to be honest. It was very hard and still is to reconcile the 'new' me with the image I had of myself in my mind. I wasn't prepared for how much pregnancy and birth would alter my body and the number of stretch marks I'd get. I also have a huge cesarean scar on my stomach that's very hard to get over emotionally."

—*Jennifer, 31, mother of two*

- Heavy vaginal bleeding. The term "lochia" is used to describe the bleeding that occurs as your uterus sheds its lining after the birth. You'll experience it whether you end up delivering vaginally or by cesarean section. Typically lasting anywhere from 10 days to 6 weeks or even longer, it gradually tapers down from a bright red, heavy flow to an almost colorless or yellowish discharge. Any activity that causes the uterus to empty (e.g., standing, walking, or breastfeeding) will result in an increase in flow. You may be surprised by the amount of bleeding and the size of the blood clots you pass. "It was a lot heavier than I thought it would be," recalls Tina, a 32-year-old mother of one. "It was much heavier than even the heaviest menstrual period." While this can be alarming, there's generally cause for concern only if you soak more than one pad over the course of an hour, you're passing blood clots that are larger than lemons, or your lochia develops an extremely unpleasant odor. These are the symptoms of a possible postpartum hemorrhage or uterine infection.

- Perineal pain. You can expect your perineum to be sore and tender after a vaginal birth, even if you didn't end up having an episiotomy or a tear. Stephanie was shocked by how swollen her perineum looked and felt: "I did not recognize parts of my own anatomy, they were so swollen," the 33-year-old mother of one recalls. "The biggest surprise came one day after I delivered. I was going to the bathroom and when I took the toilet paper to wipe, I was in utter shock at how swollen and odd my vaginal area felt. I immediately got a handheld mirror so I could take a closer look. Between the swelling and the hemorrhoids, I did not recognize myself. It was awful." If you find yourself experiencing a lot of perineal pain, you might want to try placing ice in a washcloth or rubber glove and applying it to the area, soaking in a warm tub (either a bathtub or a sitz bath), inserting chilled witch-hazel pads between your perineum and your sanitary pad, or carefully using a blow dryer to dry and warm your sore perineum. You might also want to try sitting on one of those doughnut-shaped cushions that hemorrhoid sufferers use. To minimize the risk of developing a perineal infection, you should make a point of changing your sanitary pad at least every couple of hours and of wiping yourself from front to back each time you use the bathroom.

📣 MOM'S THE WORD

"Soak some sanitary pads in water and freeze them. Wear these for the first little while postpartum. They help to soothe the perineum."

— *Carrie, 34, currently pregnant with her second child*

- Changes to the tone and feel of your vagina. If you delivered your baby vaginally, your vagina may feel stretched and tender after the delivery. Kegel exercises (pelvic floor muscle exercises) will help your vagina return to its pre-pregnant state and can also help to ward off incontinence and other gynecological problems. Note: If you are breastfeeding, you may experience some vaginal dryness — something that can cause discomfort during intercourse unless you use a water-soluble vaginal lubricant. If your problems are particularly severe, you might want to ask your doctor to prescribe a topical estrogen cream to help with lubrication.

- Difficulty urinating. It's not unusual to experience a decreased urge to urinate after you give birth. This can be caused by a low fluid intake prior to and during labor, combined with an excessive loss of fluids during the delivery (think perspiration, vomiting, and bleeding); bruising to the bladder or the urethra during labor; the effects of drugs and anesthesia during the delivery (they can temporarily decrease the sensitivity of your bladder or interfere with your ability to tell when you need to urinate); perineal pain that can cause reflex spasms in the urethra (the tube that transports urine from the bladder); and a fear of urinating on your oh-so-tender perineum. You can encourage the urine to start flowing again by contracting and releasing your pelvic muscles, upping your intake of fluids, and placing hot or cold packs on your perineum (whichever triggers your urge to urinate). If it's good old-fashioned fear that's holding you back, you might want to try drinking plenty of liquids to dilute the acidity of your urine, straddling the toilet saddle-style when you urinate, urinating while you pour water across your perineum (you can use either a peri-bottle or a bowl), or — if you really get desperate — urinating when you're standing in the shower. The problem will resolve itself over time. In fact, you'll soon be making extra trips to the bathroom as your body goes about its postpartum housekeeping, getting rid of all the excess fluids you accumulated during pregnancy. Note: If you experience intense burning after urination or an intense, painful, and unusually frequent urge to urinate, it could be because you've developed a urinary tract infection, in which case you'll want to drink plenty of unsweetened cranberry juice and contact your caregiver to arrange for treatment.

- Urinary incontinence. Some women experience the opposite problem when it comes to urination: incontinence. Incontinence usually improves during the first six weeks after the delivery (particularly if you do your Kegels religiously), but it can be rather disconcerting and inconvenient in the meantime. (Thank goodness you're going to be wearing a pad anyway.)

- Difficulty having bowel movements. The lack of food during labor and the temporarily decreased muscle tone in your intestines may mean that you don't end up having a bowel movement for a few days after the delivery. And when the urge to have a bowel movement finally hits, you may find it hard to relax and let nature takes its course, out of fear of hurting your tender perineum and/or painful hemorrhoids or of popping the stitches on your episiotomy site (you can scratch this last worry off the list, by the way). The best way to cope with this problem is to increase your intake of fluids and fiber (e.g., prune, pear, or apricot nectar; fresh fruit and vegetables; and whole grains), to avoid food and beverages that contain caffeine (e.g., coffee, cola, and chocolate), and to remain as active as possible. This will help to keep your stools soft and regular.

MOM'S THE WORD

"After a few days, I had to have a suppository. I found it embarrassing to ask for and doubly embarrassing to have it put in, but that was my own hang-up. The nurse was very professional and caring, and in the end, the relief was worth the embarrassment."

— *Jennifer, 32, mother of one*

- Afterpains. You can expect to experience afterpains, which can range in intensity from virtually unnoticeable to downright painful. The afterpains are most intense when you're nursing because your baby's sucking triggers the release of oxytocin, the hormone that causes the uterus to contract. While afterpains tend to be relatively mild after the birth of your first baby, they can be quite painful after your second or subsequent birth, something 36-year-old Marguerite discovered after giving birth to her second child last year: "I was shocked by the strength of the afterpains after my second delivery. I had vaguely remembered reading about them, but hadn't noticed anything after the first delivery, so I wasn't particularly worried about them. I found them almost as bad as labor the second time around. I couldn't believe they could be so painful!" If you're experiencing a lot of discomfort from your afterpains, you may want to ask your caregiver to prescribe a pain medication that's safe to take while you're breastfeeding. Or you can grin and bear it and wait for the afterpains to disappear on their own. (They'll decrease in both frequency and intensity over the next few weeks.)

- A flabby belly. You may also be surprised by the tone (or rather, lack thereof) of your stomach muscles. "I was completely unprepared for the jelly-belly," recalls Carrie, 34, who is currently pregnant with her second child. "It seemed so flabby and fat." Speaking of bellies, don't be surprised if you still look five to six months pregnant. This is because your uterus is just starting to return to its pre-pregnant size (a process known as involution, whereby the uterine muscles alternately relax and contract). By the time you show up for your six-week checkup, however, your uterus will be back to normal. (Whether or not the rest of you will be, however, is another matter entirely!)

- Separation of the abdominal muscles. Some women experience diastasis recti (a separation of the abdominal muscles that extend from the chest to the symphysis pubis). This muscle separation can be corrected by doing abdominal exercises (e.g. abdominal tightening, head lifts, and pelvic tilts) during the postpartum period.

- Stretch marks. They've been there all along, but you might not have been able to see the stretch marks on the underside of your belly or your upper thighs. (After all, there was a baby in the way!) It can come as a bit of a shock to see all those red-crayon-like lines. While they won't disappear entirely, they will fade from reddish purple to silver over time. Fortunately, there's better news where the linea nigra (the brown line down your belly) and the "mask of pregnancy" (the butterfly-shaped tan area around your eyes and cheeks) are concerned: as the pregnancy hormones leave your body, these two side effects of pregnancy will disappear spontaneously.

- Hair loss. Thanks to a crash in estrogen levels after the birth, your body finally gets around to doing a little housekeeping in the hair department, getting rid of all the extra hair it should have been shedding while you were pregnant. (During pregnancy, your body stopped losing hair at its usual rate of 100 hairs per day, leaving your hair looking every bit as lush as the hair on any shampoo commercial model.) Since natural regrowth can't possibly keep up with the rate at which you're shedding this excess hair, you go from lush to limp overnight. (Just think of it as The Mother of All Bad Hair Days.) Fortunately, the hair nightmare that you're experiencing will be relatively short-lived. While your hair won't look quite as lush as it did during pregnancy, it'll look a heck of a lot better than it does right now in about six months' time. Until then, ask your hairdresser to suggest a cut that will be flattering and easy to maintain. Your days of spending a half hour or more fussing with a blow dryer and a bottle of mousse are over for now!

- Breast changes. You can also expect to notice some dramatic changes to your breasts after you give birth. While your breasts already contain nutrient- and immunity-rich colostrum when you give birth, within two to three days your actual milk will come in. Your breasts may become flushed, swollen, and engorged during the 24 to 48 hours after that, whether or not you're actually planning to nurse your baby. Bevin, a 27-year-old mother of one, was surprised by the sheer size of her post-baby breasts: "We had a couple of Christmas parties to go to about a month after the delivery. I wanted to wear a dress, but everything I tried on looked bizarre. I thought I looked like a drag queen with a petite bottom and a huge chest!"

MOM'S THE WORD

"I was getting dressed one morning right after my milk had come in and my partner walked into the room. I heard a gasp. He stood staring at my breasts. When I looked in the mirror, I understood his amazement. They were huge! Unfortunately, he quickly learned that they were also extremely sore. I guess you have to take the bad with the good."

— *Tracey, 31, mother of one*

- Leaky breasts. Don't be surprised, by the way, if you find yourself leaking milk both during and between feedings. You may leak milk from one breast when you're nursing on the other side. (The leaking will tend to taper off after a minute or so but, in the meantime, you'll want to keep some breast

pads handy.) You may also find yourself leaking milk whenever you think of your baby or if you go for a particularly
long stretch between feedings. "I remember thinking that
I didn't need breast pads," confesses Jenny, 31, a first-time
mother. "Ha! I was soaked in a matter of seconds. I hadn't
ever believed that the sound of a baby crying or just thinking
about your baby could make you leak, but it was true!"

- Sore nipples. Even if you're doing everything "right," you
  may find that your nipples feel a bit sore during the first
  week of breastfeeding. The cause of the soreness if obvious:
  Your nipples aren't accustomed to being in use for hours
  every day, and it can take a little time to break them in.
  Unfortunately, most breastfeeding books don't prepare you
  for the fact that there can be some initial soreness, particularly if you're fair-haired and fair-skinned, and so it's easy to
  worry that you're experiencing a positioning problem or
  other breastfeeding problem if you feel any tenderness at all.
  Even if your baby is positioned perfectly, it's hardly surprising
  that a certain amount of soreness can occur, given how often
  and how vigorously babies suck. "I had no idea how hard a
  baby can suck. I swear it felt like she was going to suck my
  toes out through my nipples!" recalls Bevin. The best way to
  treat sore nipples is to expose your nipples to air and sunlight. (You can settle for a heat lamp, if you're not into nude
  sunbathing, but be very careful not to burn your breasts.)
  Also, to ensure maximum air flow to your nipples, avoid
  breast pads with plastic backings and clothing made out of
  synthetic fibers.

MOM'S THE WORD

"I had no problems with breastfeeding other than the usual nipple soreness: not the cracked, raw feeling, but that soreness that comes from 'overuse.' Once my nipples 'toughened up' a little, the pain was gone."

— *Lori, 29, mother of four*

- Faintness. Don't be surprised if you find yourself feeling a little faint for a day or so after the birth. Body fluid levels shift suddenly when pregnancy ends and it can take a bit of time for your cardiovascular system to adjust. If the faintness continues for more than a few days, ask your caregiver to test you for anemia (iron deficiency).

- Shivers and shakes. It's not unusual to experience shivers and shakes right after you've given birth. Researchers believe this occurs because of a resetting of the body's temperature-regulating system as your pregnancy comes to an end.

- Sweating. One of the ways your body gets rid of all the extra fluids accumulated during your pregnancy is by sweating. You can expect to perspire more heavily than usual, especially at night. You might want to cover your sheet and pillow with a towel to absorb some of the excess perspiration. Experts also believe that the sweating may be caused by the sudden decrease in your estrogen levels — something that can have you experiencing menopause-like "hot flashes" during the first week or two postpartum.

- Weight loss. Everyone knows at least one woman who was able to slip back into her pre-pregnancy jeans before she left the hospital, but women like this are the exception rather than the rule. Most of us find we still have at least a few pounds left to lose after giving birth. As a rule, you can expect to lose between 17 and 20 pounds immediately. How quickly you lose the rest of your pregnancy weight will depend on both your post-baby lifestyle and whether you decide to breastfeed. While breastfeeding can actually help you lose weight — you'll burn an extra 500 calories a day while you're nursing — most women find they aren't able to lose the last few pounds they put on during their pregnancy until after they stop breastfeeding. (Just plop one of your breasts on the nearest postal scale and you'll see why!) Unfortunately, some women find that they gain weight while they're breastfeeding since the extra energy requirements of nursing can trigger an increase in appetite. Bottom line? If you eat more food than your body needs and don't up your exercise output accordingly, you could find yourself back in gain mode again.

FACTS AND FIGURES

Don't expect to automatically feel like a million bucks once you reach the magic six-week mark. A study of more than 1,300 Australian women found that most were still experiencing a variety of aches and pains eight weeks after their babies' births. The most common complaints included exhaustion and extreme tiredness (60%), backache (53%), bowel problems (37%), hemorrhoids (30%), lack of sleep (30%), perineal soreness (22%), problems with sex (19%), urinary incontinence (19%), and frequent migraines or headaches (19%).

As you can see, your body has a tremendous amount of work to do to recover from the birth. While you might think that your body will never get back to normal, you'll be surprised to see just how much progress it has made by the time your six-week checkup rolls around. While it's unlikely that you'll be mistaken for any of the pencil-thin supermodel moms, you will be ready to do at least a decent impression of your pre-pregnancy self.

Cesarean recovery

If you gave birth via cesarean section, you can expect a few additional discomforts during the postpartum period: Tenderness around your incision, gas buildup in your upper chest and shoulders, and fatigue. Here are some tips on dealing with these common post-cesarean complaints:

- Don't be afraid to go into couch potato mode for a while. You need plenty of rest in order to heal properly, so make caring for your baby and caring for yourself your top priorities for at least the first few weeks.

- Learn how to minimize pain around your incision site. Hold a pillow against your incision when you cough, sneeze, or laugh in order to provide some gentle support to your midsection. Avoid heavy lifting and limit the number of times you trek up and down the stairs in a day. And keep your incision clean and dry and expose it to air as often as possible.

- Don't be surprised if you experience some numbness around your incision until the nerves regenerate (something that typically happens about six to nine months after the birth). You should also be prepared for the fact that your scar may continue to be bright red for up to a year. (It will fade in time, but sometimes the fading process takes longer than you'd like.)

- Don't be alarmed if you experience pressure and uncomfortable urination for a week or two afterward as a side effect of your surgery. This problem will disappear as your body heals.

- You should also expect to have a few problems with gas pains. Mother Nature's reaction to abdominal surgery is to call all intestinal activity to a halt. That's why it's normal for women who've been through a cesarean section to experience uncomfortable gas pains during the first three days (until the intestinal tract starts working again). Try taking short walks, changing your position frequently, and rocking in a chair. These techniques will help to get rid of any trapped gas, thereby relieving the gas pains that are causing you so much grief.

While the first few weeks can be a little rough, you won't feel this beat up for very long. You'll see significant improvements from day to day, and — within a couple of weeks — you'll be practically good as new and ready to tackle whatever challenges motherhood tosses your way.

Getting Back into Shape: What's Realistic and What's Not

We all know at least one Cindy Crawford type: a new mom who was able to slip into her skin-tight workout leotard within days of giving birth. What we sometimes forget, however, is that the Cindy Crawfords of the world are the exception rather than the rule; it takes most of us a whole lot longer than a couple of days to get back in shape after giving birth!

That's not to say the situation is all doom and gloom, of course. (If it were, those slim-and-trim moms you see carrying babies would be on the endangered species list!) Here are some tips on designing a workout program that will work for you during this exciting but busy time in your life:

- Give your body the credit it deserves. Rather than beating yourself up for being "out of shape," remind yourself that your body is actually in perfect shape for having just had a baby. There's a reason why your abdominal muscles are flabby and you're carrying around extra pounds: You've just sublet your uterus to your baby for the last nine months!

- Don't get too hung up on the number on the scale. You're likely to weigh a little more at least until you finish breastfeeding.

FACTS AND FIGURES

Before you fall into the trap of being too hard on yourself, heed these words of caution: You could be sabotaging your fitness success by focusing on all the things you don't like about your postpartum body. Researchers at the Stanford University School of Medicine have discovered that you're actually twice as likely to succeed at losing weight if you feel reasonably good about your body.

- Focus on boosting the amount of exercise you do rather than cutting back on your food intake. Your body needs a steady stream of nutritious food, particularly if you're breastfeeding. (This might be a good time to flip back to the sections on healthy eating in Chapters 2 and 6.)

- Stop viewing exercise as a polite euphemism for torture. If you're not in the habit of working out regularly, it's easy to treat exercise as just one more thing you have to do. Instead, try to convince yourself that you actually want to exercise because of all the good things it'll do for you, both body and soul. (You may have to lie to yourself a bit at first, but over time you'll start believing it!)

- Be realistic about what you can expect to accomplish at this stage in your life. It's better to set a series of small, achievable fitness goals for yourself than to aim so high that you throw in the towel after just a couple of days. Besides, studies have shown that people who aim for moderate rather than high-intensity workouts are only half as likely to abandon their fitness programs.

- Look for fitness activities you can enjoy with your baby in tow. Walking is a natural, of course: You simply pop the wee one into her stroller or baby carrier and hit the pavement. But so are such activities as dancing (with or without a baby in your arms), jogging (provided you buy a decent-quality jogging stroller), and weight-lifting. (Believe it or not, there are even postnatal fitness workout tapes that show you how to use your baby as a free weight!)

- Choose a fitness activity that you genuinely like. That way you'll be far more motivated to follow through on your workout, be it walking, biking, swimming, or something else entirely. (Hey, it's hard enough to convince yourself to spend what little free time you have working out. Don't make it harder on yourself by committing to an activity that triggers painful flashbacks to your sixth-grade phys ed class!)

- Choose an activity that's easy to fit into your schedule. If you're breastfeeding a baby who's colicky in the evenings, it may not make sense to sign up for an after-dinner water fitness class at your local gym. (On the other hand, if that's the only time you can squeeze in a workout and it's the one thing that's keeping you sane, then go for it.)

- Wear a sports bra or two nursing bras while you're working out to give your breasts the support they need. If you're nursing, you'll probably feel more comfortable if you breastfeed your baby right before your workout.

- If you're having trouble with incontinence, urinate before you start your workout and then wear a panty liner to guard against leakage. (If you make a point of including Kegel exercises in your workout — exercises that can help to tone your pelvic floor muscles — you'll probably find that your incontinence becomes less of a problem.)

- Don't overdo it. Joint laxity (looseness) can be a problem for months after you give birth. To minimize the risk of injury, perform all movements with caution and control when you're exercising and avoid jumping; rapid changes of direction; jerky, bouncing, or jarring motions; and deep flexion or extension of joints.

- Skip your workout if you're feeling particularly exhausted. The more tired you are, the more likely you are to injure yourself.

- Drink plenty of liquids before, during, and after your workout. It's important to keep your body fully hydrated.

- Stop exercising immediately if you experience pain, faintness, dizziness, blurred vision, shortness of breath, heart palpitations, back pain, pubic pain, nausea, difficulty walking, or a sudden increase in vaginal bleeding. You should report any of these exercise-related symptoms to your caregiver.

- Make sure your workout is suitable for someone who's just had a baby. Most fitness experts advise you to pass on knee-chest exercises, full sit-ups, and double leg lifts during the postpartum period.

- Spend your fitness dollars wisely. Before you fork over a small fortune on a gym membership, be realistic about how often you're actually going to make it there to work out. Unless they offer on-site childcare or you have someone who can come into your home a few times a week so that you can get out, you may find that it's such a hassle to get to the gym and back that you rarely step foot in the place!

- Don't pooh-pooh the benefits of working out at home. A recent Stanford University study revealed that people who exercise in their own homes are more likely to stick with their fitness programs than people who work out elsewhere. What's more, a University of Florida study confirmed what many exercise physiologists have long suspected: People who exercise at home tend to lose more weight over the course of a year than people who exercise at other locations.

- Don't allow yourself to get into a fitness rut. It's easy to allow boredom to sabotage your workout program. Either rotate fitness activities on a regular basis or find a workout buddy who can help you stay motivated. Your body will thank you for it!

- Reward yourself for sticking to your fitness program. Treat yourself to some workout clothes, a new workout video, or a new piece of exercise equipment — anything that will encourage you to build on your fitness success.

- Stick with it. Fitness should remain a priority for you long after those extra pregnancy pounds are gone. Not only will it help to ensure that your body is in the best possible physical condition, it will also help you to combat some of the day-to-day stresses that seem to go along with the whole motherhood turf!

Up until now we've been focusing on the physical challenges of the postpartum period. Now we're going to talk about the emotional challenges of becoming a mother.

FACTS AND FIGURES

Wondering if it's safe to lose weight while you're breastfeeding? According to a recent study at the University of North Carolina at Greensboro, breastfeeding moms can safely lose up to a pound a week without affecting the quality or quantity of their breastmilk.

How You May Feel About Becoming a Mother

After months of looking forward to having her baby, Maria, a 35-year-old mother of two, was hit with a bad case of stage fright when the moment of truth finally arrived. "I said to the nurse when we left the hospital, 'How can you send this tiny baby home with us? We don't know how to be parents.'"

The feelings of insecurity that Maria experienced are very common among first-time mothers. Janet, a 32-year-old first-time mother, remembers feeling more than a little shell-shocked after her daughter arrived: "I felt completely ready for the baby before the birth," she confides. "Once she was born, however, I felt less ready. I guess reality set in and I realized I had to spend 24 hours a day with a real, live baby."

MOM'S THE WORD

"Giving birth gave my life a whole new meaning. Raising children is the most difficult thing a person can ever do. I've never been happier in my entire life since I became a 'Mommy.' I've also never been so busy, tired, drained, and fulfilled."

— *Susan, 34, mother of five*

Jennifer remembers feeling awestruck that she was actually capable of giving birth to such a perfect human being: "I think through it all we both had doubts as to whether we were capable of such a miraculous act," the 32-year-old mother of one recalls. "Even now, we're still in awe of the whole process of conception, gestation, and birth, and find it hard to believe that our bodies are actually made to do that."

Her confidence in her mothering abilities was badly shaken, however, in the weeks that followed, thanks to a difficult breastfeeding experience. She persevered and managed to partially breastfeed her son until he was 6 months old, but she still remembers the anger and frustration she experienced during those early weeks of motherhood: "There can be no greater pain than knowing that your child is hungry and feeling powerless to feed him. It still angers me that I had to defend my actions to those who argued that breast is best. I agree wholeheartedly. But breastmilk is only best if it's actually in the baby. No one told me that a baby might not breastfeed. None of the stack of books and pamphlets I was given in prenatal class even mentioned the possibility that a baby might refuse the breast. As a result, I was unprepared emotionally and physically (not a bottle in the house) for being unable to feed my child in this 'oh-so-natural' way."

Joyce, a 41-year-old mother of two, found that becoming a mother changed her priorities and her view of the world. "Having the girls has made me look at life in such a different way — much less selfishly. I'm no longer the most important person in my world. They are! It's also made me much more conscious of my own mortality, partly because their growing up makes you more aware of the passing of time, but also because life is so much more precious to me. I worry about dying young because I want to be their mother for a long time — to be here for them as they grow up."

Chris, a 36-year-old mother of three, believes that becoming a mother has opened her up to a whole new world of love, but a whole world of heartache as well. "A good friend once warned me that once you become a mother, you become a mother to the whole world. That is so true. Any kind of news that has to do with children suddenly becomes personalized and the child in question is compared to your own child. The pain this can bring is excruciating when the news is bad. Famine. Murder. The loss of a child through illness."

Lori, a 29-year-old mother of four, feels that becoming a mother is the best thing that ever happened to her: "It's amazing. In some ways, it's changed my life in negative ways — there's not a lot of quiet time for me, I'm not able to be as spontaneous as I once was, there's more cleaning and cooking to do. But that doesn't even compare to the positive ways my life has changed. I feel a bond — a love that nothing can compare to. I have a pride that comes from knowing I created this wonderful life and that I'm responsible for it. I'm learning as much as I'm teaching. Not a day goes by that I don't laugh at something they say or do. I look forward to the future so that I can see their science experiments, their graduations, their weddings, their children. But I'm also desperately holding onto the past so that I don't forget that innocent look of theirs when they look right into your eyes and deep into your heart; that hearty laugh they give when they're playing hide-and-seek and have just been found; the look of amazement when they see something new or the look of pure happiness and delight when they open a birthday present or blow out their candles. I can't even begin to explain how having a baby has changed my life. It's the most rewarding experience I'll ever have."

More than the baby blues?

As wonderful as motherhood can be, it's not unusual to be hit with the "baby blues" — that hormone-driven wave of emotion that tends to come crashing over you one to three days after the birth. In fact, studies have shown that 50 to 80% of women are hit with a brief episode of mild depression at some point during the first week as their hormones return to their pre-pregnancy levels. If you find, however, that you continue to feel exhausted, anxious, and depressed for weeks after the birth, you could be suffering from postpartum depression.

Postpartum depression occurs in as many as one in five women who have recently given birth. It generally appears during the first six to eight weeks after the delivery, but can show up at any time during the year after birth. It can last anywhere from several weeks to several months, with 4% of cases lasting for a full year. In one to two out of every 1,000 births, a woman will develop a more serious form of postpartum depression known as postpartum psychosis. It's characterized by delusions, hallucinations, and anxiety, and can cause the affected woman to become a threat to both herself and her baby.

Postpartum depression is particularly common in first-time mothers and women who have suffered from it in the past. You face a higher-than-average risk of experiencing postpartum depression if

- you have a family history of postpartum depression

- you've experienced major depressive episodes in the past

- you have a history of hormonal problems (e.g., PMS)

- you experienced fertility problems prior to conceiving and/or repeated pregnancy losses, something that can cause your expectations of parenthood to be sky-high, leading to almost inevitable disappointment

- you just delivered your first baby prematurely or by cesarean section

- you just delivered multiples

- you had either a very short or very long gap between pregnancies

- you left the hospital within 24 hours of the birth

- you're experiencing a lot of financial stress

- you and your partner are having relationship problems

- you're not used to spending a lot of time at home (e.g., you've just quit your full-time job and are at home for the very first time)

- you're alone a lot or otherwise lack family support

- you experienced the death of a parent during childhood or adolescence

You may be suffering from postpartum depression if you experience one or more of the following symptoms on an ongoing basis:

- difficulty making decisions

- feelings of inadequacy (e.g., feeling incapable of caring for your baby)

- a fear of being left alone

- a fear of an impending disaster

- feeling like you don't want the baby

- a powerful desire to run away

- panic attacks and/or extreme anxiety

- feeling like your life is out of control

- a lack of interest in activities you've always enjoyed

- insomnia

- eating disturbances

- nightmares

- feeling helpless or suicidal

If you suspect you're experiencing postpartum depression, it's important to seek help from your caregiver. He or she may suggest that you go on an antidepressant drug such as sertraline (Zoloft) or fluoxetine (Prozac). (Note: According to an article in the *American Journal of Psychiatry*, it may also be safe for nursing mothers to use paroxetine [Paxil], so if you've had good results with this drug in the past, you might want to talk to your doctor about the benefits of taking Paxil again.)

You may also want to consider going for counseling or joining a postpartum depression support group so that you can share your experiences with other moms who are struggling with the same problem. It's also important to get plenty of rest and to eat properly (since inadequate sleep or nutrition will only make you feel worse), and to avoid caffeine, alcohol, and cigarettes.

Fortunately, the prognosis for women who develop postpartum depression is good: Approximately 95% of women will experience an improvement within three months of starting treatment and 65% will recover within a year. The key is to identify the problem early on: Studies have indicated that health-care professionals frequently fail to pick up the signs of postpartum depression in new mothers and, consequently, many women struggle unnecessarily with this highly debilitating disorder.

FROM HERE TO MATERNITY

You can find detailed information about the latest research on postpartum depression at the Postpartum Support International Directory Web site: www.chss.iup.edu/postpartum/.

How Your Relationship with Your Partner May Change

Feel as though there's something coming between you and your partner? You're right! It's a tiny, 8-pound human who needs to be fed and changed every two to three hours!

There's no denying it. The postpartum period can be a time of incredible adjustment for couples. Not only are both partners trying to wrap their heads around the whole idea of becoming a parent, they're also trying to work out new ways of relating to one another. And given that they're trying to accomplish these tasks in a sleep-deprived zombie-like state, it's no wonder that so many couples end up experiencing a bit of a marital meltdown during the weeks after the birth.

Here are tips on weathering the postpartum period as a couple:

FACTS AND FIGURES

A recent study at the University of Washington revealed that couples who are good friends before they start their families are better able to adjust to the stresses of early parenthood than couples who are less satisfied with their relationships.

MOM'S THE WORD

"When you see a man you love with tears in his eyes as he thanks you for giving birth to his baby, when you see him up at night comforting a crying infant, or cleaning up vomit without even mentioning it, or sitting with your child reading his favorite book again, your feelings for him change in so many ways and it's wonderful."

— *Lori, 29, mother of four*

- Accept the fact that there may be some difficult times ahead. The postpartum period is a time of tremendous adjustment for both of you. It's easy for tempers to flare and for feelings to get hurt when you're both feeling exhausted and overwhelmed by the responsibilities of parenthood. "Be nice to your husband," advises Janet, a 32-year-old mother of one. "Remember that he's also overwhelmed by the baby's arrival and is suffering from sleep deprivation, even if you're the only one who's suffering from the physical after-effects of the birth."

- Recognize that your partner may also end up being hit with the baby blues. Studies have shown that up to 3% of fathers exhibit signs of depression after their babies are born and that men whose partners experience postpartum depression are at particular risk of experiencing some sort of depression themselves.

- Make a conscious effort to invest in your relationship. It's easy to start feeling resentful and out of touch if you haven't had so much as a stolen kiss in weeks. "Take time for your marriage," recommends Nicole, a 29-year-old mother of one. "It's hard to do when the little one is consuming all your time, but it's important to still find ways to connect as a couple. We were told in prenatal class to set a date for two months after the baby's birth and go out for coffee, a drive, or even for dinner — to do something. As a new mom, this really gives you a feeling of freedom, even if all you do is talk about the baby!"

- Realize that it may take time to get your sexual relationship back on track. You may be too exhausted or too sore to think of anything but sleep during the early weeks and months after the birth. And if you're not exactly feeling terrific about your postpartum body, you may find that your libido nosedives for a while — one of the side effects of the hormone prolactin, which is produced while you're breastfeeding. You may also be reluctant to have sex for fear that you might become pregnant again. "We had sex for the first time about three weeks after giving birth," recalls one new mother. "It was kind of awkward as I was a little leery about doing the very thing that had caused me to go through such pain. And as for my sexual desire, it was like a switch had been turned off completely." Not everyone feels this way about sex, however. One first-time mom found that she felt so good about her body after giving birth that she couldn't wait to become intimate with her partner. "My hormones must have been raging after my son was born because I was interested in sex almost immediately after the delivery," she recalls. "I think I was high on the thrill of giving birth to this amazing baby. I felt almost omnipotent and was so pleased that my body was doing everything it was designed to do — get pregnant, grow a healthy baby, give birth, and breastfeed this perfect baby. I felt an overwhelming desire to make love with my husband."

- Allow your shared love for your baby to bring you closer together. "Having a baby made my relationship with my partner even stronger," says Carrie, 34, who is currently pregnant with her second child. "Watching him take care of our son and seeing what a great dad he is made me love him even more, if that's possible." Christina agrees that having a baby can enrich your relationship tremendously: "Birth is one of the most life-altering experiences you'll ever have and share as a couple," the 25-year-old mother of two explains. "Enjoy every moment and let it bring you closer together as a couple and as a family."

The Postpartum Survival Guide

Feeling exhausted by the demands of caring for your new baby? Having difficulty remembering why you wanted to become a parent in the first place? Here are some tips on surviving this wonderful yet challenging time in your life:

MOM'S THE WORD

"Everyone tells you their labor stories and neglects to mention that the truly trying times are ahead! Until I spoke to other women about it, I thought I was a failure because I found the first two months of my baby's life to be exhausting, frustrating, and emotionally draining."

— *Carole, 33, mother of two*

- Expect to feel like a rank amateur at first. It takes time to learn how to decode your baby's signals and to figure out what she does and doesn't like. And don't assume you'll get off easy if this is your second or subsequent baby. Since no two babies are exactly alike, you'll still face a bit of a learning curve as you attempt to decipher the whims of the latest arrival.

- Accept the realities of parenting a newborn. You may not be thrilled that you haven't had an uninterrupted meal or a decent night's sleep since your baby was born, but you'll do yourself and your baby a favor if you simply accept the fact that your life is going to be topsy-turvy for the foreseeable future.

- Be prepared to roll with the punches. Newborns are notoriously unpredictable. Just when you think you've figured out your baby's eating and sleeping patterns, she'll change her schedule dramatically. Rather than trying to force your new baby into adopting patterns she's not yet ready for — which will only serve to frustrate the two of you — focus your energies on trying to enjoy this special time in your lives.

- Don't worry about spoiling your baby. Ignore any well-meaning or not-so-well-meaning relatives who warn you about the evils of indulging your infant. It isn't possible to spoil a newborn. Responding quickly to his cries teaches him to trust the world around him — something that will ultimately lead to a much happier baby! (A study conducted at Johns Hopkins University during the early 1970s revealed that babies whose cries were responded to quickly cried less at 1 year of age than those babies whose cries were not responded to quite so quickly.)

- Master the art of cutting corners. This is no time to play Martha Stewart. Let the dishes accumulate in the sink until you can't stand looking at them any more. Give your vacuum cleaner an extended sabbatical. Your top priorities at this point should be taking care of your baby and yourself.

- Accept any and all offers of help. If friends and family members express a willingness to pitch in, take them up on the offer. Keep a running list of jobs that need to be done (e.g., cooking, cleaning, or picking up stamps for the baby announcements) so that you'll have a list of jobs to delegate when people ask what they can do to help. "A girlfriend of mine picked up groceries for us," recalls Tina, a 32-year-old mother of one. "Some other friends brought over supper. These things mean so much during the first few weeks."

• Get out of the house. Nothing can add to your stress level more than being housebound day after day with a newborn — especially if she is trying out for the position of Town Crier. Whether you decide to take the baby for a walk or to hit the local parent resource center, it's important to do whatever you can to avoid getting cabin fever. "Go for walks with the baby as soon as you can," suggests Janet, 32, who recently gave birth to her first baby. "You'll feel much better physically and the baby's cries will seem that much quieter in the great outdoors!"

• Connect with other parents. Keep in touch with the other new parents you met at prenatal class and compare notes on your babies' sleeping, eating, and crying patterns. You might also consider joining an online bulletin board or mailing list for women who gave birth the same month as you did. (See Appendix E for leads on some terrific online resources for parents.)

📢 **MOM'S THE WORD**

"I feel a bond with any woman who has ever given birth. When I see a woman with a baby, I feel as if I should become her friend: After all, we went through the same things and have so much in common."

— *Lori, 29, mother of four*

- Resist the temptation to compare your baby to other babies. No two babies are alike, so there's no need to hit the panic button just because your baby's spitting up a bit more than the babies of the other couples in your prenatal class.

- Accept the fact that there can be a few potholes on the road to breastfeeding success. Don't feel inadequate if breastfeeding doesn't come easily to you at first; it doesn't for everyone. "Breastfeeding is more difficult than giving birth," says Carrie, 34, who is currently pregnant with her second child. "My body did what it was made to do during the birth. Breastfeeding required some thought and learning on my part." If you run into breastfeeding difficulties, get support from an experienced nursing mother or a lactation consultant. The benefits of breastfeeding are tremendous, so it's worth persevering. If, however, breastfeeding is making your life absolutely miserable, don't be afraid to move to Plan B. Here's some sensible advice from Carolin, a 31-year-old mother of three: "If you have problems nursing, don't feel like a failure. After I felt so miserable when breastfeeding didn't work out with my first baby, my doctor gave me these words of wisdom. She said, 'A good bottlefeeding experience far outweighs a bad breastfeeding experience.' Yes, breast is best, as I have so constantly been reminded by some of the militant breastfeeding league, but bottlefeeding can be great too."

MOM'S THE WORD

"Sometimes breastfeeding can be a drag. It prevents you from getting very much else done and it deprives you of sleep — particularly when baby has a growth spurt and feeds every two hours for several days. However, most of the time it's a thoroughly enjoyable experience. Your baby will never be as happy as when she's on your breast. Sometimes she looks into your eyes with so much love. The feeling is just incredible."

—*Janet, 32, mother of one*

MOM'S THE WORD

"Nothing prepared me for the baby who wouldn't wake up to nurse and who would scream in protest at the late afternoon feeding, for breasts that didn't ever seem to live up to my expectations, or for the emotional turmoil I went through — feeling as though I was failing my baby because I couldn't seem to feed her adequately.

"It took a while for my husband to realize how emotionally involved I was in the process. To him, at first, it was just a matter of breastmilk versus formula. As time progressed, he began to understand that it was so much more than that, and he was very supportive of my decision to persevere, even though he occasionally wondered if it was worth the emotional toll it took on me."

— *Joyce, 41, mother of two breastfed babies*

- Recognize that it may take your older child time to warm up to the new baby. Even if you do all the right things, you can expect to experience the odd rough spot as your child learns how to share you and your partner with the newborn. Jane recalls how frustrated she felt when her older child refused to accept the new baby: "We talked about the baby, we read books, we made a special 'I'm a big brother' T-shirt, and we brought suckers for him to distribute at daycare. We even brought a present from the baby home from the hospital for him. It didn't really help, though. He was nearly 3 at the time and had had lots of attention before Emma's arrival. It was an event that really, truly rocked his world. He was very jealous of her and tried to hit, poke, bite, and so on. The only thing that seemed to help was when I finally clued in that he needed some time alone with me."

- Expect your worry-o-meter to go into overdrive. Now that you're responsible for ensuring the health and well-being of another human being, you'll suddenly find a million and one things to worry about. "I worried about finding a good day-care for her when I returned to work, especially after reading a lot of horror stories in the news," recalls Bevin, a 27-year-old mother of one. "I worried about getting into an accident, dropping the baby, all kinds of silly things."

- Don't expect to feel Madonna-like 24 hours a day. If you're expecting to feel totally euphoric all the time, you could be in for a major disappointment. Hey, even the women I'd personally consider nominating for the Motherhood Hall of Fame have days when they feel like running away from home! "I had many guilt feelings about not bonding instantly with my first baby," recalls Jane, a 33-year-old mother of two. "I expected overwhelming feelings of love, and I didn't have them. I didn't dislike him, but I just didn't feel the gushiness I expected. When I was finally brave enough to talk about these feelings with other moms, I was so relieved to find out how common this is. I wish I'd read about that beforehand! It could have saved me so much grief. Eventually, probably several months down the road, I did feel overwhelming love for him."

- Savor every moment of this very special time in your life. "This is a strange and magical time, but it's so very fleeting," says Maria, a 35-year-old mother of two. "Take a million photos and write everything down — every feeling, every thought. Time really does pass so quickly, and you can't remember everything."

I can't believe we've already come to the end of this book. I still feel as though I have so much left to say. But given that the book is already 50,000 words over length, my publisher would like me to turn off my computer! I hope you'll e-mail me with your comments about the book (pageone@kawartha.com) and that you'll drop by the official Web site for this book (www.having-a-baby.com) for updates and news on other related titles, including *The Mother of All Baby Books,* which is coming soon. In the meantime, I wish you and your baby all the best in your journey to birth and beyond.

Glossary

Active labor   The period of labor during which the cervix dilates from four to ten centimeters.

Adrenal gland   A small gland situated above each kidney that secretes sex hormones and other hormones, including cortisone and adrenaline.

Afterbirth   Another name for the placenta — your baby's physiological support system in utero.

Alphafetoprotein (AFP) testing   A prenatal blood test performed between 15 and 18 weeks of pregnancy to screen for both neural tube defects (high levels of AFP) and Down syndrome (low levels of AFP). If it's combined with measurements of both human chorionic gonadotropin (hCG) and unconjugated estriol, the test is referred to as maternal serum screening. These tests are screening tests rather than diagnostic tests. In other words, they can't definitely state whether or not your baby is affected by a particular problem; they can only state the likelihood that your baby is affected.

Amniocentesis   A procedure that involves inserting a needle through the abdominal wall and removing a small quantity of amniotic fluid from the sac surrounding the developing baby. The amniotic fluid is then used to test for fetal abnormalities, to determine the baby's sex, or to assess lung maturity and overall fetal well-being. Alphafetoprotein levels can also be measured using a sample of amniotic fluid.

Amniotic fluid   The protective liquid, consisting mostly of water, that surrounds the baby inside the amniotic sac.

Amniotic sac (or amnion)   The thin-walled sac within the uterus that houses the baby and the amniotic fluid.

Androgens   The name given to a general class of male sex hormones, one of which is testosterone.

Andrology   The study of the male reproductive system.

Anencephaly   A birth defect involving a malformed brain and skull. Anencephaly leads to stillbirth or death soon after birth.

Anomaly   A malformation or abnormality in any part of the body. Some anomalies are relatively minor; others can be serious, even fatal.

Anovulation   The total absence of ovulation. It's still possible to menstruate during an anovulatory cycle.

Anovulatory bleeding   The type of menstruation most often associated with anovulatory cycles. It tends to be either scanty and of short duration or abnormally heavy. The pattern of bleeding tends to be irregular.

Apgar score   An assessment of a newborn's early response to the stress of birth and life outside the womb. The test is performed one minute and five minutes after birth. A poor test result on the one-minute test can be affected by the stress of the delivery process. The result on the five-minute test is more meaningful in terms of the infant's long-term outcome. An infant with a poor Apgar score is re-tested every five minutes until a score of at least six is obtained.

Areola   The flat, pigmented area encircling the nipple of the breast.

Artificial insemination (AI)   Any method of insemination other than sexual intercourse.

Assisted insemination   The process of inserting sperm from a woman's partner into her vagina or uterus by means other than sexual intercourse.

Assisted reproduction   The use of any new reproductive technology (NRT) for the purpose of overcoming infertility to produce a child (e.g., in vitro fertilization, assisted insemination, donor insemination).

Baby blues   The term used to describe the mild depression that can occur after having a baby. Sometimes called the postpartum blues, this type of depression tends to last only a few days and typically occurs within one to two weeks of the delivery. If the feelings of depression last longer than this or are particularly severe, you may be suffering from postpartum depression.

Basal body temperature (BBT)   The female partner's temperature taken upon rising first thing in the morning. In 95% of cases, BBT readings can be used to determine if ovulation has occurred.

Binovular twins   See Fraternal twins.

Biophysical profile   A test designed to assess the well-being of the developing baby. It involves an ultrasound plus a fetal-monitoring test known as a non-stress test.

Biopsy   Surgical removal of a sample of tissue for analysis.

Blastocyst   The name given to the cluster of cells that will eventually form the fetus.

Blood pressure   There are two readings: the systolic pressure (the upper figure) and the diastolic pressure (the lower figure). You're generally considered to have high blood pressure if the reading exceeds 140/90. (Generally, elevations in diastolic pressure are considered to be most dangerous.)

Bloody show   The mucus discharge — often tinged with blood — that may indicate the cervix is effacing and/or dilating.

Braxton Hicks contractions   Irregular contractions of the uterus that occur during pregnancy and that are felt most strongly during the late third trimester. Braxton Hicks contractions neither efface nor dilate the cervix.

Breech presentation   When the fetus is positioned buttocks or feet down rather than head down.

Bromocriptine (Parlodel)   A drug that inhibits the secretion of the hormone prolactin.

CBC   Complete blood count: hemoglobin, red and white cells (red blood cells and white blood cells, respectively), and blood platelets.

Cephalopelvic disproportion   When the presenting part of the baby's head is too large for the mother's pelvis and birth canal.

Cervical dilation   A measure of how wide the cervix has opened up prior to or during labor. Cervical dilation is measured in centimeters (from 0 to 10). When you're 10 centimeters dilated, you're fully dilated and ready to push.

Cervical effacement   The thinning out of the cervix before and during labor. When the cervix is fully effaced, it is paper thin.

Cervical incompetence   A congenital defect or injury to the cervix that causes it to open prematurely during pregnancy, resulting in miscarriage or a premature birth without labor.

Cervical mucus   Mucus produced by the cervix. Cervical mucus aids in the movement of sperm from the cervix to the uterus and fallopian tubes. The mucus increases in volume and acquires an egg white–like consistency during the days leading up to ovulation.

Cervix   The entrance to the uterus.

Cesarean section   A surgical procedure used to deliver a baby via an incision made in the mother's abdomen and uterus.

Chadwick's sign   A dark-blue or purple discoloration of the vagina and cervix during pregnancy. In the days before pregnancy tests, it provided your doctor with an important clue that you could be pregnant.

Chlamydia   A common sexually transmitted disease that can render a woman infertile if left untreated. Antibiotics can be used to treat the disease.

Chloasma   Extensive brown patches of irregular shape and size on the face or other parts of the body that can occur during pregnancy. Sometimes referred to as the "mask of pregnancy."

Chorioamnionitis   An inflammation of the membranes surrounding the fetus.

Chorion   The outer sac enclosing the fetus within the uterus.

Chorionic villus sampling (CVS)   A prenatal diagnostic test in which a few placental cells are extracted via a fine hollow needle or catheter inserted into the womb via the abdomen or the cervix. Like amniocentesis, CVS can be used to detect a variety of genetic disorders and to determine the sex of the fetus. CVS can be done as early as the eighth or ninth week of pregnancy, and the results are usually known within a week.

Chromosomal abnormalities   Problems which result from errors in the duplication of the chromosomes — the thread-like structures in the nucleus of a cell that transmit genetic information.

Circumcision   Surgical removal of the foreskin of the penis.

Clomiphene citrate (Clomid or Serophene) A synthetic drug used to stimulate the hypothalamus and pituitary gland to increase FSH and LH production.

Colostrum The first substance secreted from the breasts following childbirth. Colostrum is high in protein and antibodies.

Conception When the sperm penetrates the egg.

Congenital defect A defect that is present at birth. A congenital defect is acquired during pregnancy but is not necessarily hereditary.

Conjoined twins Identical twins who have not separated completely. More commonly known as Siamese twins.

Contraction A painful, strong, rhythmic squeezing of the uterus.

Contraction stress test A test that assesses the baby's well-being by monitoring its response to uterine contractions. If you're not already in labor when the test is performed, you will be given enough synthetic oxytocin to cause three contractions in a ten-minute period. A "positive" result on the test means that your baby's heartbeat dropped near the end of or after a contraction.

Cord prolapse A rare obstetrical emergency that occurs when the umbilical cord drops out of the uterus into the vagina before the baby, leading to cord compression and oxygen deprivation.

Corpus luteum The cyst that forms in the ovary at the site of the released egg and that's responsible for the production of the hormone progesterone during the second half of the normal menstrual cycle.

Cryopreservation A freezing procedure used for the storage of embryos or gametes.

Cytomegalovirus (CMV) A group of viruses from the herpes virus family that can affect and harm the unborn baby.

Diastasis recti Separation of abdominal muscles.

Diethylstilbestrol (DES) A synthetic form of estrogen that was given to women between the 1940s and 1970s to inhibit miscarriage. DES was later discovered to have serious effects on women and children, including cancer, infertility, and miscarriage. Both male and female offspring can be affected.

Dilatation and Curettage (D & C)   A surgical procedure in which the cervix is dilated and the lining of the uterus is scraped using an instrument called a curette.

Dizygotic twins   See Fraternal twins.

Donor insemination   The process of inserting donor sperm into a woman's vagina or uterus by means other than sexual intercourse.

Doppler (doptone)   A hand-held device that uses ultrasound technology to enable the caregiver to monitor the fetal heart rate.

Doula   Someone who assists a woman and her family during labor and the postpartum period.

Due date   The date on which a baby's birth is expected, calculated by adding 279 days to the first day of the woman's last menstrual period (LMP) or 265 days to the date of ovulation, if known. Medically known as the estimated date of confinement (EDC). A simpler way to estimate your due date is to subtract three months and add five days to the date of the first day of your last menstrual period (a calculation known as Nagle's rule).

Dysmenorrhoea   Painful menstruation.

Early neonatal death   A liveborn infant who dies before the seventh day following birth is classified as having experienced an "early neonatal death."

Eclampsia   A serious but rare condition that can affect pregnant or laboring women. It is a severe form of pre-eclampsia. Symptoms of eclampsia include hypertension, edema, and protein in the urine. An emergency delivery may be necessary if the eclampsia is severe enough.

Ectopic pregnancy   A pregnancy that occurs outside the uterus, most often in the fallopian tube.

EDC/EDD   Estimated date of confinement or estimated date of delivery. Medical jargon for your due date.

Edema   The accumulation of fluid in the body's tissues, resulting in swelling.

Egg donation   The donation of one woman's egg(s) to another woman.

Ejaculate   Sperm plus fluid from the seminal vesicles and prostate gland that is ejaculated through the penis.

Electronic fetal monitoring (EFM) An electronic instrument used to record the heartbeat of the fetus as well as the mother's uterine contractions. Fetal monitors can be either external (placed on the abdomen) or internal (attached to the baby's scalp via the vagina).

Embryo The term used to describe the early stages of fetal growth, from conception through the third month of pregnancy.

Embryo transfer A procedure that involves introducing an embryo into a woman's uterus. Part of IVF treatment.

Endometrial biopsy The extraction of a small sample of endometrial tissue (tissue from the uterine lining) for examination.

Endometriosis Presence of endometrial tissue (the uterine lining) in abnormal locations such as the ovaries and the fallopian tubes. May cause painful menstruation and infertility.

Endometrium The mucus membrane lining the uterus.

Engagement When the baby's presenting part (usually the head) settles into the pelvic cavity.

Engorgement Congested or filled with fluid. This term refers to the fullness or swelling of the breasts, which can occur between the second and seventh postpartum day when a woman's breasts first start to produce milk.

Epididymis The organ that stores and nourishes sperm as they develop and make their way from the testes to the vas deferens. Sperm acquire motility (the ability to move) within the epididymis.

Epidural A local anesthetic that is injected into the epidural space at the level of the spinal cord that you wish to numb. The most popular form of pharmacological pain relief during labor and often used for cesarean sections as well.

Episiotomy A small incision made into the skin and the perineal muscle at the time of delivery to enlarge the vaginal opening and make it easier for the baby's head or body to emerge or to insert birthing instruments such as forceps.

Estimated date of confinement (EDC) The medical term for due date.

Estradiol   A type of estrogen that is released by developing follicles in the ovary. Plasma estradiol levels can be measured to assess the growth of the follicle during ovulation induction.

Estrogen   A group of hormones that are produced in the ovaries and that work with progesterone to regulate the reproductive cycle. Estrogen is produced in all phases of the cycle, whether or not you ovulate.

External version   A procedure in which the doctor turns the baby or babies in the uterus by applying manual pressure to the outside of the mother's abdomen.

Face presentation   A labor presentation that occurs when the baby's head is down but its neck is extended as if it were looking down through the birth canal.

Fallopian tubes   The long, narrow tubes that carry eggs from the ovaries to the uterus.

False labor   When you experience regular and/or painful contractions that neither dilate nor thin the cervix.

Fertilization   See Conception.

Fetal hypoxia   When the fetus is deprived of oxygen.

Fetal monitor   See Electronic fetal monitor.

Fetus   The medical term used to describe the developing baby from the end of the third month of pregnancy until birth.

FH or FHR   Fetal heart or fetal heart rate.

Fibroid tumor   A benign tumor of fibrous tissue that may occur in the uterine wall. It may be totally without symptoms or it may cause abnormal menstrual patterns, abdominal pressure and swelling (if the tumors are very large), infertility problems, and recurrent miscarriage.

Fimbria   The finger-like outer ends of the fallopian tubes that seek to capture the egg when it's released from the ovary.

Floating   The baby's head is not yet engaged.

Follicle   The structure in the ovary that has nurtured the ripening egg and from which the egg is released.

Follicle-stimulating hormone (FSH)   A hormone produced in the anterior pituitary gland that stimulates the ovary to ripen a follicle for ovulation.

Forceps A tong-like instrument that may be placed around the baby's head to help guide it out of the birth canal during a vaginal delivery.

Fraternal twins Twins who are the result of the union of two eggs and two sperm.

FSH (Follicle-stimulating hormone) A hormone produced in the anterior pituitary gland that stimulates the ovary to ripen a follicle for ovulation.

Fundal height The distance from the upper, rounded part of a pregnant woman's uterus to her pubic bone. On average, the measurement is equal to the number of weeks of pregnancy, but it may vary by as many as three to four centimeters or more, depending on the mother's height, weight, and body shape; the position of the baby; and, of course, the size of the baby and the amount of amniotic fluid. Note: Measuring fundal height is a rather inexact science. Different caregivers can get different measurements on the same day. The measurement is most reliable when it is consistently taken by the same caregiver. Also called symphysis fundal height.

Gamete The mature male or female reproductive cell (sperm are the male gametes; eggs are the female gametes).

Genetic screening Screening tests designed to indicate which couples may be at increased risk of passing along an inherited trait or disease to their baby.

Genetic surrogacy A woman is artificially inseminated, carries the pregnancy to term, and then relinquishes custody of the baby to the father (and his partner, if he's married).

Gestational diabetes Diabetes that is triggered by pregnancy. It typically occurs after the 24th week of pregnancy.

Gestational surrogacy A woman undergoes IVF to receive and carry to term an embryo made up of another woman's egg. She is not the genetic mother of the child. The couple whose egg and sperm produced the embryo then adopt the baby.

Gland A hormone-producing organ.

Glucose tolerance test A blood test used to detect gestational diabetes. Blood is drawn at specified intervals after you drink a sugary beverage. Unfortunately, the test isn't considered to be terribly useful: You can get different results by taking the test on different days.

Gonadotropin   A hormone capable of stimulating the testicles or the ovaries to produce sperm or an egg, respectively.

Gonadotropin releasing hormone (GnRH)   A hormone released from the hypothalamus that controls the synthesis and release of pituitary hormones FSH and LH.

Gonadotropin releasing hormone agonist (GnRHa)   A medication given via injection or nasal spray to suppress the release of hormones that stimulate the development of eggs.

Gonadotropins   Hormone medications given by injection to stimulate the development of eggs.

Gonorrhea   A bacterial infection spread through sexual contact that can lead to infection of the reproductive tract, infertility, serious illness in the mother, and injury to the developing baby.

Group B strep   A bacteria found in the vagina and rectum of approximately 15% of pregnant women. Women who test positive for group B strep may require antibiotics during labor to protect their babies from picking up this potentially life-threatening infection.

hCG   See Human chorionic gonadotropin.

HELLP syndrome   A severe form of pre-eclampsia which can be associated with liver dysfunction and clotting abnormalities. The syndrome can be life-threatening to both mother and baby and won't disappear until after the delivery.

Hemorrhoids   Swollen blood vessels around the anus or in the rectal canal which may bleed and cause pain, especially after childbirth.

Hirsutism   The presence of excessive body and facial in women. Hirsutism is frequently seen in patients with polycystic ovarian syndrome (PCOS), but it can also be related to hypersensitivity to normal levels of male hormones in the female body or heredity.

HIV test   A blood test to detect the presence of antibodies to the AIDS virus.

Human chorionic gonadatropin (hCG)   The hormone manufactured by the placenta in early pregnancy that causes your pregnancy test to be positive.

Hydramnios   See Polyhydramnios.

Hyperemesis gravidarum   Very severe nausea, dehydration, and vomiting during pregnancy.

Hyperstimulation   A problem that can arise during fertility treatments designed to stimulate ovulation. Symptoms include ovarian enlargement, gastrointestinal problems, abdominal distension, and weight gain. Severe cases may be further complicated by cardiovascular, pulmonary, and electrolyte disturbances, and may require hospitalization. In rare cases, heart failure or blood clot formation caused by hyperstimulation can lead to death.

Hypothalamus   The portion of the base of the brain that controls the release of hormones from the pituitary.

Hysterosalpingogram (HSG)   An X-ray that involves injecting dye into the uterus to examine the shape of the uterus and to check the fallopian tubes for any possible blockages or abnormalities.

Identical twins   When twins are the result of the fertilization and subsequent splitting of a single egg and single sperm.

Idiopathic infertility   The term used to describe unexplained infertility.

Implantation   The embedding of an embryo into the endometrium (the lining of the uterus).

Incomplete abortion   A miscarriage in which part, but not all, of the contents of the uterus are expelled.

Infertility   The inability to conceive a child.

Internal version   The act of adjusting a baby's position in the uterus by placing one hand in the mother's vagina and the other on her abdomen.

Intracytoplasmic sperm injection (ICSI)   The injection of a single sperm nucleus into the center of an egg using a microscopic needle. ICSI improves the odds that an inferior or immature sperm will be able to fertilize an egg. The technique is controversial because it's not known whether there are any long-term effects on children produced in this manner.

Intrauterine contraceptive device (IUCD or IUD)   A plastic or metal birth control device inserted into the uterus to prevent fertilization or implantation.

Intrauterine death   The death of a fetus within the uterus.

Intrauterine growth restriction (IUGR)   When the baby's growth is less than what would normally be expected for a baby of that gestational age. It can be symmetric (e.g., both the head and the body are small) or asymmetric (e.g., just the body is small).

Intrauterine insemination (IUI)   The placement of washed sperm (from partner or donor) into the uterus via a fine tube.

In vitro fertilization (IVF)   A procedure wherein a number of eggs are removed from the ovary and fertilized by sperm outside of the body. The resulting embryos are given the opportunity to divide in a protected environment for three to five days before being transferred to the uterus. Note: The embryo may also be transferred to another woman.

Kegels   Exercises that work the muscles of the pelvic floor, including those of the urethra, vagina, and rectum.

Labor   The process of childbirth, including the dilation of the cervix and the delivery of the baby and the placenta.

Laparoscopy   A surgical procedure which permits direct visual examination of the ovaries, the exterior of the fallopian tubes, and the uterus by inserting a small fiber-optic instrument through an incision made below the navel while the patient is under general anesthesia.

Late neonatal death   A liveborn infant who dies on or after the seventh day following birth, but before the 28th day.

LhRH   Luteinizing hormone. See Gonadotropin releasing hormone.

Lightening   A change in the shape of the pregnant woman's uterus a few weeks before labor. It generally occurs when the presenting part of the baby engages in the mother's pelvis.

Linea nigra   A dark line running from navel to the pubic area that may develop during pregnancy.

LMP   The first day of your last menstrual period.

LOA   Left occipito-anterior. A term that refers to the position of the crown of the baby's head (i.e., occiput) in relation to your body. In this case, your baby is "left" and "anterior" (toward your front). See also LOP, ROA, ROP.

Lochia The discharge of blood, mucus, and tissue from the uterus following childbirth. Lochia can last anywhere from a few weeks to six weeks or longer. It tends to be heaviest right after the birth and may contain large clots — some as large as a small orange.

LOP Left occipito-posterior. A term that refers to the position of the crown of the baby's head (i.e., occiput) in relation to your body. In this case, your baby is "left" and "posterior" (toward your back). See also LOA, ROA, ROP.

Low birthweight Babies who weigh less than 2,500 grams or 5 pounds 8 ounces at birth. A baby who weighs less than 1,500 grams or 3 pounds at birth is considered to be a very low-birthweight baby.

Luteal phase The phase of the menstrual cycle that lasts from ovulation through the start of menstruation.

Luteal phase defect A shortened luteal phase or one in which there is inadequate progesterone production.

Luteinizing hormone (LH) A hormone produced by the pituitary gland. It plays an important role in ovulation and implantation.

Mask of pregnancy See Chloasma.

Mastitis A painful infection of the breast characterized by fever, soreness, and swelling.

Maternal serum screening A screening test used to determine the probability that a particular woman is carrying a fetus with certain types of abnormalities. It involves taking a blood sample.

Meconium The greenish substance that builds up in the bowels of a growing fetus and that is normally discharged shortly after birth. A baby who passes meconium before birth may be in distress, so it's important to let your caregiver know immediately if your membranes rupture and the amniotic fluid that leaks out has a greenish tinge.

Menotropins (human menopausal gonadotropin or hMG) An extract of menopausal urine that contains both FSH and LH.

Miscarriage Spontaneous loss of the fetus or embryo from the womb, usually during the first trimester of pregnancy, but at any point prior to the 20th week of pregnancy, or when the baby weighs less than 500 grams. The medical term for a miscarriage is "spontaneous abortion" — a term that many couples find offensive.

Missed abortion   A situation that arises when the embryo or fetus dies in utero but the body fails to expel the contents of the uterus. It is typically diagnosed by ultrasound.

Mittelschmerz   Pain that coincides with release of an egg from the ovary.

Molar pregnancy   A pregnancy that results in the growth of abnormal placental cells rather than a fetus. Also known as a hydatidiform mole or gestational trophoblastic disease.

Monovular twins   See Identical twins.

Monozygotic twins   See Identical twins.

Mucus plug   The plug of thick and sticky mucus that blocks the cervical canal during pregnancy, protecting the baby from infection.

Multigravida   You're pregnant for the second or subsequent time.

Multipara   You've given birth one or more times before your current pregnancy.

Neonatal death   The death of a liveborn infant between birth and four weeks of age.

Neonatal intensive care unit (NICU)   An intensive care unit that specializes in the care of premature, low-weight babies and seriously ill infants.

Neural tube defects   Abnormalities in the development of the spinal cord and brain in a fetus, including anencephaly, hydrocephalus, and spina bifida.

Newborn jaundice   The yellowish tinge of a newborn's skin caused by too much bilirubin in the blood. Jaundice typically develops on the second or third day of life and lasts until the baby is 7 to 10 days old. Newborn jaundice can usually be corrected by special light treatment.

NRT   New reproductive technology.

Non-stress test   A non-invasive test in which fetal movements are monitored and recorded using an electronic fetal monitor, along with changes in fetal heart rate.

Oligohydramnios   A shortage of amniotic fluid.

Oocyte   The reproductive world's term for the egg that's produced by the ovary.

Oocyte retrieval   A surgical procedure that involves collecting eggs from the ovarian follicles.

Ovarian failure   The inability of the ovary to respond to any gonadotropic hormone stimulation. Ovarian failure is usually the result of a congenital problem (e.g., the absence of follicular tissue) or menopause. If it occurs before age 40, it is described as premature ovarian failure.

Ovaries   The female sexual glands responsible for producing estrogen and progesterone and for housing the developing egg prior to its release at ovulation. There are two ovaries: one on either side of the pelvis.

Ovulation   The point in the menstrual cycle in which a mature egg is released from the ovaries into the fallopian tubes.

Ovulation induction   The use of hormone therapy to stimulate egg development and release.

Ovum   The egg cell produced in the ovaries each month. Another word for oocyte.

Oxytocin   The naturally occurring hormone that causes uterine contractions. A synthetic form of this hormone (Pitocin) is often used to induce or augment labor.

Pap test   The popular name for the Papanicolaou test, which involves examining cervical cells under a microscope to look for any abnormalities.

Pelvic floor muscles   The group of muscles at the base of the pelvis that help support the bladder, uterus, urethra, vagina, and rectum.

Pelvic inflammatory disease (PID)   An infection that can affect the uterus, fallopian tubes, ovaries, and other parts of the reproductive system. It can be caused by sexually transmitted diseases or other organisms and can lead to infertility.

Percutaneous umbilical cord sampling (PUBS)   A diagnostic test that involves drawing blood from the fetus's umbilical cord prior to birth to test for abnormalities and genetic conditions.

Perineum   The name given to the muscle and tissue located between the vagina and the rectum.

Phenylketonuria (PKU)   A recessive genetic disorder in which a liver enzyme is defective, making it impossible for an individual to digest an amino acid known as phenylalanine. PKU is detected through a blood test done at birth and may be controlled by a special diet. If untreated, PKU results in mental retardation.

Pituitary   A gland located at the base of the human brain that is responsible for secreting a number of important hormones related to normal growth and development of fertility.

Placenta   The organ that develops in the uterus during pregnancy, providing nutrients for the fetus and eliminating its waste products.

Placental abruption   The premature separation of the placenta from the uterus.

Placental infarction   The death of part of the placenta. It is caused by a loss of blood supply to part of the placenta, which, if extensive enough, can cause stillbirth.

Placenta previa   A condition in which the placenta partially or completely blocks the cervical opening. It necessitates delivery by cesarean section and can be associated with pregnancy loss and massive hemorrhaging. (In rare cases, a hysterectomy may be required to control the bleeding.)

Polycystic ovarian syndrome (PCO)   A condition that involves the development of multiple cysts in the ovaries. Its cause is uncertain, but it appears to be linked to insulin resistance.

Polyhydramnios   An abnormal condition of pregnancy characterized by an excess of amniotic fluid.

Post-coital test   An infertility test that involves collecting cervical secretions following intercourse and analyzing them to see if the man's sperm are able to make their way through the woman's cervical mucus. Intercourse is timed to occur at the time of the menstrual cycle when the woman's cervical mucus is likely to be most receptive to sperm — around ovulation.

Post-mature baby   A baby born after 42 completed weeks' gestation. Note: The terms "post-term" or "post-dates" are preferred.

Post-menopausal pregnancies   The use of IVF and donor eggs to produce a pregnancy in a woman who is past the age of menopause.

Postpartum blues   The term used to describe the mild depression that can occur after having a baby. Sometimes called the baby blues.

Postpartum depression (PPD)   Clinical depression that can occur following the delivery. Postpartum depression is characterized by sadness, impatience, restlessness, and — in particularly severe cases — an inability to care for the baby. Severe cases in which the mother suffers hallucinations or a desire to hurt the baby are classified as postpartum psychosis.

Postpartum hemorrhage The loss of more than 15 ounces (450 ml) of blood during a vaginal delivery or 1,000 mL during a cesarean section.

Pre-eclampsia/toxemia A serious condition marked by sudden edema, high blood pressure, and protein in the urine.

Pregnancy-induced hypertension (PIH) A pregnancy-related condition in which a woman's blood pressure is temporarily elevated. Her blood pressure returns to normal shortly after she gives birth.

Pre-implantation diagnosis The diagnosis of genetic disorders or the determination of the sex in an embryo formed through IVF before it's transferred to the uterus.

Premature baby A baby born before 37 completed weeks of pregnancy.

Premature menopause Menopause that occurs before a woman reaches age 40.

Premature rupture of the membranes (PROM) When the membranes rupture before the onset of labor.

Prenatal diagnosis (PND) Testing before birth to determine whether a fetus has a particular type of malformation or disorder and/or to determine the sex of the fetus.

Presenting part The part of the baby's body that is likely to come through the cervix first.

Primigravida You are pregnant for the first time.

Primipara You are giving birth for the first time.

Progesterone A hormone secreted by the ovary after ovulation has occurred. It helps to prepare the uterus for pregnancy and maintains the endometrium in early pregnancy until the placenta takes over progesterone production.

Prolactin The hormone responsible for milk production and for suppressing ovulation in a nursing mother. Prolactin is released following the delivery of the placenta and the membranes. Elevated levels of prolactin in a non-pregnant woman can contribute to fertility problems by interfering with ovulation.

Prostate   The gland responsible for producing much of the seminal fluid.

Psychoprophylaxis   Intellectual, physical, and emotional preparation for childbirth. The term psychoprophylaxis is associated with the Bradley Method of husband-coached labor.

Quickening   The term used to describe the moment when a pregnant woman first detects fetal movement (typically between the 20th and 24th weeks if you're having your first baby and between the 16th and 20th week of pregnancy if you're having your second or subsequent baby).

Rh antibodies   Antibodies capable of crossing the placenta and destroying the baby's red blood cells. Rh antibodies can be produced if your blood type is Rh negative and the baby's blood type is Rh positive, and some of your baby's blood leaks into your circulation during pregnancy, birth, or in the event of a miscarriage. This sensitization doesn't cause a problem in the first pregnancy, but it can cause a problem during the next pregnancy. That's why you'll require an Rhogam injection immediately following delivery, a miscarriage, an abortion, or amniocentesis. Note: Some caregivers give RhoGam injections at 28 weeks to prevent early sensitization.

ROA   Right occipito anterior. A term that refers to the position of the crown of the baby's head (i.e., occiput) in relation to your body. In this case, your baby is "right" and "anterior" (toward your front). See also LOA, LOP, ROP.

ROP   Right occipito posterior. A term that refers to the position of the crown of the baby's head (i.e., occiput) in relation to your body. In this case, your baby is "right" and "posterior" (toward your back). See also LOA, LOP, ROA.

Round-ligament pain   Pain caused by the stretching of ligament on the sides of the uterus during pregnancy. It increases in severity with each pregnancy.

Rubella (German measles)   A mild, highly contagious viral disease that can cause serious birth defects in the developing baby, particularly if contracted during the first trimester. Most people are immunized against this disease as children, but it's possible to lose your immunity to the disease, which is why your caregiver will check your immunity if you're planning a pregnancy.

Ruptured membranes   The loss of fluid from the amniotic sac. Also called breaking of waters.

Sciatica   Pain in the leg, lower back, and buttock caused by irritation of the sciatic nerve.

Scrotum   The pouch of skin and thin muscle tissue that holds the testes.

Semen analysis   The examination of fresh ejaculate under the microscope to assess the number (count), shape (morphology), and ability to move (motility) of a sample of sperm.

Seminal fluid   Fluid produced by the prostate and seminal vesicle that contains sperm.

Serum thyroid stimulating hormone (sTSH)   Diagnostic test for thyroid function.

Show   See Bloody show.

Siamese twins   See Conjoined twins.

Sickle cell anemia   An inherited blood disease.

Spermatozoa (sperm)   The fully developed male reproductive cells.

Spina bifida   A congenital birth defect that occurs when the tube housing the central nervous system fails to close completely. It can result in malformations of the spinal cord or brain.

Spinal anesthesia   A regional anesthetic that is injected into the spinal fluid. Generally used for cesarean sections.

Spontaneous abortion   See Miscarriage.

Station   An estimate of the baby's progress in descending into the pelvis. Generally, negative numbers mean that the presenting part is unengaged and positive numbers mean it is engaged.

Stillbirth   A fetal death that occurs after the 20th week of gestation.

Stress test   A test that records the fetal heart rate in response to induced mild contractions of the uterus.

Stretch marks   Reddish streaks on the skin of the breasts, abdomen, legs, and buttocks that are caused by the stretching of the skin during pregnancy. Stretch marks fade over time but don't disappear entirely.

Teratogens   Agents such as drugs, chemicals, and infectious diseases that can cause birth defects in the developing baby.

Terbutaline A medication used to stop contractions in preterm labor.

Testes The male sexual glands. Contained in the scrotum, they produce the male hormone (testosterone) and the male reproductive cells (sperm).

Testosterone A male sex hormone produced in the testicles.

Thalassemia An inherited blood disease.

Threatened abortion Bleeding during the first trimester of pregnancy which is not accompanied by either cramping or contractions.

Thyroid gland A gland located at the base of the neck that secretes thyroid. Too much or too little thyroid can contribute to fertility problems.

Toxoplasmosis A parasitic infection that can cause stillbirth or miscarriage in pregnant women and congenital defects in babies.

Transition The third or final phase of the first stage of labor when the cervix goes from 7 to 10 centimeters dilation. When transition ends, the pushing stage begins.

Transverse lie When the fetus is lying horizontally across the uterus rather than in a vertical position.

Tubal ligation A permanent sterilization procedure that involves blocking off a woman's fallopian tubes to prevent conception.

Tubal pregnancy A pregnancy that occurs in the fallopian tube.

Ultrasound A technique that uses high-frequency sound waves to create a moving image, or sonogram, on a television screen.

Umbilical cord The cord that connects the placenta to the developing baby, removing waste products and carbon dioxide from the baby and bringing oxygenated blood and nutrients from the mother through the placenta to the baby.

Uterus The hollow muscular organ that protects and nourishes the fetus prior to birth.

Vacuum extraction A process in which a suction cup is attached to a vacuum pump placed on a baby's head to aid in delivery.

Vaginal birth after cesarean (VBAC) A vaginal delivery that occurs when a woman has previously delivered a baby or babies by cesarean section.

Varicocele A collection of varicose veins in the scrotum. Varicoceles can elevate scrotal temperature, contributing to fertility problems.

Varicose veins   Abnormally swollen veins, usually on the legs.

Vas deferens   The tube connecting the epididymis with the seminal vesicles.

Vasectomy   A minor surgical procedure that involves cutting the vas deferens to block the passage of sperm.

VBAC   See Vaginal birth after cesarean.

VDRL test   Test of syphilis (also referred to as RPR).

Vena cava   The major vein in the body that returns unoxygenated blood to the heart for transport to the lungs.

Vernix caseosa   A greasy white substance that coats and protects the baby's skin in utero.

Vertex   Head-down presentation.

Zygote   A cell formed by the union of egg and sperm.

Birth Plan

Feeling a bit unsure about what to put in your birth plan? Despite what some over-zealous childbirth instructors would have you believe, there's no such thing as a "right" or "wrong" way to write a birth plan. You can either write an informal letter that highlights the most important points you'd like to make about the birth, or — if you're not big on letter writing — you can simply fill in the blanks of the birth plan that follows. If there's an issue you feel strongly about and there isn't enough room for you below to go into a lot of detail, simply attach an extra page or two to your plan.

Regardless of which route you decide to go (starting from scratch or using the template below), you need at least three copies of your plan:

- a copy to give to your doctor or midwife

- a copy to attach to the pre-registration form that you fill out at the hospital (assuming, of course, that you're planning a hospital birth)

- a copy to tuck into your labor bag (if you're giving birth in the hospital) or your night-table drawer (if you're planning to give birth at home) so that you'll have an extra copy handy during labor

Note: Even if you're planning to give birth at home, you should still make a point of filling out the hospital-related section of this birth plan. It's always possible that you may end up delivering in the hospital after all, so it's best to be clear about your thoughts on any hospital-related procedures ahead of time.

Birth Plan

Personal information

Name: _____

Partner's name: _____

Home phone number: _____

Due date: _____

____ We have attended or are planning to attend prenatal classes.
____ We have taken or are planning to take a hospital tour.

About your labor support team

Name and phone number of doctor/midwife:

_____

_____

Name and phone number of doula or other labor support person(s):

_____

_____

Name and phone number of baby's doctor:

_____

_____

Names and ages of any children who will be attending the birth:

_____

_____

Laboring environment

While I am in labor, I would like (check as many as apply)
____ to have the lights dimmed.
____ to have noise and distractions in the area where I am laboring kept to a minimum.
____ to labor in the bathtub, Jacuzzi, or shower (circle the appropriate choices).
____ to have access to the following birthing equipment during labor:
    ____ birthing bed
    ____ birthing stool
    ____ birthing chair
    ____ squatting bar
    ____ birthing pool/tub
    ____ a mirror so that I can view my baby's birth.
____ to be able to listen to music.
____ to be able to wear my own clothes or no clothing at all.
____ to have my partner and/or other support person(s) with me at all times, unless an emergency situation arises.
____ to leave my contact lenses in place throughout my labor, unless it becomes necessary for me to undergo anesthesia.
____ to be permitted to have photographs and/or videos taken of my labor and my baby's birth.

Choices about the labor

If my labor
____ has not yet started when my water breaks, I'd like to wait at least 24 hours before an induction is attempted.
____ has not yet started and I'm two weeks overdue, I'd like to be induced.
____ has not yet started and I'm two weeks overdue, I'd prefer not to be induced.
____ has not progressed very far when I arrive at the hospital, I'd like to be given the option of returning home until my labor is further along.

Laboring positions

While I am in labor, I would like
____ to walk around as much as possible, and to be free to experiment with a number of different laboring positions.
____ to labor on my side.
____ to labor in a squatting position (either using a squatting bar or sitting on the toilet).
____ to be offered the option of having a massage.
____ to be given the opportunity to consume clear fluids and ice chips during my labor.

Pain relief

I'm planning to use the following pain-relief measures during my labor:

____ Relaxation
____ Breathing techniques/distraction
____ Changing positions
____ Laboring in water (shower and/or bathtub):
 ____ alone or ____ with my partner
____ Heat or cold therapy
____ Massage
____ Acupressure
____ Acupuncture
____ Hypnosis
____ Pain medications such as Stadol, Nubain, or Demerol
____ Anesthetic gases such as Nitronox
____ An epidural
____ Other (please specify): _____

_____

_____

Induction/augmentation of labor

If it becomes necessary to induce or augment my labor, I would prefer that the following technique(s) be used, if possible:

____ Natural methods of getting labor started (walking and sexual intercourse)
____ Nipple stimulation
____ Prostaglandins gel
____ Synthetic oxytocin (Pitocin)
____ Stripping membranes
____ Amniotomy (rupturing the membranes)

Delivery

I am intending to deliver my baby in the following position:

____ sitting
____ on my side
____ squatting
____ on all fours
____ on my back
____ Other (please specify): _____

After the birth

Once the baby has been delivered, I would like
___ to have my baby placed on my chest as soon as possible.
___ to have my baby wrapped in a blanket before he or she is handed to me.
___ to have my partner cut the umbilical cord.
___ to breastfeed my baby as soon as possible.
___ to avoid any unnecessary separation from my baby.
___ to have 24-hour rooming in (sharing a room) with my baby.
___ to be present myself or have my partner present for any tests my baby may require (e.g., PKU/TSH heel prick blood test).
___ to receive instruction on routine baby care procedures such as diapering, bathing, and so on.

Cesarean section

If I have a cesarean, I would like to have
___ my partner present at the delivery.
___ my labor support person present at the delivery.
___ a screen placed in front of my face to block my view of the delivery.
___ as much information as possible about what's happening on the other side of the screen.
___ as little information as possible about what's happening on the other side of the screen.
___ the delivery photographed or videotaped.
___ to touch my baby as soon as possible after the delivery.
___ to have my partner cut the cord.
___ to breastfeed as soon as possible.

Feeding

I'm intending to
___ breastfeed.
___ bottlefeed.

Circumcision

If my baby is a boy, I am intending to
___ have him circumcised.
___ not have him circumcised.

Length of stay (if you're having a hospital birth)

I'm intending to leave the hospital within
___ 6 hours of the delivery
___ 12 hours of the delivery
___ 24 hours of the delivery
___ 48 hours of the delivery
___ 3 to 5 days of the delivery.

We have written this birth plan according to our wishes for our baby's birth. We understand that medical emergencies may force us to deviate from this plan, but, as much as possible, we would like everyone who is present at our baby's birth to respect the choices we have outlined here.

Your signature   _____

Your partner's signature _____

Date   _____

Emergency Childbirth Procedures

How to deliver your baby if you're alone and without assistance

Getting help

- Try to remain calm.
- Call the emergency response number in your community and ask the person who takes the call to send out an emergency response team and to notify your doctor or midwife that you're about to deliver your baby.
- Ask a friend or neighbor to stay with you until the emergency response team arrives. (If you're able to find someone, they should follow the tips below on helping a mother who's about to give birth.)

Preparing for the birth

- Wash your hands and your vulvar area with mild detergent or soap and water.
- Spread a shower curtain, a plastic tablecloth, clean towels, newspapers, or sheets on a bed, sofa, or the floor, and then lie down until someone arrives to assist you.

Coping during labor

- If you feel the urge to push, try panting instead. It will help you to hold off on pushing until someone arrives to help deliver your baby.

- If your baby starts coming before help arrives, gently ease the baby out of your body by pushing each time you feel the urge and catching the baby with your hands.

After the birth

- Lay the baby across your abdomen or put the baby to your breast If the umbilical cord is long enough to reach.
- Don't try to pull the placenta out. If the placenta is delivered before help arrives, wrap it in towels or a newspaper and keep it elevated above the level of the baby.
- Do not try to cut the cord on your own. Wait until help arrives.

How to assist a woman who's about to give birth

What to do first

- Remain calm. Instead of panicking, focus your energies on comforting and reassuring the mother.
- Call the emergency response number in your community and ask the person who takes the call to send out an emergency response team and to notify the mother's doctor or midwife that she's about to deliver her baby.

Preparing for the delivery

- Wash your hands and the mother's vulvar area with mild detergent or soap and water.
- Spread a shower curtain, a plastic tablecloth, clean towels, newspapers, or sheets on a bed or table.
- Help the mother sit at the edge of the bed or table with her buttocks hanging off and her knees apart. Support her head with one or two pillows.
- If she's in active labor and in too much pain to climb onto the bed or table, place a stack of newspapers or folded towels under her buttocks so that she'll be far enough off the floor for you to be able to deliver the baby's shoulders easily.

- If you're in a vehicle, help the mother lie down on the seat. Then help her to position herself so that she has one foot on the floor and the other on the seat.

Assisting the mother during labor

- If the mother needs to vomit, help her turn her head to the side so that her mouth and airway will remain clear.
- Use a dishpan or basin to catch the amniotic fluid and blood.
- Encourage the mother to start panting if she feels the urge to push. This may help to delay the birth until help arrives.

Delivering the baby

- Once the baby's heard starts to crown (i.e., to emerge through the tissues at the opening of the vagina), encourage the mother to pant or blow. This will help to slow the baby's exit from the birth canal. Then, to keep the baby's head from emerging too quickly, you should apply gentle counterpressure to the baby's head.
- If you see a loop of umbilical cord around the baby's neck, gently pull on it and lift it over the baby's head.
- If the baby's amniotic sac is intact when the baby's head emerges, puncture the sac with a clean fingernail or a ballpoint pen, being sure to hold the pen away from the baby's face, and carefully move the sac away from the baby's mouth.
- Take the baby's head in your hands and press it slightly downward, asking the mother to push at the same time. Then help to ease the baby's shoulders out one at a time. Once the baby's shoulders have been delivered, the rest of the baby should slip out easily.
- Clear the baby's mouth and nose immediately after the birth, using a bulb syringe and gauze pad (if you have them) or by gently stroking the sides of the baby's nose in a downward direction, and the neck and underside of the chin in an upward direction to help expel mucus and amniotic fluid. You can also try holding the baby's head lower than its body to use gravity to drain away the fluid. Once the baby starts crying vigorously, you can return the baby to an upright position.

After the birth

- Wrap the baby in a clean blanket or towel and lay the baby across the mother's abdomen or place it at her breast if the cord is long enough.

- Don't try to pull the placenta out. If the placenta is delivered before help arrives, wrap it in towels or a newspaper and keep it elevated above the level of the baby.

- Do not try to cut the cord before help arrives.

- Keep the mother comfortable and the baby warm and dry until help arrives.

Directory of Organizations

Adoption

American Academy of Adoption Attorneys
Box 33053
Washington, DC 20033-0053
Phone: 202-832-2222
Fax: 202-293-2309
Web site: www.adoptionattorneys.org
E-mail: trustees@adoptionattorneys.org

National Adoption Center
1500 Walnut Street, Suite 701
Philadelphia, PA 19102
Phone: 800-TO-ADOPT
(800-862-3678)
215-735-9988
Fax: 215-735-9410
Web site: www.adopt.org
E-mail: nac@adopt.org

National Adoption Information Clearinghouse
330 C Street SW
Washington, DC 20447
Phone: 888-251-0075
703-352-3488
Fax: 703-385-3206
Web site: www.calib.com/naic
E-mail: naic@calib.com

National Resource Center for Special Needs Adoption
Spaulding for Children
Crossroad Office Center
16250 Northland Drive, Suite 120
Southfield, MI 48075
Phone: 248-443-7080
Fax: 248-443-7099
Web site: www.spaulding.org
E-mail: sfc@spaulding.org

North American Council on Adoptable Children
970 Raymond Avenue, Suite 106
St. Paul, MN 55114-1149
Phone: 651-644-3036
Fax: 651-644-9848
Web site: www.nacac.org
E-mail: info@nacac.org

Birth centers

The National Association of Childbearing Centers
3123 Gottschall Road
Perklomenville, PA 18074-9546
Phone: 215-234-8068
Fax: 215-234-8829
Web site: www.birthcenters.org
E-mail: reachnacc@
   birthcenters.org

Breastfeeding

International Board of Lactation Consultant Examiners
7309 Arlington Blvd., Suite 300
Falls Church, VA 22042-3215
Phone: 703-560-7330
Fax: 703-560-7332
Web site: www.iblce.org
E-mail: iblce@erols.com

International Lactation Consultant Association
1500 Sunday Drive, Suite 102
Raleigh, NC 27607
Phone: 919-787-5181
Fax: 919-787-4916
Web site: www.ilca.org/
E-mail: ilca@erols.com

LaLeche League International
1400 North Meacham Road
P.O. Box 4079
Schaumberg, IL 60168-4079
Phone: 800-LALECHE
   (800-525-3243)

847-519-7730
Fax: 847-519-0035
Web site: www.lalecheleague.org
E-mail: llli@llli.org

Nursing Mothers Counsel
P.O. Box 50063
Palo Alto, CA 94303
Phone: 650-599-3669
Fax: 831-421-0661
Web site: www.nursingmothers.org

Caregivers

American Academy of Family Physicians
11400 Tomahawk Creek Parkway
Leawood, KS 66211-2672
Phone: 913-906-6000
Fax: 913-906-6077
Web site: www.aafp.org
E-mail: fp@aafp.org

American College of Nurse-Midwives
818 Connecticut Avenue NW,
   Suite 900
Washington, DC 20006
Phone: 888-MIDWIFE
   (888-643-9433)
202-728-9860
Fax: 202-728-9897
Web site: www.acnm.org
E-mail: info@acnm.org

American College of Obstetricians and Gynecologists (ACOG)
Resource Center
409 12th Street SW
P.O. Box 96920
Washington, DC 20090-6920
Phone: 202-638-5577
Web site: www.acog.org
E-mail: resources@acog.org

Cesarean birth

Cesareans/ Support, Education, and Concern
22 Forest Road
Framingham, MA 01701
Phone: 508-877-8266

International Cesarean Awareness Network, Inc.
1304 Kingsdale Avenue
Redondo Beach, CA 90278
Phone: 310-542-6400
Fax: 310-542-5368
Web site: www.ican-online.org
E-mail: info@ican-online.org

Childbirth education

The Academy of Certified Childbirth Educators
2001 E. Prairie Circle, Suite I
Olathe, KS 66062
Phone: 800-444-8223
913-782-5116
Fax: 913-397-0933
Web site: www.acbe.com
E-mail: acbe@acbe.com

American Academy of Husband-Coached Childbirth (The Bradley Method)
P.O. Box 5224
Sherman Oaks, CA 91413-5224
Phone: 800-4-A-Birth
(800-422-4784)
818-788-6662
Fax: 818-788-1580
Web site: www.bradleybirth.com
E-mail: marjiehathaway@
bradleybirth.com

Association of Labor Assistants and Childbirth Educators (ALACE)
P.O. Box 390436
Cambridge, MA 02139
Phone: 617-441-2500
Fax: 617-441-3167
Web site: www.216.36.255.91
E-mail: alacehq@aol.com

Association of Women's Health, Obstetric, and Neonatal Nurses
2000 L Street NW, Suite 740
Washington, DC 20036
Phone: 202-261-2400
Fax: 202-728-0575
Web site: www.awhonn.org

Childbirth Without Pain Education Association
20134 Snowden
Detroit, MI 48235-1170
Phone: 313-341-3816
Fax: (as above)

Coalition for Improving Maternity Services, Inc.
P.O. Box 2346
Ponte Vedra Beach, FL 32004
Phone: 888-282-CIMS
(888-282-2467)
Fax: 904-285-2120
Web site: www.motherfriendly.org
E-mail: info@motherfriendly.org

International Association of Parents and Professionals for Safe Alternatives in Childbirth
Route 4, P.O. Box 646
Marble Hill, MO 63764
Phone: 573-238-2010
Fax: 573-238-2010
Web site: www.napsac.org
E-mail: napsac@clas.net

International Childbirth Education Association & Bookcenter (ICEA)
P.O. Box 20048
Minneapolis, MN 55420
Phone: 800-624-4934
  (for Book Center)
952-854-8660
Fax: 952-854-8772
Web site: www.icea.org
E-mail: info@icea.org

Lamaze International
2025 M Street NW, Suite 800
Washington, DC 20036
Phone: 800-368-4404
202-367-1128
Fax: 202-367-2128
Web site: www.lamaze.org
E-mail: lamaze@dc.sba.com

National Childbirth Education Foundation
P.O. Box 251
Oxford, PA 19363
Phone: 717-529-2561
E-mail: jpncef@aol.com

Doulas

Doulas of North America
13513 North Grove Drive
Alpine, Utah 84004
Phone: 801-756-7331
Fax: 801-763-1847
Web site: www.dona.org
E-mail: Doula@dona.org
referrals@dona.org
certification@dona.org

Endometriosis

Endometriosis Association International Headquarters
8585 North 76th Place
Milwaukee, Wisconsin 53223
Phone: 800-992-3636
414-355-2200
Fax: 414-355-6065
Web site: www.endometriosisassn.
  org
E-mail: endo@endometriosisassn.
  org

Genetic counseling

Genetic Alliance
4301 Connecticut Avenue NW,
  Suite 404
Washington, DC 20008-2304
Phone: 800-336-GENE
  (800-336-4363)
202-966-5557
Fax: 202-966-8553
Web site: www.geneticalliance.org
E-mail: info@geneticalliance.org

National Society of Genetic Counselors
233 Canterbury Drive
Wallingford, PA 19086-6617
Phone: 610-872-7608 (Mailbox#7)
Fax: 610-872-1192
Web site: www.nsgc.org
E-mail: nsgc@aol.com

High-risk pregnancy: Medical information and support

American Cancer Society, Inc.
1599 Clifton Road, NE
Atlanta, GA 30329
Phone: 800-231-5355
Web site: www.cancer.org

American Diabetes Association National Service Center
1701 N. Beauregard Street
Alexandria, VA 22311
Phone: 800-DIABETES
(800-342-2383)
Fax: 703-549-6995
Web site: www.diabetes.org
E-mail: customerservice@
diabetes.org

American Kidney Fund
6110 Executive Blvd., Suite 1010
Rockville, MD 20852
Phone: 800-638-8299
301-881-3052
Fax: 301-881-0898
Web site: www.kidneyfund.org
E-mail: helpline@akfinc.org

American Lung Association
1740 Broadway, 14th Floor
New York, NY 10019-4374
Phone: 800 LUNG USA
(800-586-4872)
212-315-8700
Fax: 212-265-5642
Web site: www.lungusa.org
E-mail: info@lungusa.org

Asthma & Allergy Foundation of America
1233 20th Street, Suite 402
Washington, DC 20036
Phone: 800-7ASTHMA

(800-727-8462)
202-466-7643
Fax: 202-466-8940
Web site: www.aafa.org
E-mail: info@aafa.org

Center for Sickle Cell Disease
Howard University
2121 Georgia Avenue, NW
Washington, DC 20059
Phone: 202-806-7930
Fax: 202-806-4517
Web site: www.huhosp.org/
sicklecell/default/htm

The Confinement Line
P.O. Box 1609
Springfield, VA 22151
Phone: 703-941-7183

Cooley's Anemia Foundation, Inc
129-09 26th Avenue, Suite 203
Flushing, NY 11354
Phone: 800-522-7222
718-321-CURE (718-321-2873)
Fax: 718-321-3340
Web site: www.cooleysanemia.org
E-mail: info@cooleysanemia.org

Crohn's Disease and Colitis Foundation of America
386 Park Avenue S, 17th Floor
New York, NY 10016
Phone: 800-932-2423
212-685-3440
Web site: www.ccfa.org
E-mail: info@ccfa.org

Cystic Fibrosis Foundation
6931 Arlington Road
Bethesda, MD 20814
Phone: 800-FIGHT CF
(800-344-4823)
301-951-4422
Fax: 301-951-6378
Web site: www.cff.org
E-mail: info@cff.org

DES Action USA
610 16th Street, Suite 301
Oakland, CA 94612
Phone: 800-DES-9288
   (800-337-9288)
Fax: 510 465 4815
Web site: www.desaction.org
E-mail: desaction@earthlink.net

Epilepsy Foundation
4351 Garden City Drive
Landover, MD 20785
Information & Referral:
   800-332-1000
301-459-3700
Fax: 301-577-2684
Web site: www.epilepsyfoundation.
   org
E-mail: Webmaster@efa.org

Family Empowerment Network:
Supporting Families Affected by
Fetal Alcohol Syndrome and
Related Disorders
University of Wisconsin-Madison
517 Lowell Center
610 Langdon Street
Madison, WI 53703
Phone: 800-462-5254
608-262-6590
Fax: 608-265-2329
Web site: www.dcs.wisc.edu/pda/
   hhi/fen
E-mail: fen@dcs.wisc.edu

Group B Strep Association
P.O. Box 16515
Chapel Hill, NC 27516
Phone: 919-932-5344
Fax: 919-932-3657
Web site: www.groupbstrep.org

**Huntington's Disease Society
of America**
158 W. 29th Street, 7th Floor
New York, NY 10001
Phone: 800-345-HDSA
   (800-345-4372)
Fax: 212-239-3430
Web site: www.hdsa.org
E-mail: hdsainfo@hdsa.org

Intensive Caring Unlimited (ICU)
P.O. Box 563
Newton Square, PA 19073
Phone: 610-876-7872
National Cancer Institute
Cancer Information Service
Room 3036A
6116 Executive Blvd., MSC 8322
Bethesda, MD 20892-8322
Phone: 800-4-CANCER
   (800-422-6237),
   800-332-8615 (TTY)
Web site: www.cancer.gov
E-mail: info@cancer.gov

**National Diabetes Information
Clearinghouse**
1 Information Way
Bethesda, MD 20892-3560
Phone: 800-860-8747
301-654-3327
Fax: 301-907-8906
Web site: www.niddk.nih.gov/
   health/diabetes/ndic.htm
E-mail: ndic@info.niddk.nih.gov

**National Foundation for Jewish
Genetic Diseases, Inc.**
250 Park Avenue, Suite 1000
New York, NY 10177
Phone: 212-371-1030

Web site: www.nfjgd.org
E-mail: info@nfjgd.org

National Hemophilia Foundation
116 West 32nd Street, 11th Floor
New York, NY 10001
Phone: 800-424-2634
212-328-3700
Fax: 212-328-3777
Web site: www.hemophilia.org
E-mail: info@hemophilia.org

National Kidney Foundation
30 E. 33rd Street, Suite 1100
New York, NY 10016
Phone: 800-622-9010
212-889-2210
Fax: 212-689-9261
Web site: www.kidney.org
E-mail: info@kidney.org

National Organization on Fetal Alcohol Syndrome
216 G Street, NE
Washington, DC 20002
Phone: 202-785-4585
Fax: 202-466-6456
Web site: www.nofas.org
E-mail: information@nofas.org

Organization of Teratology Information Services
c/o Pregnancy Riskline
P.O. Box 144270
Salt Lake City, UT 84114-4270
Phone: 888-285-3410
520-626-6796
Fax: 520-626-5115
Web site: www.otispregnancy.org

Sickle Cell Disease Association of America, Inc.
National Office
200 Corporate Pointe, Suite 495
Culver City, CA 90230-8727

Phone: 800-421-8453
310-216-6363
Fax: 310-215-3722
Web site: www.sicklecelldisease.org
E-mail: scdaa@
   sicklecelldisease.org

Sidelines National Support Network
P.O. Box 1808
Laguna Beach, CA 92652
Phone: 888-447-4754
949-497-2265
Fax: 949-497-5598
Web site: www.sidelines.org
E-mail: sidelines@sidelines.org

Substance Abuse & Mental Health Services Administration (SAMHSA)
U.S. Department of Health & Human Services
12-95 Parklawn
5600 Fishers Lane
Rockville, MD 20857
Phone: 301-443-4795
Fax: 301-443-0247
Web site: www.samhsa.gov/
E-mail: info@samhsa.gov

HMOs

The American Association of Health Plans
1129 20th Street NW, Suite 600
Washington, DC 20036-3421
Phone: 202-778-3200
Fax: 202-331-7487
Web site: www.aahp.org

Joint Commission on Accreditation of Healthcare Organizations
One Renaissance Boulevard
Oakbrook Terrace, IL 60181

Phone: 630-792-5000
Fax: 630-792-5005 or 630-792-5645
Web site: www.jcaho.org
E-mail: webmaster@jcaho.org

**National Committee for
Quality Assurance**
2000 L. Street NW, Suite 500
Washington, DC 20036
Phone: 202-955-3500
Fax: 202-955-3599
Web site: www.ncqa.org
E-mail: webmaster@ncqa.org

Fax: 301-984-1473
Web site: www.nichd.nih.gov/
E-mail: nichdclearinghouse@
    mail.nih.gov

**ZERO To THREE: National Center
for Infants, Toddlers, and Families**
2000 M Street NW, Suite 200
Washington, DC 20036
Phone: 202-638-1144
Fax: 202-638-0851
Web site: www.zerotothree.org
E-mail: oto3@zerotothree.org

Infant Health

American Academy of Pediatrics
141 Northwest Point Blvd.
Elk Grove Village, IL 60007-1098
Phone: 847-434-4000
Fax: 847-434-8000
Web site: www.aap.org

**National Association of Pediatric
Nurse Practitioners**
1101 Kings Highway North,
    Suite 206
Cherry Hill, NJ 08034-1912
Phone: 856-667-1773
Fax: 856-667-7187
Web site: www.napnap.org
E-mail: info@napnap.org

**Sudden Infant Death Syndrome
(SIDS) "Back to Sleep" Campaign**
c/o National Institute of Child
Health and Human Development
Clearinghouse
Box 3006
Rockville, MD 20847
Phone: 800-370-2943

Infertility

**American Society for
Reproductive Medicine**
1209 Montgomery Highway
Birmingham, AL 35216-2809
Phone: 205-978-5000
Fax: 205-978-5505
Web site: www.asrm.org
E-mail: asrm@asrm.org

American Society of Andrology
2950 Buskirk Avenue, Suite 170
Walnut Creek, CA 94596
Phone: 925-472-5910
Fax: 925-472-5901
Web site: www.andrologysociety.
    com/hom.cfm
E-mail: asa@hp-assoc.com

**American Urological Association
Headquarters**
1120 North Charles Street
Baltimore, MD 21201
Phone: 410-727-1100

Fax: 410-468-1835
Web site: www.auanet.org
Fertility Research Foundation
875 Park Avenue
New York, NY 10021
Phone: 212-744-5500
Fax: 212-744-6536
Web site: www.frfbaby.com
E-mail: frfbaby@msn.com

**International Council on Infertility
Information Dissemination, Inc.**
P.O. Box 6836
Arlington, VA 22206
Phone: 703-579-9178
Fax: 703-379-1593
Web site: www.inciid.org
E-mail: INCIIDinfo@inciid.org

RESOLVE, Inc.
1310 Broadway
Somerville, MA 02144-1731
Phone: 617-623-1156
Help Line: 617-623-0744
Fax: 617-623-0252
Web site: www.resolve.org
E-mail: resolveinc@aol.com

Surrogates by Choice
P.O. Box 05257
Detroit, MI 48205
Phone: 313-839-4946
Maternal-infant health

**American Dietetic Association
National Center for Nutrition
and Dietetics**
216 West Jackson Boulevard
Chicago, IL 60606
Phone: 312-899-0040 Ext 4853
Fax: 312-899-4739
Web site: www.eatright.org
E-mail: knowledge@eatright.org

**American Foundation for Maternal
and Child Health, Inc.**
439 E. 51st St
New York, NY 10022
Phone: 212-759-5510

**Association of Maternal and
Child Health Programs**
1220 19th Street NW, Suite 801
Washington, DC 20036
Phone: 202-775-0436
Fax: 202-775-0061
Web site: www.amchp.org
E-mail: info@amchp.org

**Center for Nutrition Policy and
Promotion, U.S. Department of
Agriculture**
1120 20th Street, NW, Suite 200,
     North Lobby
Washington, DC 20036-3406
Phone: 202-418-2312
Fax: 202-208-2321
Web site: www.usda.gov/fcs/
     cnpp.htm

**Centers for Disease Control
and Prevention**
1600 Clifton Road
Atlanta, GA 30333
Phone: 800-311-3435
404-639-3534
Web site: www.cdc.gov

**Food and Nutrition Information
Center, Agricultural Research
Service**
U.S. Department of Agriculture
National Agricultural Library
10301 Baltimore Avenue, Room 105
Beltsville, MD 20705-2351

Phone: 301-504-5719
301-504-6856 (TTY)
Fax: 301-504-6409
Web site: www.nal.usda.gov/fnic/
    general/general.html
E-mail: fnic@nalusda.gov

Maternity Center Association
281 Park Avenue South, 5th Floor
New York, NY 10010
Phone: 212-777-5000
Fax: 212-777-9320
Web site: www.maternity.org
E-mail: mcabirth@aol.com

**National Center for Education
in Maternal and Child Health**
Georgetown University
2000 15th St. N
Suite 701
Arlington, VA 22201-2617
Phone: 703-524-7802
Fax: 703-524-9335
Web site: www.ncemch.org
E-mail: info@ncemch.org

**National Healthy Mothers,
Healthy Babies Coalition**
121 North Washington Street,
    Suite 300
Alexandria, VA 22314
Phone: 703-836-6110
Fax: 703-836-3470
Web site: www.hmhb.org
E-mail: info@hmhb.org

**National Maternal and Child
Health Clearinghouse**
2070 Chain Bridge Road, Suite 450
Vienna, VA 22182-2536
Phone: 888-434-4624
703-821-8955
Fax: 703-821-2098

Web site: www.nmchc.org
E-mail: nmchc@circsol.com

National Perinatal Association
3500 East Fletcher Avenue,
    Suite 205
Tampa, FL 33613-4712
Phone: 888-971-3295
813-971-1008
Fax: 813-971-9306
Web site: www.nationalperinatal.org
E-mail: npa@nationalperinatal.org

**National Perinatal
Information Center**
144 Wayland Avenue, Suite 300
Providence, RI 02906
Phone: 401-274-0650
Fax: 401-455-0377
Web site: www.npic.org
E-mail: npic@npic.org

National Women's Health Network
514 10th Street, NW, Suite 400
Washington, DC 20004
Phone: 202-347-1140
Fax: 202-347-1168
Web site: www.
    womenshealthnetwork.org
E-mail: jaulwes@
    womenshealthnetwork.org

**National Women's Health
Resource Center**
120 Albany Street, Suite 820
New Brunswick, NJ 08901
Phone: 877-98-NWHRC
    (877-986-9472)
Fax: 732-249-4671
Web site: www.healthywomen.org
E-mail: info@healthywomen.org

New Parents Network
P.O. Box 64237
Tucson, AZ 85728
Phone: 520-327-1451
Fax: 520-881-7104
Web site: www.newparentsnetwork.
org
E-mail: moreinfo@
newparentsnetwork.org

U.S. Department of Agriculture Supplemental Food Programs Division
3101 Park Center Drive, 5th Floor
Alexandria, VA 22302
Phone: 703-305-2746
Fax: 703-305-2196
Web site: www.usda.gov

Midwifery organizations

American College of Nurse-Midwives
818 Connecticut Avenue NW,
Suite 900
Washington, DC 20006
Phone: 888-MIDWIFE
(888-643-9433)
202-728-9860
Fax: 202-728-9897
Web site: www.acnm.org
E-mail: info@acnm.org

Informed Homebirth
P.O. Box 1733
Fair Oaks, CA 95628
Phone: 916-961-6923
Fax: 916-961-6923
E-mail: ihibp@softcom.net

Midwives Alliance of North America (MANA)
4805 Lawrenceville Hwy.,
Suite 116-279
Lilburn, GA 30047

Phone: 800-923-MANA
(800-923-6262)
Fax: 801-720-3026
Web site: www.mana.org
E-mail: info@mana.org

Miscarriage, stillbirth, and infant death

A.M.E.N.D. (Aiding a Mother and Father Experiencing Neonatal Death
1559 Ville Rosa
Hazelwood, MO 63042
Phone: 314-291-0892
Web site: www.amendgroup.org
E-mail: martha@amendgroup.org

American Sudden Infant Death Syndrome Institute
National Headquarters
2480 Windy Hill Road, Suite 380
Marietta, GA 30067
Phone: 800-232-7437
770-612-1030
Fax: 770-612-8277
Web site: www.sids.org
E-mail: prevent@sids.org

Association of SIDS and Infant Mortality Programs
c/o MN SID Center, Childrens'
Hospitals and Clinics
2525 Chicago Ave., South
Minneapolis, MN 55419
Phone: 612-813-6285
Fax: 612-813-7344
Web site: www.asip1.org/
contact.html
E-mail: kathleen.fernbach@
childrenshc.org

Bereavement Services
(formerly Resolve Through
Sharing)
1910 South Avenue
La Crosse, Wisconsin 54601-5400
Phone: 800-362-9567 Ext. 4747
Web site: www.gundluth.org/
     bereave/
E-mail: berservs@gundluth.org

**Center for Loss in Multiple Birth,
Inc. (CLIMB)**
P.O. Box 91377
Anchorage, AK 99509
Phone: 907-222-5321
Web site: www.climb-support.org
E-mail: climb@pobox.alaska.net

The Compassionate Friends
P.O. Box 3696
Oak Brook, IL 60522-3696
Phone: 877-969-0010
Fax: 630-990-0246
Web site: www.
     compassionatefriends.org
E-mail: nationaloffice@
     compassionatefriends.org

**Minnesota Center for Twin and
Adoption Research University of
Minnesota**
Department of Psychology
Room N218 Elliott Hall
75 East River Road
Minneapolis, MN 55455-0344
Phone: 612-625-4067
612-625-2818
Fax: 612-626-2079
Web site: www.psych.umn.edu/
     psylabs/

**National Fetal-Infant Mortality
Review Program American College
of Obstetricians and Gynecologists**
409 12th Street, SW,
     P.O. Box 96920
Washington, DC 20090 6920
Phone: 202-863-2587
Fax: 202-484-3917
Web site: www.acog.org/goto/nfimr
E-mail: NFIMR@ACOG.ORG

National SIDS Resource Center
2070 Chain Bridge Road, Suite 450
Vienna, VA 22182
Phone: 866-866-7437
703-821-8955 ext. 249
Fax: 703-821-2098
Web site: www.sidscenter.org
E-mail: sids@circsol.com

Pails of Hope Newsletter
Pregnancy and Parenting After
     Infertility and/or Loss Support
Pen Parents, Inc.
P. O. Box 8738
Reno, NV 89507-8738
Phone: 775-826-7332
Web site: www.penparents.org
E-mail: penparents@aol.com

Perinatal Loss
2116 NE 18th Avenue
Portland, OR 97212
Phone: 503-284-7426
Fax: 503-282-8985
Web site: www.tearsoup.com
E-mail: grieving@tearsoup.com

A Place to Remember
de Ruyter-Nelson Publications, Inc.
1885 University Avenue, Suite 110
St. Paul, MN 55104

Phone: 800-631-0973
651-645-7045
Fax: 651-645-4780
Web site: www.aplacetoremember.com
E-mail: aptr@aplacetoremember.com

Pregnancy and Infant Loss Center
1421 E. Wayzata Boulevard, Unit 70
Wayzata, MN 55391
Phone: 952-473-9372
Fax: 952-473-8978
Web site: www.pilc.org

Pregnancy Loss Support Program
National Council of Jewish Women
820 Second Avenue
New York, NY 10017-4504
Phone: 212-687-5030
Fax: 212-687-5032
Web site: www.ncjwny.org/
services_support.htm
E-mail: actionline@ncjw.org

Share Pregnancy & Infant Loss
Support Inc. St. Joseph Health
Center
300 First Capitol Drive
St. Charles, MO 63301-2893
Phone: 800-821-6819
636-947-6164
Fax: 636-947-7486
Web site: www.nationalshareoffice.com
E-mail: share@nationalshareoffice.com

SIDS Alliance
1314 Bedford Avenue, Suite 210
Baltimore, MD 21208
Phone: 800-221-SIDS
(800-221-7437)
410-653-8226

Fax: 410-653-8709
Web site: www.sidsalliance.org
E-mail: info@sidsalliance.org

Sudden Infant Death Syndrome
(SIDS) "Back to Sleep" Campaign
c/o National Institute of
Child Health and Human
Development Clearinghouse
Box 3006
Rockville, MD 20847
Phone: 800-370-2943
Fax: 301-984-1473
Web site: www.nichd.nih.gov/
E-mail: nichdclearinghouse@
mail.nih.gov

Twinless Twins
P.O. Box 980481
Ypsilanti, MI 48198-0481
Phone: 219-627-5414
Web site: www.fwi.com/twinless
E-mail: twinworld1@aol.com

Wintergreen Press
3630 Eileen Street
Maple Plain, MN 55359
Phone: 952-476-1303
Web site: www.wintergreenpress.com
E-mail: wpress@wintergreenpress.com

Wisconsin Stillbirth Service Project
University of Wisconsin-Madison
Clinical Genetics Center
1500 Highland Avenue
Madison, WI 53705-2280
Phone: 608-262-9722
Fax: 608-263-3496
Web site: www.wisc.edu/wissp
E-mail: modaff@waisman.wisc.edu

Multiple births

Center for the Study of Multiple Birth
333 E. Superior Street, Room 464
Chicago, IL 60611
Phone: 312-266-9093
Fax: 312-908-5800
Web site: www.multiplebirth.com
E-mail: lgk395@northwestern.edu

MOST (Mothers of Supertwins) (Triplets or more)
P.O. Box 951
Brentwood, NY 11717-0627
Phone: 631-859-1110
Fax: 631-859-3580
Web site: www.mostonline.org
E-mail: Maureen@mostonline.org

National Organization of Mothers of Twins Clubs, Inc.
P.O. Box 438
Thompson Station, TN 37179-0438
Phone: 877-540-2200
Web site: www.NOMOTC.org
E-mail: NOMOTC@aol.com

Triplet Connection
P.O. Box 99571
Stockton, CA 95209
Phone: 209-474-0885
Fax: 209-474-9243
Web site: www.tripletconnection.
   org
E-mail: tc@tripletconnection.org

Twin Hope Inc.
2592 W 14th Street
Cleveland, OH 44113
Phone: 502-243-2110, 24-hour
   hotline
Web site: www.twinhope.com
E-mail: twinhope@twinhope.com

The Twins Foundation
P.O. Box 6043
Providence, RI 02940-6043
Phone: 401-751-TWIN
   (401-751-8946)
Fax: 401-751-4642
Web site: www.twinsfoundation.
   com
E-mail: twins@twinsfoundation.
   com

Twin to Twin Transfusion Syndrome Foundation
411 Longbeach Parkway
Bay Village, OH 44140
Phone: 800-815-9211
440-899-TTTS (440-899-8887)
Fax: 440-899-1184
Web site: www.tttsfoundation.org
E-mail: info@ttts.foundation.org

Natural family planning organizations

Couple to Couple League
P.O. Box 111184
Cincinnati, OH 45211-1184
Phone: 513-471-2000
Fax: 513-557-2449
Web site: www.ccli.org
E-mail: ccli@ccli.org

Parent support

National Association of Mothers' Centers
64 Division Avenue
Levittown, NY 11756
Phone: 800-645-3828
516-520-2929
Fax: 516-520-1639

Web site: www.motherscenter.org
E-mail: info@motherscenter.org

Postpartum Support International
927 North Kellogg Avenue
Santa Barbara, CA 93111
Phone: 805-967-7636
Fax: 805-967-0608
Web site: www.postpartum.net
E-mail: jhonikman@earthlink.net

Premature infants

**American Association of
Premature Infants**
P.O. Box 46371
Cincinnati, OH 45246-0371
Phone: 513-956-4331
Web site: www.aapi-online.org
E-mail: feedback@aapi-online.org

Prenatal health

**Registry of Pregnancies Exposed to
Chemotherapeutic Agents**
Department of Human Genetics
940 NE 13th Street, Room 2B2418
Oklahoma City, OKLA 73104
Phone: 405-271-8685
Fax: 405-271-8697

Reproductive health

**American Society for Colposcopy
and Cervical Pathology**
20 West Washington St., Suite 1
Hagerstown, MD 21740
Phone: 800-787-7227
301-733-3640
Fax: 301-733-5775

Web site: www.asccp.org
E-mail: khall@asccp.org

Safety

The Danny Foundation
1451 Danville Blvd., Suite 202
P.O. Box 680
Alamo, CA 94507
Phone: 800-83-DANNY
(800-833-2669)
925-314-8130
Fax: 925-314-8133
Web site: www.dannyfoundation.
org
E-mail: info@dannyfoundation.org

**Juvenile Products Manufacturers
Association**
17000 Commerce Parkway, Suite C
Mt. Laurel, NJ 08054
Phone: 856-439-0500
Fax: 856-439-0525
Web site: www.jpma.org
E-mail: jpma@ahint.com

National Safety Council
1121 Spring Lake Drive
Itasca, IL 60143-3201
Phone: 630-285-1121
Fax: 630-285-1315
Web site: www.nsc.org
E-mail: webmaster@nsc.org

U.S. Consumer Information Center
1800 F Street NW, Room G-142
Washington, DC 20405
Phone: 202-501-1794
Fax: 202-501-4281
Web site: www.pueblo.gsa.gov/
E-mail: catalog.pueblo@gsa.gov

U.S. Consumer Product Safety Commission
4330 East-West Highway
Bethesda, MD 20814-4408
Phone: 800-638-2772
Fax: 301-504-0399
Web site: www.cpsc.gov
E-mail: info@cpsc.gov

U.S. Department of Labor Occupational Safety and Health Administration
Office of Public Affairs
200 Constitution Avenue,
    Room N-3647
Washington, DC 20210
Phone: 202-693-1999
Fax: 202-693-1634
Web site: www.osha.gov

Sexually transmitted diseases

American Social Health Association (ASHA)
P.O. Box 13827
Research Triangle Park, NC
    27709-3827
Phone: 919-361-8400
Fax: 919-361-8425
Web site: www.ashastd.org

National Herpes Hotline
c/o American Social Health
    Association
P.O. Box 13827
Research Triangle Park, NC 27709
Phone: 919-361-8488
Fax: 919 361-8425
Web site: www.ashastd.org

Special needs/birth defects

The Arc of the United States
(The National Organization of and for People with Mental Retardation and Related Developmental Disabilities and their Families)
1010 Wayne Avenue, Suite 650
Silver Spring, MD 20910
Phone: 301-565-3842
Fax: 301-565-5342
Web site: www.thearc.org
E-mail: info@thearc.org

Autism Research Institute
4182 Adams Avenue
San Diego, CA 92116
Phone: 619-281-7165
Fax: 619-563-6840
Web site: www.autism.com/ari

Autism Society of America
7910 Woodmont Avenue, Suite 300
Bethesda, MD 20814-3067
Phone: 800-328-8476
301-657-0881
Fax: 301-657-0869
Web site: www.autism-society.org
E-mail: info@autism-society.org

Birth Defect Research for Children, Inc.
930 Woodcock Road, Suite 225
Orlando, FL 32803
Phone: 407-895-0802
Fax: 407-895-0824
Web site: www.birthdefects.org
E-mail: abdc@birthdefects.org

Brain Injury Association, Inc.
105 North Alfred Street
Alexandria, VA 22314

Phone: 800-444-6443
703-236-6000
Fax: 703-236-6001
Web site: www.biausa.org
E-mail: FamilyHelpline@biausa.org

Cleft Palate Foundation
104 South Estes Drive, Suite 204
Chapel Hill, NC 27514
Phone: 800-24-CLEFT
   (800-242-5338)
919-933-9044
Fax: 919-933-9604
Web site: www.cleftline.org
E-mail: cleftline@aol.com

Easter Seals
230 West Monroe Street,
   Suite 1800
Chicago, IL 60606
Phone: 800-221-6827 Ext. 7153
312-726-6200
Fax: 312-726-1494
Web site: www.easter-seals.org
E-mail: info@easter-seals.org

**Federation for Children
with Special Needs**
1135 Treemont Street, Suite 420
Boston, MA 02120
Phone: 800-331-0688 (Mass. Only)
617-236-7210
Fax: 617-572-2094
Web site: www.fcsn.org
E-mail: fcsninfo@fcsn.org

Hydrocephalus Association
870 Market S, Suite 705
San Francisco, CA 94102
Phone: 415-732-7040
Fax: 415-732-7044
Web site: www.hydroassoc.org
E-mail: hydroassoc@aol.com

**Juvenile Diabetes Research
Foundation International**
120 Wall Street, 19th Floor
New York, NY 10005-4001
Phone: 800-533-CURE
   (800-533-2873)
212-785-9500
Fax: 212-785-9595
Web site: www.jdrf.org
E-mail: info@jdrf.org

**March of Dimes Birth
Defects Foundation**
1275 Mamaroneck Avenue
White Plains, NY 10605
Phone: 888-MODIMES
   (888-663-4637)
914-428-7100
Fax: 914-428-8203
Web site: www.modimes.org
E-mail: resourcecenter@
   modimes.org

**Muscular Dystrophy
Association-USA**
3300 E. Sunrise Drive
Tucson, AZ 85718
Phone: 800-572-1717
520-529-2000
Fax: 520-529-5300
Web site: www.mdausa.org,
   www.mdaenespanol.org
E-mail: mda@mdausa.org

**National Center on Birth Defects
and Developmental Disabilities**
4770 Buford Highway, N.E.
Atlanta, GA 30341
Phone: 770-488-7150
Fax: 770-488-7156
Web site: www.cdc.gov/ncbddd

National Down Syndrome Congress
7000 Peachtree-Dunwoody Road
Building #5 - Suite 100
Atlanta, Georgia 30328
Phone: 800-232-NDSC
    (800-232-6372)
770-604-9500
Fax: 770-604-9898
Web site: www.NDSCcenter.org
E-mail: NDSCcenter@aol.com

National Down Syndrome Society (NDSS)
666 Broadway
New York, NY 10012-2317
Phone: 800-221-4602
212-460-9330
Fax: 212-979-2873
Web site: www.ndss.org
E-mail: info@ndss.org

National Fathers Network
(For Fathers/Men and Families
raising children with special
healthcare needs and/or
developmental disabilities)
16120 NE 8th Street
Bellevue, WA 98008-3937
Phone: 425-747-4004, ext. 218
Fax: 425-747-1069
Web site: www.fathersnetwork.org
E-mail: jmay@fathersnetwork.org

National Information Center for Children and Youth with Disabilities (NICHCY)
P.O. Box 1492
Washington, DC 20013-1492
Phone: 800-695-0285 (V/TTY)
202-884-8200 (V/TTY)
Fax: 202-884-8441

Web site: www.nichcy.org
E-mail: nichcy@aed.org

National Organization for Rare Disorders (NORD)
P.O. Box 8923
100 Route 37
New Fairfield, CT 06812-8923
Phone: 800-999-NORD
    (800-999-6673)
203-746-6518
Fax: 203-746-6481
Web site: www.rarediseases.org
E-mail: orphan@rarediseases.org

National Reye's Syndrome Foundation
P.O. Box 829
Bryan, OH 43506
Phone: 800-233-7393
Fax: 419-636-9897
Web site: www.reyessyndrome.org
E-mail: nrsf@reyessyndrome.org

Parents Helping Parents
3041 Olcott St.
Santa Clara, CA 95054
Phone: 408-727-5775
Fax: 408-727-0182
Web site: www.php.com
E-mail: info@php.com

Spina Bifida Association of America
4590 MacArthur Blvd. NW,
    Suite 250
Washington, DC 20009-4226
Phone: 800-621-3141
202-944-3285
Fax: 202-944-3295
Web site: www.sbaa.org
E-mail: sbaa@sbaa.org

Through the Looking Glass
National Resource Center for
Parents with Disabilities
2198 Sixth Street, Suite 100
Berkeley, CA 94710
Phone: 800-644-2666
510-848-1112
Fax: 510-848-4445
Web site: www.lookingglass.org
E-mail: TLG@lookingglass.org

United Cerebral Palsy Associations
1660 L Street NW, Suite 700
Washington, DC 20036
Phone: 800-872-5827
202-973-7197 (TDD)
Fax: 202-776-0414
Web site: www.ucp.org
E-mail: national@ucp.org

Waterbirth

**Waterbirth International Resource
and Referral Service**
Global Maternal/ Child Health
Association
P.O. Box 1400
Wilsonville, OR 97070
Phone: 800-641-2229
503-673-0026
Fax: 503-673-0029
Web site: www.waterbirth.org
E-mail: waterbirth@aol.com

Work and family

Families and Work Institute
267 Fifth Avenue
New York, NY 10016
Phone: 212- 465-2044
Fax: 212-465-8637
Web site: www.familiesandwork.org
E-mail: ebrownfield@
   familiesandwork.org

Web Site Directory

S o many Web sites, so little time. As you've no doubt discovered by now, there are thousands of pregnancy-related sites to visit. Since you've only got nine months to surf, I've hand-picked the best ones for you.

Note: While the Web sites in this directory represent the crème de la crème of what was out there when this book went to press, it's likely that other equally good pregnancy Web sites will emerge over time. If you know of a Web site that should be included when this book is revised, please drop me a line to let me know. You can e-mail me at pageone@kawartha.com or contact me via my Web site: www.having-a-baby.com.

By the way, don't forget to check out the dozens of useful sites that are listed in the Directory of Organizations in Appendix D. To save space, I haven't bothered repeating those Web site addresses here.

WEB SITE	HIGHLIGHTS
Breastfeeding	
Dr. Hale's Breastfeeding Pharmacology Page: neonatal.ttuhsc.edu/lact	A good source of information on drug use during pregnancy.
La Leche League: www.lalecheleague.org	The official Web site of the international breastfeeding organization.
Fertility/Infertility	
American Society for Reproductive Medicine: www.asrm.com	Contains a wealth of valuable information on a wide range of fertility-related topics, including full-text versions of countless booklets.
Atlanta Reproductive Health Center: www.ivf.com	Contains detailed information on fertility and infertility, including an online photo gallery that illustrates various high-tech fertility methods.
Centers for Disease Control and Prevention's Assisted Reproductive Technologies Success Rates: www.cdc.gov/nccdphp/drh/art.htm	Contains the full text of the CDC's annual report on fertility clinics. Essential information for anyone who's thinking of using the services of a U.S. fertility clinic.
Fertile Thoughts: www.fertilethoughts.net	An excellent way to connect with other couples who are struggling with fertility problems. An excellent source of information and support.
Fertilitext: www.fertilitext.org	Contains useful information on ovulation predictor kits, fertility drugs, and more. Sponsored by a pharmacy.
Infertility Resources: www.ihr.com/infertility	Provides detailed information on infertility, surrogacy, and related topics.
International Council on Infertility Information Dissemination: www.inciid.org	An excellent starting point for research on any infertility-related topic. Features articles, bulletin boards, and more.
IVF.com — A Couple's Guide to Overcoming Infertility: www.ivf.com/fert.html	Detailed information on a variety of infertility-related topics.
Organization of Parents Through Surrogacy: www.opts.com	A Web site dedicated to the complex issues surrounding surrogate parenthood.
RESOLVE, Inc.: www.resolve.org	The Web site of the national fertility organization of the same name.

Fitness During Pregnancy

Fit Pregnancy: www.fitpregnancy.com — Contains articles from the print publication of the same name. A good source of information on prenatal fitness.

Health Information (General)

Centers for Disease Control and Prevention: www.cdc.gov — The site is packed with information and statistics on every health topic imaginable, including the *Assisted Reproductive Technology Success Rates* report, which is published annually.

HealthAnswers.com: www.healthanswers.com — Contains articles on fertility, infertility, pregnancy, and more.

Intelihealth: www.intelihealth.com — A leading health Web site featuring information from Harvard Medical School.

Mayo Health Oasis (Mayo Clinic): www.mayohealth.org — Features meticulously researched articles on a wide variety of health-related topics, including fitness and nutrition.

PubMed — National Library of Medicine: www.ncbi.nlm.nih.gov/entrez/query.fcgi — A database that allows you to search for abstracts from the latest medical journals.

Reuters Health: www.reutershealth.com — An excellent source of breaking news on the health front.

WebMD: www.Webmd.com — One of the top health Web sites. Features an entire area devoted to pregnancy.

Infant Health and Safety

American Academy of Pediatrics: www.aap.org — Wondering about the American Academy of Pediatrics' (AAP) stand on a particular issue? This is the site to visit. You'll also want to check out Familydoctor.org, the AAP's consumer health Web site (see below).

Consumer Product Safety Commission: www.cpsc.gov — The site to visit for information on product recalls of baby gear. You can sign up for e-mail notification of such recalls.

continued

HIGHLIGHTS (Continued)

WEB SITE	HIGHLIGHTS
Infant Health and Safety	
Dr. Greene.com: www.drgreene.com	The brainchild of the California pediatritican of the same name, DrGreene.com is one of the friendliest and most parent-friendly pediatric health Web sites. Definitely worth a visit.
Family Doctor.org (American Academy of Pediatrics): www.familydoctor.org	The American Academy of Pediatrics' consumer health Web site. Reliable information on a variety of pediatric health topics.
Federal Consumer Information Center: www.pueblo.gsa.gov	A good source for health and safety information, parenting advice, and much more.
Food Guide Pyramid: www.nal.usda.gov:8001/py/pmap.htm	An online copy of the Food Guide Pyramid.
Juvenile Products Manufacturers Association: www.jmpa.org	In the consumer portion of the site, you'll find detailed safety information on shopping for baby gear. You'll also find contact information for the major U.S. juvenile products manufacturer — something that can come in handy if you need replacement parts for your child's stroller.
March of Dimes: www.modimes.org	Detailed information on giving your baby the healthiest possible start in life.
Maternal and Child Health State Resource Sheets: www.nmchc.org/html/states.htm	Features contact information for maternal and child health authorities for each state.
Sesame Street Parents: www.sesameworkshop.org/parents	The tag line for the site says it all: "Parenting essentials for moms and dads who grew up on Sesame Street."
Zero to Three: www.zerotothree.org	Comprehensive information on all aspects of infant and toddler development, including detailed information from the Johnson & Johnson Pediatric Institute on what you can do to promote your baby's social, emotional, and intellectual development.

Labor and Postpartum Support

Childbirth and Postpartum Professionals Association: www.postpartumdoula.com

Contains information about using the services of a labor support or postpartum support professional.

Doulas of North America: www.dona.com

Contains information about the benefits of using the services of a doula.

Nutrition During Pregnancy

American Dietetic Association: www.eatright.org

Comprehensive information on a variety of nutrition-related topics.

Tufts University Nutrition Navigator: www.navigator.tufts.edu

Provides links to the best online sites.

Pregnancy (General)

American College of Nurse-Midwives: www.midwife.org

Features a detailed consumer health area that addresses common questions about midwifery care.

American College of Obstetricians and Gynecologists: www.acog.com

Features a patient information brochure of the month on such topics as breastfeeding and infertility, as well as other useful information on a variety of reproductive health topics.

BabyCenter.com: www.babycenter.com

One of the leading U.S. pregnancy and baby sites. Packed with useful information on a variety of pregnancy and parenting-related topics.

BabyCorner.com: www.thebabycorner.com

A friendly parenting Web site run by parents for parents. Features a dedicated areas for dads and dads-to-be.

BabyZone.com: babyzone.com

A great place to swap pregnancy and parenting tips with other parents. Very grassroots.

Baby Science: www.babyscience.com

Practical tips on preparing your older child for the birth of a new baby. The official site for my children's books *Baby Science: How Babies Really Work* and *Before You Were Born: The Inside Story*.

continued

HIGHLIGHTS (Continued)

WEB SITE	HIGHLIGHTS (Continued)
Pregnancy (General)	
ePregnancy: www.epregnancy.com	Part of a network of Web sites created by two Web-savvy moms. Definitely worth a visit.
Family.com: www.family.com	Disney's Web site for parents. Features articles on a variety of pregnancy- and parenting-related topics.
First Nine Months: www.pregnancycalendar.com/firstgmonths	An amazing online film about the wonders of conception, pregnancy, and birth.
Having-a-Baby.com: www.having-a-baby.com	My official pregnancy Web site.
Intelihealth: www.intelihealth.com	The health site developed by Johns Hopkins University. Contains plenty of useful pregnancy-related information.
iParenting.com: www.iparenting.com	Part of a network of more than 30 Web sites devoted to preconception, pregnancy, and parenting.
The Labor of Love: www.thelaboroflove.com	A parenting Web site that has all kinds of fun and unusual extras: belly photos, baby shower planning tools, and much more.
Mayo Health O@sis: www.mayohealth.org	The official site of the Mayo Clinic. Contains detailed information on a variety of health-related topics, including pregnancy.
MedicineNet: www.medicinenet.com	Contains detailed information on a variety of health-related topics, including pregnancy. Features an online medical dictionary and more.
Medscape: www.medscape.com	Another major health site that offers detailed information on a variety of health-related topics, including pregnancy.
The Merck Manual www.merck.com/pubs/mmanual/section18/sec18.htm	Contains the entire text of this highly respected medical manual. Features detailed information on a variety of pregnancy-related topics.
Midlife Mommies: www.midlifemommies.com	A Web site for women who are embarking on motherhood a little later in life.

Pregnancy (General)

MidwiferyToday.com — The Homebirth Choice:
www.midwiferytoday.com/articles/default.asp?t=homebirthchoice

An article from *Midwifery Today* magazine that makes a compelling case for homebirth.

The New York Times — Women's Health: http://www.nytimes.com/pages/health/womenshealth/index.html

An excellent source of information on a variety of topics related to women's health, including pregnancy.

Obstetric Ultrasound: www.ob-ultrasound.net

Detailed information on how ultrasounds work and what can be learned by conducting ultrasounds at various points in pregnancy. Worth a visit to see the ultrasound photos alone!

Oxygen.com — Family & Home: www.oxygen.com/topic/family

The pregnancy and parenting area of Oprah-owned Oxygen.com.

Pregnancy.org: www.pregnancy.org

A not-for-profit parenting community built by and for parents. Expect the unexpected!

Parenting.com: www.parenting.com

The official Web site of *Parenting Magazine.*

Parents.com: www.parents.com

The official Web site of *Parents* magazine.

ParentsPlace.com: www.parentsplace.com

One of two iVillage web sites devoted to parenting. ParentsPlace.com focuses on pregnancy to age three while a sister site, Parentsoup.com, deals with the concerns of parents with older children. You'll find bulletin boards, interactive tools, and more.

Sidelines National Support Network: www.sidelines.org

An excellent source of support for women experiencing a high-risk pregnancy.

Thrive Online: thriveonline.oxygen.com

The health area of Oprah-owned Oxygen.com. Features articles on a variety of health topics, including pregnancy.

TravelHealth: www.travelhealth.com

Features a number of useful articles on traveling during pregnancy.

Visual Embryo: www.visembryo.com/baby/index.html

A supremely cool site that walks you through the various stages of fetal development. A great way to share your pregnancy with your partner.

continued

WEB SITE	HIGHLIGHTS (Continued)
Pregnancy (Miscarriage, Stillbirth, or Infant Death)	
SIDS Network: www.sids-network.org	Contains information on topics related to pregnancy and infant loss. An excellent source of leads on online support groups dealing with these issues.
Subsequent Pregnancy After a Loss Support Group: www.spals.com	Explains how you can subscribe to the Subsequent Pregnancy After a Loss Support Group. Also contains a number of useful links to other related resources.
Wisconsin Stillbirth Service Program: www.wisc.edu/wissp/when.htm	Contains useful information on coping with stillbirth.
Pregnancy (Multiple Births)	
Centre for the Study of Multiple Births: www.multiplebirth.com	Resources of interest to parents of multiples.
Freebies FAQ: www.owc.net/~twins/freebie.htm	The scoop on coupons, discounts, and other bargains available to parents who are expecting twins or other multiples.
Triplet Connection: www.tripletconnection.org	A great place to connect with parents of triplets, quadruplets, and more.
Working During pregnancy	
Catalystwomen.org: www.catalystwomen.org	The official Web site of Catalyst, a non-profit organization dedicated to advancing women in the workplace. An excellent place to find statistics on the economics of being a one- or two-income family, the need for flexible working arrangements, and other hot topics of interest to women working outside the home.
Childcare Guide.com: www.childcare-guide.com	The official Web site for my book, *The Unofficial Guide to Childcare*.
Department of Labor: Pregnancy Discrimination: www.dol.gov/dol/wb/public/wb_pubs/pregnant.htm	The facts on pregnancy discrimination in the workplace.
U.S. Equal Opportunity Commission: www.eeoc.gov	An excellent source of information about pregnancy discrimination and related workplace issues.
Working Mother: www.workingmother.com	The official Web site of the print publication of the same name.

Statistics at a Glance

BIRTH-RELATED STATISTICS: UNITED STATES (1999)

Number of births	3,959,417
Place of delivery	
Hospital	3,923,059
Home	23,518
Birth center	9,642
Clinic or doctor's office	464
Other non-hospital setting	2,353
Unspecified location	381
Multiple Births, Number Of	
Twins	114,307
Triplets	6,742
Quadruplets	512
Quintuplets and other higher order multiples	67
Cesarean rate	22%
Preterm birth rate	11.8%
Low birthweight rate	7.8%

continued

Common Obstetric Procedures (Rate Per 1,000 Live Births)

Amniocentesis	26.5
Ultrasound	658.5
Labor induction	197.9

Pregnancy- and Birth-Related Complications (Rate Per 1,000 Live Births)

Breech/malpresentation	38.9
Cord prolapse	2.0
Fetal distress	39.6
Meconium, moderate/heavy	54.7
Placenta previa	3.2
Placental abruption	5.6
Premature rupture of membranes	25.6
Birth injuries	2.9

Congenital Anomalies (Rate Per 100,000 Live Births)

Central nervous system anomalies

Anencephalus	11.0
Spina bifida/meningocele	20.1
Hydrocephalus	21.5
Microcephalus	5.9
Other central nervous system anomalies	20.0

Circulatory/respiratory anomalies

Heart malformations	119.8
Other circulatory/respiratory anomalies	140.6

Gastrointestinal anomalies

Rectal atresia/stenosis	9.0
Tracheo-esophageal fistula/esophageal atresia	13.3
Omphalocele/gastroschisis	30.2
Other gastrointestinal anomalies	29.8

Congenital Anomalies (Rate Per 100,000 Live Births)

Urogenital anomalies

Malformed genitalia	76.3
Renal agenesis	13.7
Other urogenital anomalies	99.0

Chromosomal anomalies

Cleft lip/palate	80.9
Polydactyly/syndactyly/adactyly	87.9
Clubfoot	55.7
Diaphragmatic hernia	13.1
Other musculoskeletal/integumental anomalies	251.1
Down syndrome	45.5
Other chromosomal anomalies	36.9

Source: Department of Health and Human Services, Centers for Disease Control and Prevention, National Center for Health Statistics, National Vital Statistics System, National Vital Statistics Report. Volume 49, Number 1. April 17, 2001.

THE RISK OF GIVING BIRTH TO A LIVEBORN CHILD WITH DOWN SYNDROME OR ANOTHER CHROMOSOMAL ANOMALY

Age of Mother	Risk of Down Syndrome	Total Risk for All Chromosomal Abnormalities
20	1:1667	1:526
21	1:1667	1:526
22	1:1429	1:500
23	1:1429	1:500
24	1:1250	1:476
25	1:1250	1:476
26	1:1176	1:455
27	1:1111	1:455
28	1:1053	1:435

continued

Age of Mother	Risk of Down Syndrome	Total Risk for All Chromosomal Abnormalities
29	1:1000	1:417
30	1:952	1:384
31	1:909	1:384
32	1:769	1:323
33	1:625	1:286
34	1:500	1:238
35	1:385	1:192
36	1:294	1:156
37	1:227	1:127
38	1:175	1:102
39	1:137	1:83
40	1:106	1:66
41	1:82	1:53
42	1:64	1:42
43	1:50	1:33
44	1:38	1:26
45	1:30	1:21
46	1:23	1:16
47	1:18	1:13
48	1:14	1:10
49	1:11	1:8

Source: Mark H. Beers, M.D., and Robert Berkow, M.D. The Merck Manual of Diagnosis and Therapy. 17th edition., Whitehouse Station, New Jersey: Merck Publications, 1999.

INFANT DEATHS AND INFANT MORTALITY RATES FOR 130 SELECTED CAUSES (RATES PER 100,000 LIVE BIRTHS)

Cause	Number	Rate
All causes	27,953	706.3
Certain infectious and parasitic diseases	**558**	**14.1**
Certain intestinal infectious diseases	20	0.5
Diarrhea and gastoenteritis of infectious origin	0	*
Tuberculosis	2	*
Tetanus	—	*
Diphtheria	—	*
Whooping cough	7	*
Meningococcal infection	32	0.8
Septicemia	281	7.1
Congenital syphilis	2	*
Gonococcal infection	—	*
Viral diseases	**134**	**3.4**
Acute poliomyelitis	—	*
Varicella (chickenpox)	3	*
Measles	1	*
Human immunodeficiency virus (HIV) disease	14	*
Mumps	—	*
Other and unspecified viral diseases	116	2.9
Candidiasis	27	0.7
Malaria	1	*
All other and unspecified infectious and parasitic diseases	47	1.2
Neoplasms	**125**	**3.2**
Malignant neoplasms	67	1.7
Hodgkin's disease and non-Hodgkin's lymphomas	2	*
Leukemia	27	0.7
Other and unspecified malignant neoplasms	38	1.0
In situ neoplasms, benign neoplasms, neoplasms of uncertain or unknown behavior	58	1.5

continued

Cause (Continued)	Number	Rate
Diseases of the blood and blood-forming organs and certaindisorders involving the immune mechanism	93	2.3
Anemias	12	*
Hemorrhagic conditions and other diseases of blood and blood-forming organs	63	1.6
Certain disorders involving the immune mechanism	18	*
Endocrine, nutritional, and metabolic diseases	241	6.1
Short stature, not elsewhere classified	24	0.6
Nutritional deficiencies	9	*
Cystic fibrosis	12	*
Volume depletion, disorders of fluid, electrolyte and acid-base balance	53	1.3
All other endocrine, nutritonal, and metabolic diseases	143	3.6
Diseases of the nervous system	439	11.1
Meningitis	116	2.9
Infantile spinal muscular atrophy, type 1 (Werdnig-Hoffman)	41	1.0
Infantile cerebral palsy	13	*
Anoxic brain damage, not elsewhere classified	35	0.9
Other diseases of the nervous system	234	5.9
Diseases of the ear and mastoid process	4	*
Diseases of the circulatory system	667	16.9
Pulmonary heart disease and diseases of pulmonary circulation	219	5.5
Pericarditis, endocarditis, and myocarditis	20	0.5
Cardiomyopathy	131	3.3
Cardiac arrest	27	0.7
Cerebrovascular diseases	104	2.6
All other diseases of the circulatory system	165	4.2
Diseases of the respiratory system	673	7.0
Acute upper respiratory infections	10	*
Influenza and pneumonia	312	7.9
Influenza	13	*
Pneumonia	299	7.6
Acute bronchitis and acute bronchiolitis	62	1.6
Bronchitis, chronic and unspecified	19	*
Asthma	5	*
Pneumonitis due to solids and liquids	15	*

Diseases of the respiratory system	673	7.0
Other and unspecified diseases of the digestive system	249	6.3
Disease of the digestive system	499	12.6
Gastric, duodenitis, and noninfective enteritis and colitis	242	6.1
Hernia of abdominal cavity and intestinal obstruction without hernia	65	1.6
All other and unspecified diseases of digestive system	191	4.8
Diseases of the genitourinary system	191	4.8
Renal failure and other disorders of kidney	163	4.1
Other and unspecified diseases of the genitourinary system	28	0.7
Certain conditions originating in the perinatal period	14,097	356.2
Newborn affected by maternal factors and by complications of pregnancy, labor, and delivery	2,741	69.3
Newborn affected by maternal hypertensive disorders	71	1.8
Newborn affected by other maternal conditions which may be unrelated to present pregnancy	68	1.7
Newborn affected by maternal compliations of pregnancy	1,402	35.4
Newborn affected by incompetent cervix	385	9.7
Newborn affected by premature rupture of membranes	648	16.4
Newborn affected by multiple pregnancy	225	5.7
Newborn affected by other complications of pregnancy	143	3.6
Newborn affected by complications of placenta, cord, and membranes	1,025	25.9
Newborn affected by complications involving placenta	532	13.4
Newborn affected by complications involving cord	64	1.6
Newborn affected by chorioamnionitis	429	10.8
Newborn affected by other and unspecified abnormalities of membranes	1	*
Newborn affected by other complications of labor and delivery	145	3.7
Newborn affected by noxious influences transmitted via placenta or breast milk	29	0.7
Disorders related to length of gestation and fetal malnutrition	4,459	112.7
Slow fetal growth and fetal malnutrition	62	1.6

continued

Cause (Continued)	Number	Rate
Disorders related to short gestation and low birth weight, not elsewhere classified	4,397	111.1
Extremely low birth weight or extreme immaturity	3,327	84.1
Other low birth weight or extreme immaturity	1,069	27.0
Birth trauma	20	0.5
Intrauterine hypoxia and birth asphyxia	613	15.5
Intrauterine hypoxia	113	2.9
Birth asphyxia	500	12.6
Respiratory distress of newborn	1,111	28.1
Other respiratory conditions originating in the perinatal period	1,722	43.5
Congenital pneumonia	82	2.1
Neonatal aspiration syndromes	84	2.1
Interstitial emphysema and related conditions originating in the perinatal period	230	5.8
Pulmonary hemorrhage originating in the perinatal period	269	6.8
Chronic respiratory disease originating in the perinatal period	336	8.5
Atelectasis	649	16.4
All other respiratory conditions originating in the perinatal period	70	1.8
Infections specific to the perinatal period	869	22.0
Bacterial sepsis of newborn	689	17.4
Omphalitis of newborn with or without mild hemorrhage	0	*
All other infections specific to the perinatal period	180	4.5
Hemorrhagic and hematological disorders of newborn	620	15.7
Neonatal hemorrhage	508	12.8
Hemorrhagic disease of newborn	1	*
Hemolytic disease of newborn due to isoimmunization and other perinatal jaundice	16	*
Hematological disorders	95	2.4
Syndrome of infant of a diabetic mother and neonatal diabetes mellitus	8	*
Necrotizing enterocolitis of newborn	405	10.2
Hydrops fetalis not due to hemolytic disease	189	4.8
Other perinatal conditions	1,342	33.9

Congenital malformations, deformations, and chromosomal abnormalities	5,471	138.2
Anecephaly and similar malformations	311	7.9
Congenital hydrocephalus	93	2.3
Spina bifida	22	0.6
Other congenital malformations of nervous system	263	6.6
Congenital malformations of heart	1,593	40.2
Other congenital malformations of circulatory system	220	5.6
Congenital malformations of respiratory system	564	14.3
Congenital malformations of digestive system	93	2.3
Congenital malformations of genitourinary system	366	9.2
Congenital malformations and deformations of musculoskeletal system, limbs, and integument	487	12.3
Down syndrome	94	2.4
Edward's syndrome	440	11.1
Patau's syndrome	250	6.3
Other congenital malformations and deformations	508	12.8
Other chromosomal abnormalities, not elsewhere classified	166	4.2
Symptoms, signs, and abnormal clinical and laboratory findings, not elsewhere classified	3,612	91.3
Sudden infant death syndrome	2,583	65.3
Other symptoms, signs, and abnormal clinical and laboratory findings, not elsewhere classified	1,029	26.0
All other diseases (residual)	23	0.6
External causes of mortality	1,259	31.8
Accidents (unintentional injuries)	833	21.0
Transport accidents	188	4.8
Motor vehicle accidents	183	4.6
Other and unspecified transport accidents	5	*
Falls	12	*
Accidental discharge of firearms	0	*
Accidental drowning and submersion	67	1.7
Accidental suffocation and strangulation in bed	246	6.2
Other accidental suffocation and strangulation	153	3.9

continued

Cause (Continued)	Number	Rate
External causes of mortality		
Accidental inhalation and ingestion of food or other objects causing obstruction of respiratory tract	62	1.6
Accidents caused by exposure to smoke, fire and flames	40	1.0
Accidental poisoning and exposure to noxious substances	12	*
Other and unspecified accidents	52	1.3
Assault (homicide)	323	8.2
Assault (homicide) by hanging, strangulation and suffocation	33	0.8
Assault (homicide) by discharge of firearms	8	*
Neglect, abandonment and other maltreatment syndromes	122	3.1
Assault (homicide) by other and unspecified means	160	4.0
Complications of medical and surgical care	52	1.3
Other external causes	50	1.3

* Figure does not meet standards of reliability or precision.

Source: Department of Health and Human Services, Centers for Disease Control and Prevention, National Center for Health Statistics, National Vital Statistics System, National Vital Statistics Report. Volume 49, Number 1. April 17, 2001.

APPENDIX G

Recommended Reading

Andreae, Simon. *Anatomy of Desire. The Science and Psychology of Sex, Love and Marriage.* Great Britain: Little, Brown, 1998.

Angier, Natalie. *Woman. An Intimate Geography.* New York: Houghton Mifflin Company, 1999.

Baker, Robin, Ph.D. *Sperm Wars. The Science of Sex.* New York: HarperCollins, 1996.

Baker, Robin, Ph.D. and Elizabeth Oram. *Baby Wars. Parenthood and Family Strife.* Toronto: HarperCollins, 1998.

Bing, Elisabeth, and Libby Colman. *Laughter and Tears: The Emotional Life of New Mothers.* New York: Henry Holt and Company, 1997.

Cancellaro, Cecelia. *Pregnancy Stories: Real Women Share the Joys, Fears, Thrills, and Anxieties of Pregnancy from Conception to Birth.* Oakland, CA: New Harbinger Publications Inc., 2001.

Caton, Donald, M.D. *What a Blessing She Had Chloroform: The Medical and Social Response to the Pain of Childbirth from 1800 to the Present.* New Haven, Conn.: Yale University, 1999.

Clapp James F., III. *Exercising Through Your Pregnancy.* Champaign, IL: Human Kinetics, 1998.

Davis, Deborah L. *Empty Cradle, Broken Heart: Surviving the Death of Your Baby.* Colorado: Fulcrum Publishing, 1996.

Douglas, Ann. *Baby Science: How Babies Really Work.* Toronto: Owl Books/Greey de Pencier, 1998. *Before You Were Born: The Inside Story.* Toronto: Owl Books/Greey de Pencier, 2000. *The Unofficial Guide to Childcare.* New York: Hungry Minds, 1998.

Douglas, Ann, and Elizabeth Lewin. *Family Finance: The Essential Guide for Parents.* Chicago: Dearborn, 2001.

Douglas, Ann, and John R. Sussman, M.D. *Trying Again: A Guide to Pregnancy After Miscarriage, Stillbirth, and Infant Loss.* Dallas: Taylor Publishing, 2000. *The Unofficial Guide to Having a Baby.* New York: Hungry Minds, 1999.

Dunham, Carroll, and the Body Shop Team. *Mamatoto: A Celebration of Birth.* New York: Penguin Books, 1991.

Eiger, Marvin S., and Sally Wendkos Olds. *The Complete Book of Breastfeeding.* New York: Workman, 1999.

Enkin, Murray, et al. *A Guide to Effective Care in Pregnancy and Childbirth.* New York: Oxford, 1999.

Etcoff, Nancy. *Survival of the Prettiest: The Science of Beauty.* New York: Doubleday, 1999.

Fields, Denise and Alan. *Baby Bargains.* 4th edition. Boulder, Colorado: Windsor Peaks Press, 2001.

Fisher, Helen. *Anatomy of Love. A Natural History of Mating, Marriage, and Why We Stray.* New York: Fawcett, 1992.

Gardephe, Colleen Davis, and Steve Ettlinger. *Don't Pick Up the Baby or You'll Spoil the Child and Other Old Wives' Tales About Pregnancy and Parenting.* San Francisco: Chronicle Books, 1993.

Gilbert, Elizabeth Stepp, and Judith Smith Harmon. *Manual of High Risk Pregnancy.* St. Louis: Mosby, 1998.

Harris, A. Christine. *The Pregnancy Journal.* San Francisco: Chronicle Books, 1996.

Herman, Barry, and Susan K. Perry. *The Twelve Month Pregnancy.* Chicago: Lowell House, 1999.

Huggins, Kathleen. *The Nursing Mother's Companion.* Boston: Harvard Common Press, 1990.

Iovine, Vicki. *The Girlfriend's Guide to Pregnancy: Or Everything Your Doctor Won't Tell You.* New York: Simon & Schuster, 1995.

Jackson, Deborah. *With Child: Wisdom and Traditions for Pregnancy, Birth and Motherhood.* San Francisco: Chronicle Books, 1999.

Jackson, Marni. *The Mother Zone: Love, Sex, and Laundry in the Modern Family.* New York: Henry Holt, 1992.

Jansen, Robert. *Overcoming Infertility: A Compassionate Resource for Getting Pregnant.* New York: W. H. Freeman. 1997.

Jeffris, B. G., and J. L. Nichols. *Safe Counsel or Practical Eugenics.* Illinois: Nichols, 1893.

Jones, Carl. *Alternative Birth. The Complete Guide. Health Options for You and Your Baby.* Los Angeles: Jeremy P. Tarcher, Inc., 1991.

Kitzinger, Sheila. *Breastfeeding Your Baby.* Revised Edition. New York: Alfred A. Knopf, 1998. *The Experience of Childbirth.* London: Penguin, 1987. *The Complete Book of Pregnancy and Childbirth.* New York: Alfred A. Knopf., 1989.

Klaus, Marshall H., and Phyllis H. Klaus. *Your Amazing Newborn.* Massachusetts: Perseus Books, 1998.

Kohner, Nancy, and Alix Henley. *When a Baby Dies: The Experience of Late Miscarriage, Stillbirth and Neonatal Death.* London: Pandora Press, 1991.

Leach, Penelope. *Babyhood.* London: Penguin Books, 1983. *Your Baby and Child: From Birth to Age Five.* New York: Alfred A. Knopf, 1995.

Lerner, Harriet. *The Mother Dance: How Children Change Your Life*. New York: HarperCollins, 1998.

Linden, Dana Weschler, Emma Trenti Paroli, and Mia Weschler Doron. *Preemies: The Essential Guide for Parents of Premature Babies*. New York: Pocket Books, 2000.

Luke, Barbara, and Tamara Eberlein. *When You're Expecting Twins, Triplets, or Quads*. New York: Harper Perennial, 1999.

Manginello, Frank P., and Theresa Foy DiGeronimo. *Your Premature Baby: Everything You Need to Know About Childbirth, Treatment, and Parenting*. New York: John Wiley, 1998.

Mullen, Anne. *Missed Conceptions: Overcoming Infertility*. Scarborough: McGraw-Hill, 1990.

Newman, Dr. Jack, and Teresa Pitman. *The Ultimate Breastfeeding Book of Answers*. New York: Prima Publishing, 2000.

Nilsson, Lennart. *A Child Is Born*. New York: DTP, 1993.

Pasquariello, Patrick S., Jr. *The Children's Hospital of Philadelphia Book of Pregnancy and Child Care: From Before Birth Through Age Five*. New York: John Wiley and Sons, 1999.

Paulson, Richard J., and Judith Sachs. *Rewinding Your Biological Clock: Motherhood Late in Life: Options, Issues, and Emotions*. New York: W.H. Freeman, 1999.

Pennybacker, Mindy, and Aisha Ikramuddin. *Mothers and Others for a Livable Planet Guide to Natural Baby Care: Nontoxic and Environmentally Friendly Ways to Take Care of Your New Child*. New York: John Wiley and Sons, 1999.

Peoples, Debby, and Harriette Rovener Ferguson. *What to Expect When You're Experiencing Infertility: How to Cope with the Emotional Crisis and Survive*. New York: W.W. Norton, 1998.

Peppers, Larry G., and Ronald J. Knapp. *How to Go On Living After the Death of a Baby*. Georgia: Peachtree Publishers Limited, 1985.

Rosenthal, M. Sara. *The Gynecological Sourcebook*. Los Angeles: Lowell House, 1994. *The Pregnancy Sourcebook: Everything You Need to Know*. Los Angeles: Lowell House, 1995.

Sanders, Catherine M., Ph.D. *How to Survive the Loss of a Child: Filling the Emptiness and Rebuilding Your Life*. Rocklin, California: Prima Publishing, 1992.

Sears, William, Martha Sears, and Linda Hughey Holt. *The Pregnancy Book: A Month-by-Month Guide*. New York: Little Brown, 1997.

Sears, William. *The Breastfeeding Book*. New York: Little Brown and Company, 2000.

Serota, Cherie, and Jody Kozlow Gardner. *Pregnancy Chic: The Fashion Survival Guide*. New York: Random House, 1998.

Silber, Sherman, M.D. *How to Get Pregnant*. New York: Warner Books, 1980.

Small, Meredith, F. *Our Babies, Ourselves. How Biology and Culture Shape the Way We Parent*. New York: Doubleday, 1998.

Smith, Graig W. *Common Pregnancy Myths: Fact or Folklore?* Cincinnati: Woodview Publishing, 1998.

Stern, Daniel N., Nadia Bruschweiler-Stern. and Alison Freeland. *The Birth of a Mother: How the Motherhood Experience Changes You Forever.* New York: Basic Books, 1998.

Stoppard, Miriam. *Conception, Pregnancy, and Birth.* New York: DK Publishing, 2000.

Sussman, John R., and B. Blake Levitt. *Before You Conceive.* New York: Bantam, 1989.

Thompson, Lana. *The Wandering Womb.* New York: Prometheus Books, 1999.

Vaughan, Christopher. *How Life Begins. The Science of Life in the Womb.* New York: Dell, 1996.

Weschler, Toni. *Taking Charge of Your Fertility.* New York: HarperCollins, 1995.

Yalom, Marilyn. *A History of the Breast.* New York: Ballantine Books, 1997.

Index

What's a new mother to do?

the mother of all baby books

The Ultimate Guide to Your Baby's First Year

ANN DOUGLAS

Author of The Mother of All Pregnancy Books

If you think pregnancy is bewildering, wait until your bundle of joy arrives! Where can you go for straight answers to baby-care questions? *The Mother of All Baby Books* delivers just what you need—a fresh, fun, non-bossy guide to baby's first year. From breastfeeding vs. bottlefeeding to dealing with colic and diaper rash, this must-have book helps you make the right decisions, worry less, and keep your baby happy and healthy.